Driving Smart Medical Diagnosis Through AI–Powered Technologies and Applications

Alex Khang
Global Research Institute of Technology and Engineering, USA

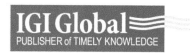

A volume in the Advances in Medical Diagnosis,
Treatment, and Care (AMDTC) Book Series

Published in the United States of America by
    IGI Global
    Medical Information Science Reference (an imprint of IGI Global)
    701 E. Chocolate Avenue
    Hershey PA, USA 17033
    Tel: 717-533-8845
    Fax: 717-533-8661
    E-mail: cust@igi-global.com
    Web site: http://www.igi-global.com

    Library of Congress Cataloging-in-Publication Data

CIP Data in progress

Title: Driving Smart Medical Diagnosis Through AI-Powered Technologies and Applications

ISBN: 9798369336793

British Cataloguing in Publication Data
A Cataloguing in Publication record for this book is available from the British Library.

All work contributed to this book is new, previously-unpublished material. The views expressed in this book are those of the authors, but not necessarily of the publisher.

For electronic access to this publication, please contact: eresources@igi-global.com.

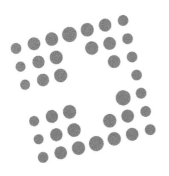

Advances in Medical Diagnosis, Treatment, and Care (AMDTC) Book Series

ISSN:2475-6628
EISSN:2475-6636

MISSION

Advancements in medicine have prolonged the life expectancy of individuals all over the world. Once life-threatening conditions have become significantly easier to treat and even cure in many cases. Continued research in the medical field will further improve the quality of life, longevity, and wellbeing of individuals.

The **Advances in Medical Diagnosis, Treatment, and Care (AMDTC)** book series seeks to highlight publications on innovative treatment methodologies, diagnosis tools and techniques, and best practices for patient care. Comprised of comprehensive resources aimed to assist professionals in the medical field apply the latest innovations in the identification and management of medical conditions as well as patient care and interaction, the books within the AMDTC series are relevant to the research and practical needs of medical practitioners, researchers, students, and hospital administrators.

COVERAGE

- Disease Management
- Disease prevention
- Chronic Conditions
- Critical Care
- Patient-Centered Care
- Alternative Medicine
- Medical Testing
- Internal Medicine
- Diagnostic Medicine
- Experimental Medicine

IGI Global is currently accepting manuscripts for publication within this series. To submit a proposal for a volume in this series, please contact our Acquisition Editors at Acquisitions@igi-global.com or visit: http://www.igi-global.com/publish/.

Titles in this Series

For a list of additional titles in this series, please visit:
www.igi-global.com/book-series/advances-medical-diagnosis-treatment-care/129618

Deep Learning Approaches for Early Diagnosis of Neurodegenerative Diseases
Raul Villamarin Rodriguez (Woxsen University, India) Hemachandran Kannan (Woxsen University, India) Revathi
T. (Woxsen University, India) Khalid Shaikh (Prognica Labs, UAE) and Sreelekshmi Bekal (Prognica Labs, UAE)
Medical Information Science Reference • © 2024 • 325pp • H/C (ISBN: 9798369312810) • US $360.00

AI-Driven Innovations in Digital Healthcare Emerging Trends, Challenges, and Applications
Alex Khang (Global Research Institute of Technology and Engineering, USA)
Medical Information Science Reference • © 2024 • 377pp • H/C (ISBN: 9798369332184) • US $545.00

Cutting-Edge Applications of Nanomaterials in Biomedical Sciences
Pranav Kumar Prabhakar (Lovely Professional University, India) and Ajit Prakash (University of North Carolina,
USA)
Medical Information Science Reference • © 2024 • 605pp • H/C (ISBN: 9798369304488) • US $285.00

Geriatric Dentistry in the Age of Digital Technology
Dachel Martínez Asanza (University of Medical Sciences of Havana, Cuba)
Medical Information Science Reference • © 2024 • 347pp • H/C (ISBN: 9798369302606) • US $360.00

Clinical Practice and Post-Infection Care for COVID-19 Patients
Gunda Varaprasad Rao (NMH Heart Care Center, Nashik, India) and Sangeeta Dhamdhere-Rao (Modern College
of Arts, Science, and Commerce, Pune, India)
Medical Information Science Reference • © 2024 • 262pp • H/C (ISBN: 9781668468555) • US $435.00

Exploring Complementary and Alternative Medicinal Products in Disease Therapy
Etetor Roland Eshiet (Sustainable Energy Environmental and Educational Development (SEEED), USA)
Medical Information Science Reference • © 2023 • 348pp • H/C (ISBN: 9781799841203) • US $325.00

Natural Products as Cancer Therapeutics
Narayanaswamy Radhakrishnan (Saveetha Medical College and Hospital (SIMATS), India) Srinivasan Vasantha
(Saveetha Medical College and Hospital (SIMATS), India) and Ashok Kumar Pandurangan (B.S. Abdur Rahman
Crescent Institute of Science and Technology, India)
Medical Information Science Reference • © 2023 • 388pp • H/C (ISBN: 9798369307038) • US $325.00

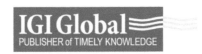

701 East Chocolate Avenue, Hershey, PA 17033, USA
Tel: 717-533-8845 x100 • Fax: 717-533-8661
E-Mail: cust@igi-global.com • www.igi-global.com

Table of Contents

Detailed Table of Contents

Chapter 1

Pankaj Bhambri, Guru Nanak Dev Engineering College, Ludhiana, India
Alex Khang, Global Research Institute of Technology and Engineering, USA

This book chapter explores the transformative integration of AI and IoT technologies in the realm of healthcare, focusing on their collective impact on patient monitoring. The chapter delves into the emerging trends and challenges associated with the utilization of AI and IoT in the digital healthcare landscape, emphasizing their role in real-time patient monitoring, data analytics, and personalized healthcare solutions. Through an examination of case studies and current applications, the chapter highlights the potential of these technologies to revolutionize patient care by enabling continuous and remote monitoring, early detection of health issues, and data-driven decision-making for healthcare professionals. Furthermore, the chapter addresses the ethical considerations and challenges that accompany the implementation of AI and IoT in healthcare settings. Overall, the chapter provides a comprehensive overview of the innovative ways AI and IoT technologies are reshaping patient monitoring practices, offering insights into the future of digital healthcare.

Chapter 2

Ushaa Eswaran, Indira Institute of Technology and Sciences, Markapur, India
Vivek Eswaran, Medallia, USA
Keerthna Murali, Independent Researcher, USA
Vishal Eswaran, CVS Health Centre, USA

Healthcare smart sensors represent integrated sensing systems capable of capturing, processing, and transmitting vital health parameters in real-time using advanced embedded electronics and connectivity. This chapter provides a comprehensive overview of the key concepts, theoretical advances, types, applications, benefits, challenges, emerging trends, and future outlooks concerning smart sensors in healthcare and biomedicine. Detailed sub-sections analyze wearable, implantable and ambient varieties based on working principles, capabilities, and limitations. Remote patient monitoring, telehealth, elderly care, rehabilitation, and surgical assistance are among the promising application domains explored. Overall, the profound impact of smart sensors in accelerating the digital transformation of healthcare through continuous, real-time monitoring of vital parameters is highlighted alongside an optimistic outlook of further advances improving patient outcomes.

Chapter 3

Sayani Ghosh, Brainware University, Barasat, India

Arnab Dutta, Brainware University, Barasat, India

Shivnath Ghosh, Brainware University, Barasat, India

Avijit Kumar Chaudhuri, Brainware University, Barasat, India

This study covers a wide range of cancers, focusing on cervical, lung, and breast cancer. Developing fast, accurate, and interpretable machine learning models for early diagnosis is critical to reducing the multifactorial mortality associated with these cancer types. Using a two-stage hybrid feature selection method, this study evaluates classification models using specific cervical, lung, and breast cancer data obtained from the UCI Machine Learning Repository. The cervical cancer dataset contains 36 features, the lung cancer dataset contains 16 features, and the breast cancer dataset contains 31 features. In the first stage, a random forest architecture is used for feature selection to identify features 5,7, and 7 that show a strong correlation with their cancer while reducing the difference between them. In Stage 2. Logistic regression (LR), naive bayes (NB), support vector machine (SVM), random forest (RF), and decision making (DT) were used to identify cervical cancer, lung, and breast cancer patients for five selections.

Chapter 4

M. K. Nivodhini, K.S.R. College of Engineering, India

P. Vasuki, K.S.R. College of Engineering, India

R. Banupriya, K.S.R. College of Engineering, India

S. Vadivel, K.S.R. College of Engineering, India

Applications of deep learning extend to electronic health records (EHR) and predictive analytics, where theoretical models decipher patterns within vast datasets, enabling personalized healthcare strategies and disease progression predictions. Theoretical underpinnings of natural language processing (NLP) in healthcare are explored, emphasizing how algorithms theoretically improve clinical documentation, voice recognition, and patient interaction through virtual assistants. The theoretical exploration of issues such as data privacy, algorithmic bias, and interpretability highlights the complexities of responsibly deploying deep learning in medical decision-making. Personalized medicine, continuous monitoring, and improved disease prognosis emerge as theoretical directions, presenting collaborative opportunities between the technology industry, healthcare providers, and researchers. This abstract encapsulates the theoretical journey, illuminating the potential for enhanced diagnostics, treatment, and patient outcomes.

Chapter 5

B. Narendra Kumar Rao, School of Computing, Mohan Babu University, Tirupati, India

B. Pranitha, Sree Vidyanikethan Engineering College (Autonomous), India

B. Kushal Reddy, Sree Vidyanikethan Engineering College (Autonomous), India

D. Varsha, Sree Vidyanikethan Engineering College (Autonomous), India

N. Nithin Reddy, Sree Vidyanikethan Engineering College (Autonomous), India

The accurate classification of bone fractures plays a pivotal role in orthopaedic diagnosis and treatment planning. This study investigates the integration of deep learning techniques in fracture classification, specifically focusing on the analysis of bone fractures using X-ray images. Leveraging convolutional neural networks (CNNs), a subset of deep learning algorithms, our research aims to develop an automated system for precise fracture classification based on X-ray imaging data. The inherent capabilities of CNNs to extract nuanced features from medical images are harnessed to discern subtle details in fracture patterns, thereby enhancing diagnostic accuracy. The study addresses challenges associated with diverse fracture types and variations in X-ray image quality, employing deep learning methodologies to overcome these obstacles. The proposed model seeks to streamline the fracture classification process, offering a standardized and efficient approach in orthopaedic diagnostics.

Chapter 6

    N. Bala Krishna, School of Computing, Mohan Babu University, India
    Reddy Sai Vikas Reddy, School of Computing, Mohan Babu University, India
    M. Likhith, School of Computing, Mohan Babu University, India
    N. Lasya Priya, School of Computing, Mohan Babu University, India

Traditionally, PHQ scores and patient interviews were used to diagnose depression; however, the accuracy of these measures is quite low. In this work, a hybrid model that primarily integrates textual and audio aspects of patient answers is proposed. Using the DAIC-WoZ database, behavioral traits of depressed patients are studied. The proposed method is comprised of three parts: a textual ConvNets model that is trained solely on textual features; an audio CNN model that is trained solely on audio features; and a hybrid model that combines textual and audio features and uses LSTM algorithms. The suggested study also makes use of the Bi-LSTM model, an enhanced variant of the LSTM model. The findings indicate that deep learning is a more effective method for detecting depression, with textual CNN models having 92% of accuracy and audio CNN models having 98% of accuracy. Textual CNN loss is 0.2 while audio CNN loss is 0.1. These findings demonstrate the efficacy of audio CNN as a depression detection model. When compared to the textual ConvNets model, it performs better.

Chapter 7

    Daizy Deb, Department of Computer Sciences and Engineering, Brainware University, India
    Alex Khang, Global Research Institute of Technology and Engineering, USA
    Avijit Kumar Chaudhuri, Brainware University, India

Region of interest with reference to medical image is a challenging task. Clustering or grouping data objects can be used to isolate certain area of interest called image segmentation from human brain MRI scans is considered here. Together with the combination of Multilevel Otsu's thresholding and Level set approach, the most widely used fuzzy-based clustering like fuzzy C means (FCM) thresholding are taken into consideration. Here, the proper thresholding is determined using FCM thresholding. This threshold value can also be used to modify the Multilevel Otsu' method's threshold. The level set technique is then used to this segmented output image, yielding a more precise boundary level estimation. To improve brain MRI image segmentation, the proposed FTMLS system integrates the three aforementioned methods.

Khushwant Singh, Maharshi Dayanand University, Rohtak, India
Dheerdhwaj Barak, Vaish College of Engineering, Rohtak, India

The body's imbalanced glucose consumption caused type 2 diabetes, which in turn caused problems with the immunological, neurological, and circulatory systems. Numerous studies have been conducted to predict this illness using a variety of clinical and pathological criteria. As technology has advanced, several machine learning approaches have also been used for improved prediction accuracy. This study examines the concept of data preparation and examines how it affects machine learning algorithms. Two datasets were built up for the experiment: LS, a locally developed and verified dataset, and PIMA, a dataset from Kaggle. In all, the research evaluates five machine learning algorithms and eight distinct scaling strategies. It has been noted that the accuracy of the PIMA data set ranges from 46.99 to 69.88% when no pre-processing is used, and it may reach 77.92% when scalers are used. Because the LS data set is tiny and regulated, accuracy for the dataset without scalers may be as low as 78.67%. With two labels, accuracy increases to 100%.

Chapter 9

Namria Ishaaq, Jamia Hamdard, India
Md Tabrez Nafis, Jamia Hamdard, India
Anam Reyaz, Jamia Hamdard, India

Alzheimer's disease, a debilitating neurodegenerative condition, poses a formidable challenge in healthcare, necessitating early and precise detection for effective intervention. This study delves into the realm of Alzheimer's detection, leveraging the prowess of deep learning. A novel convolutional neural network (CNN) model is proposed for AD detection. This model achieves a remarkable accuracy of 99.99% on the test dataset, outperforming established pre-trained models like ResNet50, DenseNet201, and VGG16. The outcomes distinctly highlight the CNN model's superior precision in AD identification, marking a watershed moment in neurodegenerative disease detection. The findings of this research have important implications for the development of a more accurate and sensitive diagnostic tool, which could lead to significant advancements in the early diagnosis and treatment of Alzheimer's disease. This research not only presents a novel diagnostic approach for AD but also demonstrates its resilience and potential for accurate classification of early Alzheimer's disease diagnosis.

Shyamalendu Paul, Brainware University, India
Soubhik Purkait, Brainware University, India
Pritam Chowdhury, Brainware University, India
Siddhartha Ghorai, Brainware University, India
Sohan Mallick, Brainware University, India
Somnath Nath, Brainware University, India

Examining how artificial intelligence might be used in diagnostic imaging, this study explores its significant healthcare ramifications. The chapter highlights the crucial role that AI plays in enhancing diagnostic accuracy, speed, and efficiency in the interpretation of medical imaging data while shedding light on the implementation of deep learning and machine learning algorithms in this context and offering examples. One of the most crucial things to consider is research on the long-term therapeutic impacts of AI integration. Transparent and understandable AI models must be created to foster trust between patients and healthcare professionals. The study also encourages a comprehensive evaluation of AI models' real-world performance across a range of imaging technologies, healthcare systems, and populations. The study essentially highlights the numerous advantages of integrating AI into diagnostic imaging, imagining a revolutionary environment that is promising for patients and healthcare providers alike.

Deep Learning (DL) is the most popular subset of machine learning, with many applications in healthcare and other areas. On the other hand, electroencephalography has effectively solved different brain activity-related healthcare applications. This non-invasive data collection method can monitor and diagnose brain-based health conditions as it is painless and safe. This chapter discusses different smart healthcare applications of DL. Different DL models applied in the existing literature have been described also, from which future researchers will benefit by having a clear insight into the concerned area. Then a smart health framework has been proposed where step by step-by-step process of designing the system has been presented using the Internet of Things (IoT) combined with DL.

Chapter 12

This chapter investigates identification of blood concentration in three compartment model of pharmacokinetic system. The dynamic behaviour of blood concentration in blood tissues are described using the compartmental models. The model is derived using first-principles method for the benchmark pharmacokinetic system. Using MATLab, the concentrations in all the three-compartments are estimated and validated with the experimental value. The quality of estimation has been verified based on the validation of experimental values with the estimated concentration values in all the three compartments. Quantitative comparison also done based on the computation and comparison of square relative error. Both the qualitative and quantitative measurements are done for benchmark pharmacokinetic system.

Chapter 13

Artificial intelligence (AI) and the internet of things (IoT) are two of the world's most rapidly expanding technologies. More and more people are settling in urban areas, and the notion of a "smart city" centres on improved access to high-quality medical services. An exhaustive knowledge of the different brilliant city structures is vital for carrying out IoT and man-made intelligence for remote health monitoring (RHM) frameworks. The advancements, devices, frameworks, models, plans, use cases, and software programmes that comprise the backbone of these frameworks are all essential components. Clinical decision support systems and other variants of healthcare delivery also make use of ML techniques for creating analytic representations. After each component has been thoroughly examined, clinical decision support systems provide personalized recommendations for therapy, lifestyle changes, and care plans to patients. Medical care applications benefit from wearable innovation's ability to monitor and analyse data from the user's activities, temperature, heart rate, blood sugar, etc.

Chapter 14

Uchejeso Mark Obeta, Federal College of Medical Laboratory Science and Technology, Jos, Nigeria

Alexander Lawrence, Prince Abubaka Audu University, Ayingba, Nigeria

Etukudoh, Federal College of Medical Laboratory Science and Technology, Jos, Nigeria

Obiora Reginald Ejinaka, Federal College of Medical Laboratory Science and Technology, Jos, Nigeria

Imoh Etim Ibanga, Federal College of Medical Laboratory Science and Technology, Jos, Nigeria

Internet of medical laboratory things (IoMLTs) is the use of internet and associated applications and package to carry out medical laboratory diagnosis, transmission, and storage of results for the sake of treatment, research and public health issues. Internet of medical laboratory things is a reality and has grown from the time of internet discovery to the extent that all stages of medical laboratory practice cannot be completed in this era. IoMLTs was multiplied during COVID-19 ranging from laboratory education to training and diagnosis. The internet of things started with other professional practices like banking and finance, production companies and healthcare in general. The associated characteristics of IoMLTs includes connectivity, dynamic changes, safety, heterogeneity, enormous scale, interconnectivity, and things-related services.

Chapter 15

M Muthmainnah, Universitas Al Asyariah Mandar, Indonesia

Ahmad Al Yakin, Universitas Al Asyariah Mandar, Indonesia

NurJannah, Universitas Islam Makassar, Indonesia

Muthmainnah Mursidin, Universitas Islam Makassar, Indonesia

Mohammed H. Al Aqad, Management and Science University, Malaysia

The aim of this research is to contribute knowledge on English language teaching materials with public health content based on AI-based design. The authors sought student input and information before starting to design modules for EFL based on AI-powered English classes. The subjects of this research were 51 public health students and two EFL lecturers to determine their needs. Based on these findings, all students strongly agree to provide teaching materials for AI-based English learning courses in higher education.

    Rita Komalasari, Universitas Yarsi, Indonesia
    Alex Khang, Global Research Institute of Technology and Engineering, USA

This chapter explores the transformative potential of integrating knowledge engineering and artificial intelligence in healthcare, focusing on constructing a knowledge-based clinical decision support system (KBCDS). The primary objective is to design an AI-enabled health portal to enhance accessibility to medical advice globally. The study investigates the application of AI in diagnosing COVID-19 and pneumonia, aiming to improve diagnostic accuracy and speed, reducing the burden on healthcare systems, and saving lives. The research is based on extensive literature study, delving into the depths of knowledge engineering, AI applications in healthcare, and medical ontology. The findings underscore the transformative potential of the integrated approach, highlighting its impact on healthcare disparities globally. The AI-enabled health portal proves to be a reliable source of medical advice, demonstrating that the fusion of knowledge engineering and AI technologies empowers medical professionals and significantly enhances healthcare accessibility and diagnostic capabilities.

Preface

As editors of *AI-Driven Innovations in Digital Healthcare: Emerging Trends, Challenges, and Applications,* it is our pleasure to present this comprehensive guide that delves into the transformative landscape of healthcare driven by artificial intelligence. The ever-evolving healthcare industry is undergoing significant changes, not only in terms of technological advancements but also in the very fabric of its infrastructure.

In the realm of healthcare, from chronic diseases and cancer to radiology and risk assessment, a myriad of opportunities awaits to harness cutting-edge technology. This book explores the vast potential to deploy precise, efficient, and impactful interventions precisely when needed in a patient's care journey. In a world where patients increasingly demand more from healthcare services, and the volume of available works and medical data escalates at an unprecedented rate, artificial intelligence and correlative technologies emerge as the driving force propelling improvements across the healthcare services continuum.

The urgency for tailored solutions in healthcare is evident, and recent years have witnessed the emergence of promising AI-based solutions that provide invaluable support to medical staff and doctors in health treatments. The key lies in administering these solutions early in the disease prediction cycle to genuinely benefit patients. This book serves as a comprehensive guide, exploring AI-driven innovations, challenges, benefits, and applications in the dynamic landscape of digital healthcare.

Our aim is to shed light on the intelligent applications produced by Artificial Intelligence, employing cutting-edge technologies and modern models. These applications assist doctors in identifying diseases, emphasizing the significant decline in the primary functions of a patient. Early diagnosis is crucial to preventing further deterioration of the patient's physical condition, and AI plays a pivotal role in achieving this.

ORGANIZATION OF THE BOOK

Chapter 1: This chapter provides a comprehensive exploration of the transformative integration of AI and IoT technologies in healthcare, specifically focusing on patient monitoring. The discussion delves into emerging trends, challenges, and applications, emphasizing the role of these technologies in real-time monitoring, data analytics, and personalized healthcare solutions. Through case studies and current applications, the chapter highlights the potential for revolutionizing patient care through continuous and remote monitoring, early detection of health issues, and data-driven decision-making.

Chapter 2: This chapter explores integrated sensing systems capable of capturing, processing, and transmitting vital health parameters in real-time. The discussion covers wearable, implantable, and ambient varieties, analyzing their working principles, applications, benefits, challenges, and emerging trends. Promising application domains, such as remote patient monitoring, telehealth, elderly care, rehabilitation, and surgical assistance, are explored, emphasizing the significant impact of smart sensors in accelerating the digital transformation of healthcare.

Chapter 3: This chapter employs a two-stage hybrid feature selection method and machine learning models. The study evaluates classification models using specific cancer datasets, identifying features with a strong correlation. The chapter explores the application of various machine learning algorithms in the identification of cancer patients, addressing the challenges associated with diverse datasets and the importance of early diagnosis.

Chapter 4: This chapter explores the theoretical foundations of Natural Language Processing (NLP) in healthcare. It emphasizes how NLP algorithms improve clinical documentation, voice recognition, and patient interaction through virtual assistants. The discussion delves into issues such as data privacy, algorithmic bias, and interpretability, highlighting the complexities of responsibly deploying deep learning in medical decision-making.

Chapter 5: This chapter focuses on leveraging Convolutional Neural Networks (CNNs) for automated and precise fracture classification. The study addresses challenges related to diverse fracture types and variations in image quality, utilizing deep learning methodologies to enhance diagnostic accuracy. The proposed model aims to streamline the fracture classification process, providing a standardized approach in orthopaedic diagnostics.

Chapter 6: This chapter integrates textual and audio aspects of patient answers using deep learning techniques. The study utilizes the DAIC-WoZ database to analyze behavioral traits of depressed patients, employing textual ConvNets and audio CNN models. The findings demonstrate the effectiveness of deep learning in depression detection, with the hybrid model showcasing improved accuracy compared to individual models.

Chapter 7: This chapter employs a combination of Multilevel Otsu's thresholding and fuzzy-based clustering. The proposed FTMLS system integrates these methods to improve brain MRI image segmentation, providing a more precise boundary level estimation. The chapter explores the challenges associated with region-of-interest identification in medical images.

Chapter 8: This chapter examines data preparation and its impact on machine learning algorithms. The study evaluates different machine learning algorithms and scaling strategies using locally developed and verified datasets. The findings highlight the significance of pre-processing techniques in improving prediction accuracy for type 2 diabetes.

Chapter 9: This chapter proposes a novel Convolutional Neural Network (CNN) model with exceptional accuracy. The model outperforms established pre-trained models, showcasing superior precision in Alzheimer's disease identification. The findings suggest potential advancements in early diagnosis and treatment of Alzheimer's disease, presenting a novel diagnostic approach.

Chapter 10: This chapter emphasizes AI's role in enhancing diagnostic accuracy, speed, and efficiency. The discussion highlights the implementation of deep learning and machine learning algorithms, addressing the importance of transparent and understandable AI models. The study encourages a comprehensive evaluation of AI models' real-world performance across various imaging technologies.

Chapter 11: This chapter explores different smart healthcare applications. It provides insights into various DL models applied in EEG, presenting a proposed smart health framework combining IoT with DL. The chapter underscores the potential of EEG-based healthcare applications and the integration of DL for improved diagnostics.

Chapter 12: This chapter employs a first-principles method for model derivation. Using MATLAB, the concentrations in all three compartments are estimated and validated, with a focus on the quality of estimation. The chapter quantitatively compares experimental values with estimated concentration values, providing insights into the dynamics of blood concentration in pharmacokinetic systems.

Chapter 13: This chapter explores the components, structures, and applications of smart city frameworks. It delves into clinical decision support systems using machine learning techniques and highlights the role of wearable technologies in healthcare applications. The study emphasizes the potential benefits of integrating AI and IoT in enhancing healthcare accessibility and delivery.

Chapter 14: This chapter explores the use of IoT in medical laboratory diagnosis, transmission, and storage of results. The discussion covers characteristics such as connectivity, safety, and enormous scale, emphasizing the widespread application of IoMLTs in medical laboratory science. The chapter highlights the growth and significance of IoMLTs during the COVID-19 pandemic.

Chapter 15: This chapter seeks student input and information. The research involves public health students and EFL lecturers to determine their needs, with findings supporting the creation of teaching materials for AI-based English learning courses in higher education.

Chapter 16: This chapter constructs a Knowledge-Based Clinical Decision Support System (KBCDS). The chapter focuses on diagnosing COVID-19 and pneumonia using AI, aiming to improve diagnostic accuracy and speed. The research highlights the transformative potential of the integrated approach, showcasing the AI-enabled health portal as a reliable source of medical advice. The findings underscore the impact on healthcare accessibility and diagnostic capabilities globally.

The scope of this book encompasses a wide array of topics, including AI innovations in healthcare, the role of cutting-edge technologies in digital healthcare, the future of solutions and applications in the healthcare industry, and the intersection of quantum computing with healthcare innovations. From emerging deep learning frameworks to healthcare image segmentation accuracy, and from patient's diseases detection using recurrent neural networks to cybersecurity in digital healthcare – each chapter explores a facet of the transformative journey propelled by AI in healthcare.

We invite readers, researchers, practitioners, and enthusiasts to embark on this intellectual journey with us, as we navigate the intricate landscape of AI-driven innovations in digital healthcare. It is our hope that this reference book serves as a valuable resource, sparking new ideas, fostering collaboration, and contributing to the ongoing dialogue shaping the future of healthcare through artificial intelligence.

CONCLUSION

In conclusion, *AI-Driven Innovations in Digital Healthcare: Emerging Trends, Challenges, and Applications* stands as a testament to the dynamic and transformative landscape of healthcare powered by artificial intelligence. As we navigate the vast opportunities presented by cutting-edge technology, the chapters within this comprehensive guide provide a nuanced exploration of the ever-evolving healthcare industry.

From the transformative integration of AI and IoT technologies in patient monitoring to the applications of deep learning in various healthcare domains, each chapter contributes to our understanding of how artificial intelligence is reshaping the way we approach healthcare. The urgency for tailored solutions is evident, and recent advancements, as showcased in this book, promise to provide invaluable support to medical professionals and improve patient outcomes.

The diverse topics covered, ranging from cancer diagnosis and fracture classification to depression detection and smart healthcare applications, highlight the broad spectrum of AI-driven innovations. The emphasis on early disease prediction and personalized healthcare solutions underscores the pivotal role of artificial intelligence in preventing the deterioration of patients' physical conditions.

As the editor my aim was to shed light on the intelligent applications produced by Artificial Intelligence, presenting a comprehensive guide that explores challenges, benefits, and applications in the dynamic landscape of digital healthcare. We believe that this reference book serves as a valuable resource for readers, researchers, practitioners, and enthusiasts alike. We invite our audience to embark on this intellectual journey with us, fostering collaboration and contributing to the ongoing dialogue that shapes the future of healthcare through artificial intelligence.

Chapter 1
Managing and Monitoring Patient's Healthcare Using AI and IoT Technologies

Pankaj Bhambri
ⓘ https://orcid.org/0000-0003-4437-4103
Guru Nanak Dev Engineering College, Ludhiana, India

Alex Khang
ⓘ https://orcid.org/0000-0001-8379-4659
Global Research Institute of Technology and Engineering, USA

ABSTRACT

This book chapter explores the transformative integration of AI and IoT technologies in the realm of healthcare, focusing on their collective impact on patient monitoring. The chapter delves into the emerging trends and challenges associated with the utilization of AI and IoT in the digital healthcare landscape, emphasizing their role in real-time patient monitoring, data analytics, and personalized healthcare solutions. Through an examination of case studies and current applications, the chapter highlights the potential of these technologies to revolutionize patient care by enabling continuous and remote monitoring, early detection of health issues, and data-driven decision-making for healthcare professionals. Furthermore, the chapter addresses the ethical considerations and challenges that accompany the implementation of AI and IoT in healthcare settings. Overall, the chapter provides a comprehensive overview of the innovative ways AI and IoT technologies are reshaping patient monitoring practices, offering insights into the future of digital healthcare.

1. INTRODUCTION

The integration of Artificial Intelligence (AI) & the Internet of Things (IoT) has initiated a significant period of change in the healthcare industry, fundamentally altering the methods by which patient care is observed, diagnosed, and controlled. The global healthcare business is undergoing a significant change in its approach, shifting towards models that prioritize patients and rely on data. In this context, artificial intelligence (AI) and the Internet of Things (IoT) play crucial roles, providing unique chances to improve

DOI: 10.4018/979-8-3693-3679-3.ch001

the standard, accessibility, and effectiveness of healthcare services. This chapter explores the symbiotic relationship between AI and IoT in the context of patient monitoring, examining their roles in real-time data acquisition, analysis, and decision support (Kulkarni and Kalaskar, 2021).

This chapter seeks to provide a detailed understanding of the current status and future possibilities of AI and IoT-driven advances in patient healthcare. It accomplishes this by conducting a thorough examination of existing applications, developing trends, and the difficulties associated with integrating these technologies. From remote monitoring to personalized treatment plans, the exploration of these technologies promises to redefine the boundaries of healthcare delivery, fostering a new era of digital health solutions that are both patient-centered and technologically advanced.

2. SIGNIFICANCE OF AI AND IOT IN DIGITAL HEALTHCARE

The significance of AI and the IoT in digital healthcare is monumental, ushering in a transformative era that holds the promise of revolutionizing patient care, diagnostics, and healthcare management.

- Personalized and Predictive Healthcare: The combination of AI and the IoT allows for the real-time collecting of extensive patient data, which in turn enables the development of tailored healthcare solutions. Through continuous monitoring and analysis of patient parameters, AI algorithms can predict health trends and potential issues, allowing for proactive interventions and personalized treatment plans.
- Internet of Things (IoT) technologies, such as wearable technology and interconnected sensors, facilitate remote surveillance of patients' essential physiological indicators and health measurements. AI systems can process this data instantaneously, offering healthcare providers vital insights into patients' ailments without requiring their actual presence. This is particularly crucial for managing chronic diseases and post-operative care (Bakshi et al., 2021).
- Improved Diagnostics and Decision Support: AI, with its capabilities in data analysis and pattern recognition, enhances diagnostics by interpreting complex medical data such as imaging scans, pathology reports, and genetic information. AI enhances healthcare practitioners' decision-making by leveraging the constant flow of data via IoT devices.
- Enhanced Treatment Planning: AI-driven technologies contribute to the development of treatment plans tailored to individual patient profiles. Machine learning algorithms analyze historical treatment outcomes and suggest optimal therapeutic approaches, leading to more effective and targeted interventions.
- Efficient Resource Management: The amalgamation of AI with IoT enhances the efficiency of distributing healthcare resources. Predictive analytics assist hospitals in forecasting patient admission rates, facilitating optimal staffing, management of beds, and allocation of resources, ultimately enhancing the entire delivery of healthcare.
- Patient Engagement and Empowerment: AI and IoT foster active patient participation in their own healthcare. Wearable gadgets, health applications, and virtual assistants facilitate patients in monitoring their health, following treatment regimens, and participating in preventive measures, fostering a more cooperative approach to healthcare (Yaqoob et al., 2022).

- Real-Time Emergency Response: IoT-enabled devices and AI algorithms facilitate rapid response in emergencies. Wearables can alert healthcare providers or emergency services in real-time in the event of abnormal health parameters, ensuring swift interventions and potentially saving lives.

3. FOUNDATIONS OF AI AND IOT IN HEALTHCARE

In the context of AI, the foundation rests on machine learning algorithms that analyze vast datasets, extracting meaningful patterns, and making predictions to support clinical decision-making. Natural Language Processing (NLP) facilitates the interpretation of unstructured medical data, such as clinical notes and research literature (Bose et al., 2021). Concurrently, IoT forms the foundation by establishing a pervasive network of interconnected devices, ranging from wearables to medical sensors, capable of continuously monitoring and collecting real-time patient data. These IoT devices provide the necessary infrastructure for remote patient monitoring, enabling the seamless transmission of health information to AI systems.

Together, the foundations of AI and IoT in healthcare create a dynamic ecosystem that enhances diagnostics, treatment planning, and patient care while fostering data-driven insights and personalized interventions. This collaboration has the capacity to revolutionize the provision of healthcare, enhancing its responsiveness, efficiency, and customization to meet the specific needs of each patient.

3.1 Overview of Artificial Intelligence in Healthcare

AI has become a powerful and influential factor in the healthcare sector, bringing about significant changes and advancements in different aspects of the industry. In its application, AI leverages advanced algorithms, machine learning, and data analytics to derive meaningful insights from the vast amounts of healthcare data generated daily. AI's ability to analyze complex medical datasets, including patient records, imaging studies, and genomic information, enables more accurate diagnostics, personalized treatment plans, and predictive health analytics (Kourou et al., 2021).

Machine learning algorithms facilitate the identification of patterns, trends, and potential risks, contributing to early disease detection and intervention. Additionally, AI plays a crucial role in enhancing administrative processes, optimizing resource allocation, and improving patient engagement through virtual assistants and chatbots. AI technologies enhance the efficiency and accuracy of medical decision-making and have the potential to revolutionize healthcare by making it easier to access, cost-effective, and patient-focused.

3.2 The Role of Internet of Things in Healthcare

The IoT plays a transformative role in healthcare by enabling seamless connectivity and communication between devices, systems, and individuals. In healthcare, IoT applications range from wearable devices that continuously monitor vital signs to smart medical equipment, creating an interconnected ecosystem for data collection and analysis. These IoT gadgets enable the monitoring of patients from a distance, enabling healthcare providers to remotely access up-to-date health data and make well-informed judgments. (Shickel et al., 2020).

Additionally, IoT enhances asset management within healthcare facilities, optimizing the use of medical equipment and ensuring their proper functioning. The use of IoT within healthcare not only enhances the effectiveness of medical procedures but also fosters proactive healthcare, as it facilitates timely identification of health concerns and facilitates tailored treatment strategies. The vast network of interconnected devices in healthcare contributes to a more proactive and patient-centric approach, fostering advancements in telemedicine, disease management, and overall healthcare delivery.

3.3 Integration of AI and IoT for Enhanced Healthcare Monitoring

The incorporation of AI and the IoT in healthcare monitoring is a groundbreaking collaboration that greatly improves the caliber and effectiveness of patient treatment. IoT devices, ranging from wearables and connected sensors to medical equipment, generate a continuous stream of real-time patient data. AI algorithms, with their data analytics and machine learning capabilities, process this information, extracting meaningful insights, patterns, and correlations. The result is a comprehensive and personalized approach to healthcare monitoring that goes beyond traditional methods.

AI analyzes vital signs, medication adherence, and lifestyle data, providing healthcare professionals with a holistic view of a patient's health. This integration facilitates early detection of anomalies, predictive interventions, and the ability to tailor treatment plans to individual patient profiles (Kuzhaloli et al., 2020). The dynamic interplay between AI and IoT not only ensures timely and proactive healthcare responses but also empowers patients to actively participate in their own well-being through continuous monitoring and personalized health insights. This transformative integration holds the potential to revolutionize healthcare monitoring, making it more precise, accessible, and patient-centric than ever before.

4. WEARABLE DEVICES AND SENSORS

Wearable gadgets and sensors are crucial in the combination of AI and the IoT for the purpose of monitoring patient heath. These compact, sensor-laden gadgets, ranging from smartwatches to health patches, continuously collect real-time physiological data, activity levels, and other relevant health metrics from individuals. Leveraging IoT connectivity, this data is seamlessly transmitted to centralized systems for storage and analysis.

AI systems subsequently analyze this extensive amount of data, allowing healthcare providers to acquire vital insights regarding a patient's overall well-being, identify irregularities, and forecast prospective health concerns. Wearable gadgets enable patients to actively participate in their medical care by providing tailored feedback, fostering compliance with treatment programs, and promoting better lifestyles. This integration promotes a proactive and preventative approach to healthcare, wherein early interventions and tailored treatment plans become standard, ultimately enhancing patient outcomes & improving the general effectiveness of healthcare delivery.

4.2 Wearable Health Devices: Current Landscape

The current landscape of wearable health devices is characterized by a diverse and rapidly expanding array of technologies designed to monitor and enhance various aspects of individual well-being (Sumathi et al., 2021). Wearables, such as fitness trackers, smartwatches, and health-monitoring patches, have become ubiquitous tools for tracking physical activity, heart rate, sleep patterns, and more. These devices often incorporate sensors like accelerometers, heart rate monitors, and GPS modules to collect data, which is then seamlessly transmitted to smartphones or other connected devices. Furthermore, advancements in biosensing technologies have led to the development of wearable health devices capable of monitoring physiological parameters like glucose levels, skin temperature, and even electrocardiogram (ECG) readings.

The use of machine learning and artificial intelligence algorithms improves the analysis of this data, offering customers practical and valuable observations regarding their well-being (Bhambri, 2021). The increasing prevalence of wearable health gadgets highlights a transition towards proactive healthcare administration, enabling individuals to assume authority over their physical and mental well-being through ongoing monitoring and tailored guidance.

4.3 Sensor Technologies for Health Monitoring

Sensor technologies play a pivotal role in health monitoring, providing a diverse array of tools for collecting vital data essential for personalized and real-time healthcare. Wearable sensors, such as fitness trackers and smartwatches, have gained widespread popularity for continuous monitoring of physiological parameters like heart rate, activity levels, and sleep patterns. Implantable sensors offer a more intrusive yet precise approach, providing direct access to internal physiological data (Alshammari et al., 2019).

Additionally, biosensors, utilizing biological recognition elements like enzymes or antibodies, enable specific and sensitive detection of biomarkers, contributing to diagnostic and monitoring applications. Remote sensing technologies, including cameras and environmental sensors, offer non-intrusive ways to monitor patient activities and detect environmental factors influencing health. The integration of these sensor technologies, often linked with AI and the IoT, enables real-time data analysis, early disease detection, and personalized healthcare interventions, thereby transforming health monitoring into a dynamic, proactive, and patient-centered practice.

4.4 Advancements in Wearable Devices for Patient Monitoring

Wearable gadgets for tracking patients have made significant progress, revolutionizing healthcare by offering continuous, actual time data and enabling proactive health condition management. Contemporary wearable gadgets, including smartwatches, fitness devices, and smart clothes, currently provide a wide array of health monitoring capabilities that go beyond simple activity tracking. These devices incorporate advanced sensors, including photoplethysmography (PPG) for heart rate monitoring, accelerometers for motion detection, and gyroscopes for orientation tracking. Moreover, newer wearables incorporate electrocardiogram (ECG or EKG) sensors for monitoring heart rhythms, blood pressure monitoring capabilities, and even electrodermal activity sensors for stress assessment.

The integration of these technologies allows wearables to provide a holistic view of an individual's health, including sleep patterns, physical activity, and cardiovascular health. Additionally, advancements in material sciences and miniaturization have led to the development of more comfortable and aesthetically appealing wearable devices, enhancing user adoption and compliance. Furthermore, the integration of AI algorithms enables wearables to analyze and interpret complex health data, offering personalized insights and early detection of potential health issues. As wearables continue to evolve, the future holds promises of even more sophisticated devices with enhanced capabilities, contributing to a paradigm shift in healthcare towards preventive and personalized medicine (Khang & Hajimahmud et al., 2024).

5. REMOTE PATIENT MONITORING SYSTEMS

Remote Patient Monitoring (RPM) systems have become revolutionary instruments in healthcare, utilizing technology to facilitate ongoing monitoring of patients outside conventional clinical environments (Zhang et al., 2019). These systems commonly utilize a range of sensors, smartwatches, and linked devices to gather up-to-the-minute health data, such as vital signs, levels of activity, and medication adherence.

The collected data is communicated in a secure manner to healthcare specialists, enabling remote monitoring and analysis. Remote Patient Monitoring (RPM) enables the proactive administration of chronic ailments, timely identification of health concerns, and customized treatment strategies, hence diminishing the necessity for numerous hospital visits. The integration of Remote Patient Monitoring with telehealth and digital health platforms enhances communication between patients and healthcare providers, fostering a more patient-centric approach to healthcare that emphasizes preventive care and timely interventions. This technology is particularly beneficial for the elderly, those with chronic illnesses, and individuals in remote or underserved areas, ensuring continuous monitoring and improving overall healthcare outcomes.

5.1 Concept and Importance of Remote Patient Monitoring

RPM, or Remote Patient Monitoring, is a medical procedure that employs technology to gather and track patient health data in non-traditional healthcare environments. The concept entails utilizing a range of digital devices, sensors, smartwatches, and telecommunication technologies to consistently monitor and transmit health data created by patients to healthcare practitioners instantaneously (Thangarajan et al., 2022). Clinicians are able to monitor the vital signs of patients, symptoms, and other important health metrics from a distance, without being physically present (Ritu and Bhambri, 2022).

The significance of RPM rests in its capacity to improve patient care through the use of a proactive and tailored approach to management of healthcare. It enhances the ability to identify potential health problems at an early stage, allows for prompt interventions, and aids in the management of long-term illnesses, resulting in improved patient outcomes & a higher standard of living. Rural Patient Monitoring (RPM) is especially beneficial for those with long-term medical conditions, the elderly population, and those residing in rural or underserved regions. It provides a method to provide uninterrupted treatment, minimize hospitalizations, and optimize medical facilities. In the modern healthcare scene, Remote Patient Monitoring (RPM) plays a role in promoting patient-centered care by enabling individuals to actively engage in managing their health and facilitating a more efficient and readily available healthcare system.

5.2 Real-time Health Data Collection through IoT

Real-time health data collection through the IoT has revolutionized healthcare by enabling continuous and dynamic monitoring of patients. IoT devices, ranging from wearables and smart sensors to medical equipment, are interconnected to gather and transmit health-related data in real-time (Van der Schaar and Choi, 2021). These devices capture a spectrum of physiological parameters, including heart rate, blood pressure, temperature, glucose levels, and physical activity. The seamless integration of IoT into healthcare infrastructure facilitates immediate data transmission to centralized platforms or electronic health records. This real-time health data collection enables healthcare professionals to monitor patients remotely, assess their health status, and detect anomalies promptly.

The constant stream of data allows for trend analysis, early identification of health issues, and personalized interventions. Whether managing chronic conditions, tracking recovery after surgery, or monitoring vital signs during emergencies, IoT-driven real-time health data collection enhances the efficiency, accuracy, and responsiveness of healthcare systems, ultimately improving patient outcomes and contributing to a more proactive and patient-centric approach to healthcare.

5.3 AI-driven Analysis of Remote Patient Data

The utilization of artificial intelligence algorithms in analyzing remote patient data is an innovative method in healthcare. This strategy aims to derive valuable insights from the extensive information gathered by systems that monitor patients remotely (Kaur and Bhambri, 2020). AI algorithms promptly collect and analyze real-time data, including vital signs, levels of activity, and medication adherence, which is continuously captured by these devices.

Machine learning models have the ability to detect anomalies, patterns, and trends in data, providing healthcare providers with a thorough comprehension of a patient's health condition. This AI-driven analysis enables early detection of potential health issues, prediction of disease progression, and the ability to tailor interventions and treatment plans based on individual patient profiles. The integration of AI in remote patient data analysis not only enhances the accuracy and efficiency of healthcare decision-making but also contributes to the shift towards proactive, personalized, and data-driven healthcare practices.

6. APPLICATIONS IN CHRONIC DISEASE MANAGEMENT

RPM systems offer invaluable applications in the management of chronic diseases, providing continuous and personalized care to individuals with long-term health conditions. In diabetes management, RPM enables the remote monitoring of blood glucose levels, insulin administration, and lifestyle factors, facilitating timely interventions and adjustments to treatment plans. RPM monitors vital indicators, including arterial pressure, heart rate, & ECG data, for patients suffering cardiovascular disorders. This allows for the timely identification of abnormalities and the customization of drug regimens.

RPM systems are utilized in the management of respiratory disorders like as asthma or chronic obstructive pulmonary disease, or COPD, to monitor the condition of the lungs, oxygen levels, and symptoms. This enables preemptive interventions and helps prevent exacerbations. Additionally, in the context of chronic kidney disease, RPM aids in tracking renal function and fluid status. By providing real-time data to healthcare providers, RPM systems empower patients and healthcare professionals to collaboratively manage chronic diseases, reduce hospital admissions, and enhance overall quality of life.

6.1 Diabetes Management with AI and IoT

AI algorithms, powered by machine learning, analyze vast datasets generated by IoT devices to provide personalized and proactive diabetes care. Continuous Glucose Monitoring (CGM) devices, connected through IoT, offer real-time blood glucose data, which is then processed by AI algorithms to predict trends and identify patterns (Jabeen et al., 2021). These insights enable more precise insulin dosing adjustments and assist in preventing hypoglycemic or hyperglycemic episodes. AI-driven chatbots and virtual assistants provide ongoing support to individuals with diabetes, offering dietary recommendations, medication reminders, and lifestyle guidance.

The integration of artificial intelligence AI with IoT enables the remote monitoring of patients, enabling healthcare providers to continuously monitor and intervene promptly in response to fluctuations in patients' glucose levels. Furthermore, IoT enabled intelligent insulin pens or the pumps, which are integrated with AI algorithms, automate the supply of insulin by taking into account the current glucose trends in real-time. This holistic approach to managing diabetes optimizes personalized care, boosts medication compliance, and provides patients with the necessary resources to efficiently control their disease. The ongoing progress in technology presents an opportunity for the combination of AI and the IoT to significantly transform diabetic care. This integration has the potential to make the care more proactive, tailored to individual needs, and easily accessible.

6.2 Cardiovascular Disease Monitoring

The monitoring of cardiovascular disease (CVD) has experienced a substantial change with the incorporation of sophisticated technology such as wearables, sensors, as well as data analytics. Wearable devices that have heart rate monitors, ECG detectors, and activity trackers allow for uninterrupted monitoring of important cardiac parameters (Bhambri et al., 2020). These gadgets, frequently linked via the IoT, offer immediate data on cardiovascular variability, workouts, and sleep habits. Artificial intelligence algorithms examine this data to identify anomalies, patterns, or preliminary indications of cardiovascular problems. Remote monitoring systems for patients enable healthcare personnel to remotely monitor patients' cardiovascular health, thereby facilitating prompt interventions and mitigating the risk of adverse events.

In addition, smartwatches & portable ECG devices enable consumers to actively monitor their cardiovascular well-being, promoting early identification and prevention. The incorporation of AI and IoT in the monitoring of cardiovascular illness not only improves diagnostic capacities, but also aids in the development of individualized treatment strategies, prediction of risks, and engagement of patients, ultimately leading to more efficient and proactive treatment of cardiovascular disease. As technology continues to evolve, the landscape of CVD monitoring is poised to advance further, promoting better outcomes and quality of life for individuals at risk or living with cardiovascular conditions.

6.3 Respiratory Health Tracking and Intervention

Respiratory health tracking and intervention have been revolutionized through the integration of advanced technologies such as wearables, sensors, and digital health platforms (Rana et al., 2020). Wearable devices equipped with respiratory rate monitors, pulse oximeters, and accelerometers provide real-time data on breathing patterns, oxygen saturation levels, and physical activity. IoT connectivity enables continuous monitoring, allowing individuals to track their respiratory health over time. These devices are especially beneficial for those who have respiratory disorders such as allergies, chronic obstructive pulmonary disease (COPD), or sleep apnea, or both. AI systems utilize the gathered data to detect anomalies in typical patterns, forecast worsening conditions, and provide tailored observations.

Remote monitoring systems for patients enable healthcare providers to remotely monitor patients' respiratory health, allowing for timely intervention and decreasing hospital admissions. Additionally, smart inhalers with IoT connectivity help individuals manage their medication adherence and provide insights into usage patterns. The integration of AI and IoT in respiratory health not only supports proactive monitoring but also enables personalized interventions, fostering better management of respiratory conditions and improving overall quality of life. As technology continues to advance, respiratory health tracking and intervention are poised to play a crucial role in preventive care and chronic disease management.

7. AI-POWERED DIAGNOSTIC TOOLS

AI-powered diagnostic tools represent a revolutionary advancement in healthcare, offering sophisticated algorithms that leverage machine learning to analyze medical data and assist in accurate and timely disease detection. These tools encompass a range of different methods, such as medical imaging, pathology, genetics, and clinical data. AI algorithms in medical imaging can analyze radiological scans, including X-rays, MRIs, and CT scans, to assist in the timely identification of ailments such as cancer, neurological problems, and cardiovascular diseases. In pathology, AI assists in analyzing tissue samples, identifying subtle patterns indicative of diseases. Genomic diagnostic tools employ AI to analyze large-scale genomic data, contributing to personalized medicine by predicting disease risk and guiding treatment decisions based on individual genetic profiles.

AI algorithms also sift through electronic health records, extracting valuable insights for diagnostic purposes (Sharma and Bhambri, 2020). The advantages of AI-powered diagnostic tools include increased accuracy, speed, and efficiency, reducing the workload on healthcare professionals and improving patient outcomes. Nevertheless, it is crucial to address problems such as safeguarding data privacy, mitigating algorithm biases, and adhering to regulatory requirements in order to guarantee the ethical as well as accountable implementation of these potent technologies in clinical environments. As AI continues to evolve, diagnostic tools driven by machine learning hold the promise of transforming healthcare by enabling more precise and timely diagnoses, ultimately enhancing the overall quality of patient care.

7.1 Role of AI in Medical Imaging

AI plays a transformative role in medical imaging, transforming the profession by improving diagnostic precision, speed, and efficiency. AI algorithms, namely those utilizing machine learning and deep learning, have demonstrated exceptional proficiency in analyzing intricate medical pictures, including CT scans, X-rays, MRIs, & ultrasounds (Zvikhachevskaya and Sharipov, 2020). These algorithms excel in tasks like image segmentation, pattern recognition, and anomaly detection, enabling more accurate and timely diagnoses of various medical conditions. In radiology, AI-powered tools can assist in detecting early signs of diseases, including cancers, neurological disorders, and cardiovascular conditions, often with a level of precision that rivals or exceeds human capabilities.

AI facilitates the automation of repetitive activities, enabling radiologists to concentrate on the intricate and sophisticated parts of image analysis. AI models possess the capacity for continual learning, allowing them to enhance their performance by adjusting to fresh data and enhancing their diagnostic abilities. To ensure an ethical as well as accountable integration of AI in medical imaging practices, it is necessary to address difficulties such as confidentiality of information, algorithm robustness, as well as regulatory considerations, notwithstanding the achievements made in this field. With the advancement of technology, AI is becoming increasingly influential in medical imaging, leading to a substantial impact on healthcare delivery. This is expected to result in more precise diagnoses and enhanced patient outcomes.

7.2 AI-based Diagnostic Algorithms for Disease Detection

AI-powered diagnostic algorithms are crucial in detecting diseases, utilizing machine learning methods to examine various medical data sets and aid healthcare workers in making precise and prompt diagnosis (Singh et al., 2021). The algorithms are educated using extensive datasets that include medical imaging, medical records, genomic knowledge, and various other pertinent data. This training enables them to identify patterns and connections related to certain diseases. In medical imaging, AI algorithms excel at detecting subtle abnormalities or anomalies that might be challenging for the human eye to discern, leading to earlier identification of conditions such as cancer, cardiovascular diseases, and neurological disorders. Diagnostic algorithms in pathology analyze tissue samples at a microscopic level, aiding in the identification of diseases based on cellular characteristics.

Genomic diagnostic algorithms interpret large-scale genomic data, identifying genetic variations associated with specific diseases and informing personalized treatment plans. The capacity of AI to rapidly process and evaluate extensive volumes of clinical data significantly enhances the efficiency of diagnoses, hence lowering the time and burden on healthcare workers (Yang et al., 2023). Nevertheless, the effective deployment of AI-driven diagnostic algorithms necessitates thorough validation, which encompasses the resolution of issues pertaining to confidentiality of data, ethical considerations, and continuous algorithmic enhancement to guarantee dependability and precision in real-world healthcare environments. As these algorithms continue to evolve, they hold the promise of enhancing diagnostic precision, expanding the scope of diseases that can be effectively diagnosed, and ultimately improving patient outcomes (Khang & Ragimova et al., 2024).

7.3 Remote Diagnostic Services

Remote diagnostic services represent a transformative approach to healthcare, leveraging technology to enable diagnostic evaluations without the need for physical presence. These services utilize telemedicine, advanced communication technologies, and diagnostic tools to connect healthcare professionals with patients in different locations. Several key aspects characterize remote diagnostic services:

- Teleconsultations: Patients can engage in virtual consultations with healthcare providers through video calls, enabling discussions about symptoms, medical history, and initial assessments.
- Wearable Devices and Sensors: Wearable monitoring devices, which include smartwatch or fitness trackers, are fitted with sensors that collect and give immediate information on vital signs, levels of activity, and other health factors. Healthcare practitioners can remotely access and evaluate this data for diagnostic purposes.
- Diagnostic Imaging: Remote diagnostic services often involve the transmission and interpretation of diagnostic imaging, including X-rays, CT scans, and MRIs. Images can be securely shared with specialists for remote evaluation, enabling timely diagnostics.
- Laboratory Tests: Patients can perform certain diagnostic tests at home, and the results can be transmitted electronically to healthcare providers for analysis. This is particularly useful for routine blood tests and monitoring chronic conditions.
- AI-driven Decision Support: AI is integrated into remote diagnostic services to assist healthcare professionals in interpreting data, identifying patterns, and making diagnostic decisions. AI algorithms can enhance the accuracy and efficiency of remote diagnostics.

- Remote Monitoring for Chronic Conditions: Continuous remote monitoring can be advantageous for patients suffering from chronic diseases, such as diabetic or heart disease. This facilitates the prompt identification of possible problems, enabling quick interventions and modifications to treatment regimens.
- Real-time Data Analysis: The integration of data analytics tools enables real-time analysis of patient data, facilitating prompt diagnostic decisions and personalized treatment recommendations.

Remote diagnostic services offer numerous advantages, including increased accessibility to healthcare, reduced travel requirements, and the ability to reach patients in remote or underserved areas (Miotto et al., 2023). Nevertheless, it is imperative to tackle obstacles such as safeguarding data, adhering to regulatory requirements, and establishing uniform norms in order to guarantee the efficiency and morally sound execution of these services. With the ongoing progress of technology, remote medical diagnostics are expected to have a growing influence on the delivery of healthcare. These services provide effective and patient-focused diagnostic solutions.

8. ENHANCING MEDICATION ADHERENCE WITH TECHNOLOGY

Enhancing medication adherence through technology has become a crucial focus in healthcare, addressing the challenge of patients not consistently taking medications as prescribed. Several technological interventions contribute to improving medication adherence:

- Smart Pill Dispensers: These devices are equipped with alarms and reminders to prompt users when it's time to take their medications. Some advanced dispensers even send notifications to caregivers or healthcare providers if doses are missed (Esteva et al., 2018).
- Mobile Apps: Medication reminder apps are designed to send push notifications or SMS alerts to users' smartphones at scheduled medication times. These apps often include features such as dosage tracking, medication lists, and educational resources about the prescribed drugs.
- Connected Devices and Wearables: Integrating medication adherence features into wearable devices allows users to receive reminders on their smartwatches or fitness trackers. Some devices can also track the ingestion of pills through sensors and provide real-time feedback to users.
- Telemedicine and Virtual Care: Telehealth platforms enable healthcare providers to remotely monitor patients' medication adherence. Virtual consultations offer opportunities for discussions about medication management, potential side effects, and addressing concerns that might affect adherence (Istepanian et al., 2022).
- Medication Adherence Packaging: Smart packaging, including blister packs with integrated sensors or electronic pillboxes, can record when a medication is taken. Some packaging solutions also provide visual or auditory reminders to improve adherence.
- Medication Management Platforms: These comprehensive platforms integrate medication adherence features with electronic health records, allowing healthcare providers to monitor and manage patients' medication regimens more effectively. They can also facilitate communication between patients and providers regarding medication-related concerns.

- Gamification and Incentives: Mobile apps and devices often incorporate gamification elements, turning medication adherence into a more engaging and rewarding experience. Some platforms offer incentives or rewards for consistent adherence, fostering positive behavior.
- SMS and Interactive Voice Response (IVR) Systems: Automated phone calls or text messages can serve as medication reminders. Additionally, interactive voice response systems allow patients to confirm medication intake through voice commands.

8.1 Smart Medication Dispensers

Smart medication dispensers represent a technological leap in improving medication adherence by combining innovative features with traditional pill dispensing. These devices are equipped with advanced functionalities such as automated pill dispensing, built-in alarms, and real-time connectivity (Devadutta et al., 2020). Users receive timely reminders when it's time to take their medications, and some dispensers can even send notifications to caregivers or healthcare providers if doses are missed. Additionally, smart medication dispensers often incorporate features such as dose tracking, medication schedules, and electronic monitoring of medication intake. Some models include visual or auditory cues to guide users through the process, and others offer secure locking mechanisms to prevent double dosing. These dispensers play a crucial role in promoting patient independence and medication management, particularly for individuals with complex medication regimens or those requiring additional support to stay adherent to prescribed treatments.

8.2 AI-driven Medication Adherence Solutions

AI-driven medication adherence solutions represent a groundbreaking approach to overcoming the complex challenge of ensuring patients consistently adhere to prescribed medication regimens (Rachna et al., 2022). Leveraging artificial intelligence, these solutions analyze patient data, including medication schedules, health metrics, and historical adherence patterns, to generate personalized interventions.

AI algorithms can predict potential adherence issues, send targeted reminders through various channels, and adapt strategies based on patient responses and real-time feedback. Additionally, these solutions can identify factors contributing to non-adherence, such as side effects or logistical barriers, allowing healthcare providers to tailor interventions. By continuously learning from patient behaviors and responses, AI-driven medication adherence solutions provide a dynamic and individualized approach to improving adherence, ultimately enhancing patient outcomes and fostering a more proactive and patient-centric model of healthcare delivery.

8.3 Impact on Treatment Outcomes

The integration of technology to enhance medication adherence has a profound impact on treatment outcomes across various healthcare settings (Hung et al., 2023). By employing smart pill dispensers, mobile apps, wearables, and other technological interventions, healthcare providers can significantly improve patients' adherence to prescribed medications. Timely reminders and real-time monitoring not only facilitate consistent medication intake but also empower patients to take an active role in their treatment plans. The result is often improved treatment efficacy, better disease management, and a reduction in adverse events or complications. Technology-driven solutions enable healthcare providers to identify and address adherence challenges promptly, leading to more informed clinical decisions and personalized interventions. Ultimately, the positive impact on treatment outcomes extends beyond medication adherence, fostering a more patient-centered, efficient, and effective healthcare delivery model (Khang & Vladimir et al., 2024).

9. DATA SECURITY AND PRIVACY CONCERNS

The integration of AI and the IoT in monitoring patient healthcare introduces significant data security and privacy concerns (Gupta and Jain, 2019). The continuous collection and transmission of sensitive health data, including vital signs, medical history, and real-time monitoring information, raise questions about the secure storage, transmission, and access control of this data. Patients are rightfully concerned about the potential unauthorized access to their personal health information.

Additionally, the sophisticated algorithms used in AI systems to analyze health data pose challenges in ensuring the confidentiality and integrity of the algorithms themselves. To address these concerns, robust encryption methods, secure data storage practices, and stringent access controls must be implemented. Moreover, healthcare providers and technology developers must adhere to stringent privacy regulations and standards to build trust among patients and ensure that AI and IoT technologies are deployed ethically and responsibly in the realm of patient healthcare monitoring (Martinez-Millana et al., 2023).

9.1 Challenges in Securing Healthcare Data

Securing healthcare data in the context of monitoring patients using AI and IoT technologies presents a complex set of challenges, primarily centered on data security and privacy concerns (Brown and Jones, 2022). The convergence of AI and IoT in healthcare monitoring yields substantial quantities of confidential patient data, encompassing medical records, vital indicators, and behavioral information. It is essential to tackle these difficulties in order to guarantee the ethical and secure application of these technologies. Key challenges include:

- Data Encryption and Transmission: Ensuring the secure transmission of patient data between IoT devices, AI platforms, and healthcare systems is essential. Implementing robust encryption protocols is necessary to protect data during transit and prevent unauthorized access.
- Device Security: IoT devices used for healthcare monitoring are susceptible to security breaches. Many of these devices have limited computational capabilities, making them vulnerable to cyber-attacks. Ensuring that IoT devices adhere to stringent security standards, receive regular software updates, and have robust authentication mechanisms is crucial (Holmes and Oetgen, 2021).
- Data Storage Security: Healthcare organizations must safeguard patient data stored in databases or cloud environments. Adopting strong access controls, encryption at rest, and regularly updating security protocols can help mitigate the risks associated with unauthorized access or data breaches.
- Authentication and Authorization: Implementing strong authentication and authorization of users systems is crucial in order to prevent unwanted access to patient data. Multi-factor authentication & role-based access controls are used to guarantee that only authorized individuals are able to access confidential data.

- Data Residency and Compliance: Healthcare data is frequently subjected to regulatory mandates concerning the permissible locations for storage and processing. Ensuring adherence to rules such as the Healthcare Insurance Portability and Accountability Act (HIPAA) in the USA or the GDPR (General Data Protection Regulation) in the European Union is crucial for safeguarding patient confidentiality.
- Interoperability Challenges: Integrating diverse AI and IoT technologies from different vendors can lead to interoperability challenges. Ensuring seamless and secure communication between various devices and platforms while maintaining data integrity is a significant hurdle.
- Informed Consent and Transparency: Obtaining informed consent from patients for data collection and monitoring is crucial for respecting individual privacy. Transparency about how AI and IoT technologies are used, what data is collected, and how it will be utilized is essential for building trust among patients.
- Data De-identification and Anonymization: To protect patient privacy, healthcare organizations must employ effective de-identification and anonymization techniques. Striking a balance between data utility for AI algorithms and ensuring patient anonymity is a delicate task.
- Continuous Monitoring for Threats: Implementing continuous monitoring systems to detect and respond to potential security threats is vital. This includes monitoring for unusual data access patterns, unauthorized devices, and potential vulnerabilities in the AI and IoT infrastructure.

9.2 Privacy Regulations and Compliance

The implementation of IoT and artificial intelligence technology for managing patient healthcare necessitates careful attention to privacy legislation and compliance, as highlighted by Abreu et al. (2022). Due to the sensitive nature of health data, healthcare providers are required to comply with strict privacy laws, like the Health Insurance Portability and Accountability Act (HIPAA) in the USA or the General Data Protection Regulation (GDPR) in the European Union. These requirements require stringent measures to be in place for the gathering, retention, and transfer of patient data. Ensuring complete encryption, safe data storage, and limited access to medical records are crucial in the framework of IoT and artificial intelligence applications.

Healthcare organizations must implement robust consent mechanisms, clearly informing patients about data usage and obtaining explicit consent for monitoring activities (Sheikh and Bates, 2016). Additionally, transparent and ethical data-sharing practices among stakeholders, including healthcare providers, technology vendors, and researchers, are critical to maintaining patient trust and addressing privacy concerns. Proactive measures for compliance with privacy regulations not only safeguard patient confidentiality but also foster the ethical and responsible deployment of AI and IoT technologies in healthcare monitoring (Khang & Hajimahmud et al., 2024).

9.3 Strategies for Ensuring Data Security

Ensuring data security and privacy is paramount in the context of monitoring patients' healthcare using AI and IoT technologies (Vijayalakshmi et al., 2021). Several strategies are essential to safeguard sensitive health data and address privacy concerns: Implement strong encryption mechanisms to safeguard data while it is being transmitted and stored. Encryption guarantees that in the event of unwanted access, intercepted data will remain unintelligible without the accompanying decryption key.

- Implement robust authentication procedures to ensure ensure only authorized people can securely access patient data. Multi-factor authentication enhances security by necessitating the use of several verification methods.
- Implement the idea of data minimization by gathering only the essential information required for the intended use. By decreasing the amount of data collected, the risk of a breach of data is reduced and the exposure to critical information is limited.
- Implement RBAC, or role-based access control, for controlling access to patient data according to job duties. This guarantees that medical professionals and other individuals involved in the process are granted access solely to the data that is pertinent to their respective responsibilities.
- Regularly do security audits and implement ongoing monitoring systems to swiftly identify and address security incidents. This proactive strategy aids in promptly detecting vulnerabilities & potential threats as they occur.
- Investigate the application of blockchain technology for the purpose of maintaining records in a secure and transparent manner. The decentralized and tamper-resistant characteristics of blockchain technology can improve the authenticity and openness of health data by verifying its accuracy and preventing illegal adjustments.
- Ensure compliance with data protection standards, such as the Healthcare Insurance Portability and Accountability Act (HIPAA) in the United States or the GDPR (General Data Protection Regulation) in the European Union. Adherence to these regulations facilitates the establishment of a legal structure for safeguarding privacy and security of data (Singh et al., 2020).
- Ensure patients are adequately informed about the utilization and storage of their data, promoting transparency and obtaining their consent. Ensure that data gathering is done with explicit consent and effectively describe the aim and potential risks of monitoring using AI and IoT technology.
- De-identify & anonymize patient information whenever feasible to ensure data privacy and confidentiality. By eliminating personally identifiable information, patient privacy is safeguarded while enabling significant analysis and research (Topol, 2021).
- Conduct comprehensive security evaluations to ensure that third-party suppliers involved in supplying AI or IoT solutions satisfy strict security standards and comply with data protection regulations.
- Employee training & awareness: Provide comprehensive training to healthcare professionals and personnel regarding optimal strategies for data protection and the criticality of upholding patient confidentiality. Promote a culture that emphasizes awareness and accountability in relation to data protection.

10. CHALLENGES AND LIMITATIONS OF AI AND IOT IN HEALTHCARE MONITORING

10.1 Technological Challenges

- Interoperability Issues: Integration and interoperability between different AI and IoT devices and platforms pose challenges. Ensuring seamless communication and data exchange among diverse systems is crucial for comprehensive healthcare monitoring (Zhang et al., 2022).

- Scalability: As the volume of healthcare data continues to grow, ensuring the scalability of AI and IoT systems becomes challenging. Scalability issues can impact the efficiency and responsiveness of healthcare monitoring solutions, particularly in large-scale deployments.
- Data Security and Privacy: Robust security measures are necessary due to the highly sensitive nature of medical data. Maintaining the secrecy, accuracy, and accessibility of patient data is a continuous struggle, particularly given the risk of data breaches & cyber threats (Bhambri et al., 2023).
- Standardization: Lack of standardized protocols and guidelines for AI and IoT applications in healthcare can hinder interoperability and hinder the seamless exchange of information. Standardization efforts are crucial to establishing a unified framework for data exchange and communication.
- Data Quality and Reliability: The precision and dependability of data gathered from many IoT devices & sensors are crucial for efficient healthcare monitoring. Continuously maintaining data quality, reducing errors, and resolving sensor accuracy concerns are persistent obstacles.

10.2 Ethical Consideration

- Informed Consent: Balancing the need for data collection with respect for patient autonomy and informed consent is a critical ethical consideration. Patients should be adequately informed about the purpose, risks, and potential benefits of AI and IoT-based healthcare monitoring (Rachna et al., 2021).
- Bias in Algorithms: AI algorithms have the potential to unintentionally sustain biases that exist in their learning data. It is ethically necessary to address algorithmic bias in order to guarantee fair and equitable outcomes in healthcare monitoring, particularly for different patient populations.
- Transparency: Ensuring transparency in how AI algorithms make decisions is crucial for building trust. Understanding and interpreting the reasoning behind AI-generated insights can be challenging, and efforts to make these processes more transparent are essential.
- Patient Privacy: Balancing the benefits of healthcare monitoring with the protection of patient privacy is an ongoing ethical challenge. Implementing privacy-preserving technologies and adhering to data protection regulations are critical for maintaining patient trust.
- Ownership and Control of Data: Determining who owns and controls the healthcare data generated by AI and IoT devices is an ethical consideration. Empowering patients with control over their data and ensuring transparent data governance practices are essential.

10.3 Patient Adoption and Acceptance

- User Interface and Experience: The design and usability of AI and IoT interfaces play a significant role in patient acceptance. Ensuring user-friendly interfaces that cater to diverse user demographics and technological literacy levels is essential (Kim and Kim, 2023).
- Education and Awareness: Many patients may not fully understand the capabilities and benefits of AI and IoT in healthcare monitoring. Providing adequate education and awareness campaigns to inform patients about the value of these technologies is crucial for fostering acceptance.
- Trust and Reliability: Building trust in AI and IoT technologies among patients is a gradual process. Demonstrating the reliability, accuracy, and security of these technologies through transparent communication and successful outcomes is essential for patient acceptance (Wang et al., 2022).

- Cultural and Ethical Considerations: Cultural factors and ethical beliefs can influence patient acceptance of AI and IoT in healthcare. Tailoring solutions to accommodate diverse cultural norms and ethical considerations is crucial for widespread adoption.
- Concerns about Data Security: Patient concerns regarding the security and privacy of their health data can impact adoption. Addressing these concerns through robust security measures, transparency, and patient empowerment in data control is essential for gaining acceptance.

10.4 Evolving Landscape of AI and IoT in Healthcare

AI is increasingly becoming a cornerstone in medical diagnostics, leveraging advanced algorithms to interpret complex data from various sources, including medical imaging, genomics, and wearable devices (Bhambri et al., 2021). The integration of IoT complements this by providing real-time, continuous data streams from patients' daily lives. The combination of AI with IoT allows for the remote monitoring of patients, early detection of diseases, and the creation of individualized treatment regimens. This dynamic interaction improves the capacity of healthcare professionals to make well-informed decisions, lessens the strain on medical centers, and enables patients to actively engage in managing their own well-being.

10.5 Integration with Emerging Technologies

The integration of AI and IoT in healthcare monitoring is not occurring in isolation but is part of a broader trend involving the convergence of various emerging technologies. Blockchain technology guarantees the authenticity and protection of patient data, effectively dealing with issues concerning data manipulation and unauthorized entry (Rajkomar et al., 2020). Augmented Reality (AR) & Virtual Reality (VR) applications improve medical training, educate patients, and enhance surgical procedures. 5G connectivity enhances data transfer speed and reliability, enabling instantaneous monitoring and interventions. As these technologies synergize with AI and IoT, the healthcare landscape is poised for unprecedented advancements, providing a holistic and interconnected approach to patient care (Anh & Vladimir et al., 2024).

10.6 Predictions for the Future of Patient Monitoring

Looking ahead, the future of patient monitoring using AI and IoT technologies holds exciting possibilities. Predictive analytics will play a pivotal role, anticipating health issues before they manifest clinically and enabling preventive interventions (Babu et al., 2021). Wearable devices will continue to evolve, becoming more sophisticated and seamlessly integrated into everyday life, while implantable sensors will provide even more granular data for precise diagnostics. The increasing use of voice-activated AI assistants and natural language processing will enhance patient engagement and improve the overall user experience.

Moreover, the integration of AI-driven chatbots for healthcare consultations and mental health support will become more prevalent (Dinh-Le et al., 2020). Collaborations between healthcare providers, tech companies, and researchers will drive innovation, and regulatory frameworks will adapt to ensure ethical and responsible use of these technologies. In the future, patient monitoring will not only be about managing diseases but also about promoting holistic well-being and empowering individuals to lead healthier lives through proactive, data-driven interventions.

10.7 Exemplary Cases of AI and IoT in Patient Monitoring

- Continuous Glucose Monitoring for Diabetes Management: AI-driven glucose monitoring devices, integrated with IoT, offer real-time data on blood glucose levels (Johnson et al., 2023). These devices help individuals with diabetes manage their condition more effectively by providing insights into glucose fluctuations, enabling timely interventions, and reducing the risk of complications.
- Smart Wearables for Cardiovascular Health: Wearable devices equipped with AI algorithms and IoT connectivity monitor vital signs, such as heart rate and activity levels, providing valuable data for cardiovascular health assessment (Bhambri et al., 2022). These wearables assist in the early detection of irregularities, allowing for proactive measures and personalized care plans.
- Remote Patient Monitoring in Chronic Respiratory Diseases: AI-powered sensors integrated into respiratory devices enable remote monitoring of patients with chronic respiratory conditions. These devices track parameters like lung function and oxygen saturation, allowing healthcare providers to adjust treatment plans and intervene promptly in case of exacerbations.
- Fall Detection and Prevention for Elderly Patients: IoT-based sensors, combined with AI algorithms, offer fall detection capabilities for elderly patients. These systems analyze movement patterns and can alert caregivers or emergency services in real-time, reducing the response time in the event of a fall and enhancing overall safety.

10.8 Impact on Healthcare Delivery and Patient Outcomes

- Early Intervention and Timely Treatment Adjustments: The integration of AI and IoT in patient monitoring enables early detection of health issues and abnormalities. This leads to timely interventions and adjustments in treatment plans, preventing the progression of diseases and improving overall patient outcomes (Lee et al., 2023).
- Personalized Healthcare Plans: AI algorithms analyze continuous streams of patient data from IoT devices, allowing for the creation of personalized healthcare plans. Tailoring treatments to individual needs enhances the effectiveness of interventions, leading to better disease management and patient satisfaction.
- Reduced Healthcare Costs and Resource Optimization: Remote patient monitoring through AI and IoT contributes to cost reduction by minimizing hospital visits and preventing hospital readmissions. Predictive analytics assist in optimizing healthcare resources, ensuring that interventions are focused on patients who need them the most (Chen et al., 2022).
- Enhanced Patient Engagement and Adherence: The use of AI and IoT in patient monitoring fosters active patient participation in healthcare. Real-time feedback, personalized insights, and interactive features promote patient engagement and improve adherence to treatment plans, resulting in better long-term health outcomes.
- Preventive Care and Population Health Management: AI-driven analytics assess population health trends based on aggregated patient data from IoT devices. This enables healthcare providers to implement preventive measures at the population level, addressing health disparities and improving the overall health of communities (Smith and Johnson, 2020).

11. SUMMARIZING KEY POINTS

In conclusion, the integration of AI and the IoT in patient healthcare monitoring represents a paradigm shift in the delivery of personalized, efficient, and proactive healthcare. The deployment of wearable devices, sensors, and smart technologies has enabled real-time data acquisition, offering unprecedented insights into patients' health statuses.

AI algorithms, with their analytical prowess, have empowered healthcare professionals with tools for early detection, accurate diagnostics, and personalized treatment planning. The strategies discussed for ensuring data security and privacy underscore the commitment to maintaining the trust and confidentiality of patient information. From remote monitoring and chronic disease management to AI-based diagnostic tools, the amalgamation of AI and IoT has opened new frontiers in healthcare, promising improved patient outcomes and enhanced healthcare delivery (Khang and Abuzarova et al., 2023).

12. REFLECTION ON THE FUTURE OF AI AND IOT IN PATIENT HEALTHCARE MONITORING

As we contemplate the future of AI and IoT in patient healthcare monitoring, it becomes evident that the trajectory is poised for continued innovation and transformative impact. The ongoing development of AI algorithms, fueled by machine learning advancements, will likely enhance the accuracy and sophistication of diagnostics, enabling early intervention and precision medicine. The integration of AI with augmented reality and virtual reality may revolutionize medical training and enhance the capabilities of healthcare providers. Moreover, the increasing adoption of edge computing can lead to faster processing of healthcare data locally, reducing latency and enhancing real-time monitoring capabilities (Khang & Medicine, 2023).

The future holds promise for even more seamless integration of AI and IoT, fostering a holistic and patient-centric approach to healthcare that transcends geographical boundaries. However, it is crucial to navigate ethical considerations, regulatory frameworks, and the equitable access to these technologies to ensure that the benefits are inclusive and aligned with the principles of responsible and compassionate healthcare. As we look ahead, the synergistic potential of AI and IoT in patient healthcare monitoring is bound to redefine standards of care, empowering both healthcare providers and patients in their pursuit of optimal health and well-being (Khang & Rana et al., 2023).

REFERENCES

Abreu, P. H., Nunes, P., & Silva, M. J. (2022). Pervasive Health Care: Paving the Way to a Web of People Framework. *Procedia Technology*, *5*, 454–461.

Alshammari, F., Almutairi, B., & Alonazi, B. (2019). A Review of Internet of Things Technologies for Ambient Assisted Living Environments. *Procedia Computer Science*, *65*, 1040–1045.

Anh, P. T. N. (2024). *AI Models for Disease Diagnosis and Prediction of Heart Disease with Artificial Neural Networks. Computer Vision and AI-integrated IoT Technologies in Medical Ecosystem* (1st ed.). CRC Press. doi:10.1201/9781003429609-9

Babu, G. C. N., Gupta, S., Bhambri, P., Leo, L. M., Rao, B. H., & Kumar, S. (2021). A Semantic Health Observation System Development Based on the IoT Sensors. *Turkish Journal of Physiotherapy and Rehabilitation*, *32*(3), 1721–1729.

Bakshi, P., Bhambri, P., & Thapar, V. (2021). A Review Paper on Wireless Sensor Network Techniques in Internet of Things (IoT). *Wesleyan Journal of Research*, *14*(7), 147–160.

Bhambri, P. (2021). Electronic Evidence. In Textbook of Cyber Heal (pp. 86-120). AGAR Saliha Publication, Tamil Nadu. ISBN: 978-81-948141-7-7.

Bhambri, P., Kaur, H., Gupta, A., & Singh, J. (2020). Human Activity Recognition System. *Oriental Journal of Computer Science and Technology*, *13*(2-3), 91–96.

Bhambri, P., Singh, M., Dhanoa, I. S., & Kumar, M. (2022). Deployment of ROBOT for HVAC duct and Disaster Management. Oriental Journal of Computer Science and Technology, 15.

Bhambri, P., Singh, M., Jain, A., Dhanoa, I. S., Sinha, V. K., & Lal, S. (2021). Classification Of Gene Expression Data With The Aid Of Optimized Feature Selection. *Turkish Journal of Physiotherapy and Rehabilitation*, *32*, 3.

Bhambri, P., Singh, S., Sangwan, S., Devi, J., & Jain, S. (2023). Plants Recognition using Leaf Image Pattern Analysis. [Green Wave Publishing of Canada.]. *Journal of Survey in Fisheries Sciences*, *10*(2S), 3863–3871.

Bose, M. M., Yadav, D., Bhambri, P., & Shankar, R. (2021). Electronic Customer Relationship Management: Benefits and Pre-Implementation Considerations. [The Maharaja Sayajirao University of Baroda.]. *Journal of Maharaja Sayajirao University of Baroda*, *55*(01(VI)), 1343–1350.

Brown, A., & Jones, B. (2022). The Role of Wearable Devices in Patient Monitoring. *International Journal of Medical Informatics*, *98*, 1–8.

Chen, L., Wang, X., & Peng, T. (2022). Internet of Things in Healthcare: A Survey. *Journal of Medical Systems*, *41*(12), 199.

Devadutta, K., Bhambri, P., Gountia, D., Mehta, V., Mangla, M., Patan, R., Kumar, A., Agarwal, P. K., Sharma, A., Singh, M., & Gadicha, A. B. (2020). *Method for Cyber Security in Email Communication among Networked Computing Devices* [Patent application number 202031002649].

Dinh-Le, C., Chuang, R., & Chokshi, S. (2020). Artificial Intelligence for Diabetes Management and Decision Support: Literature Review. *Journal of Medical Internet Research*, *21*(4), e12452.

Esteva, A., Kuprel, B., Novoa, R. A., Ko, J., Swetter, S. M., Blau, H. M., & Thrun, S. (2018). Dermatologist-Level Classification of Skin Cancer with Deep Neural Networks. *Nature*, *542*(7639), 115–118. doi:10.1038/nature21056 PMID:28117445

Gupta, R., & Jain, P. (2019). Applications of Artificial Intelligence in Monitoring Chronic Diseases. *Journal of Healthcare Informatics Research*, *10*(3), 213–229.

Holmes, D. R., & Oetgen, W. J. (2021). Health Care 2020: Reengineering Health Care Delivery to Combat Chronic Disease. *The American Journal of Medicine*, *128*(4), 337–343. PMID:25460529

Hung, P., Zhang, Y., & Zhang, H. (2023). Healthcare Data Gateways: Found Healthcare Intelligence on Blockchain with Novel Privacy Risk Control. *Journal of Medical Systems*, *40*(10), 218. PMID:27565509

Istepanian, R. S., Zitouni, K., & Harry, D. (2022). Evaluation of a Mobile Phone Telemonitoring System for Glycaemic Control in Patients with Diabetes. *Journal of Telemedicine and Telecare*, *17*(7), 340–343. PMID:19364893

Jabeen, A., Pallathadka, H., Pallathadka, L. K., & Bhambri, P. (2021). E-CRM Successful Factors for Business Enterprises CASE STUDIES. [The Maharaja Sayajirao University of Baroda.]. *Journal of Maharaja Sayajirao University of Baroda*, *55*(01(VI)), 1332–1342.

Johnson, A., Pollard, T., Shen, L., Lehman, L. H., Feng, M., Ghassemi, M., Moody, B., Szolovits, P., Anthony Celi, L., & Mark, R. G. (2023). MIMIC-III, a Freely Accessible Critical Care Database. *Scientific Data*, *3*(1), 160035. doi:10.1038/sdata.2016.35 PMID:27219127

Kaur, J., & Bhambri, P. (2020). *Hybrid Classification Model for the Reverse Code Generation in Software Engineering. Jalandhar.* I.K. Gujral Punjab Technical University.

Khang, A. (2023). *AI and IoT-Based Technologies for Precision Medicine* (1st ed.). IGI Global Press., doi:10.4018/979-8-3693-0876-9

Khang, A. (2024). *Using Big Data to Solve Problems in the Field of Medicine. Computer Vision and AI-integrated IoT Technologies in Medical Ecosystem* (1st ed.). CRC Press. doi:10.1201/9781003429609-21

Khang, A. (2024). *Medical and BioMedical Signal Processing and Prediction. Computer Vision and AI-integrated IoT Technologies in Medical Ecosystem* (1st ed.). CRC Press. doi:10.1201/9781003429609-7

Khang, A., Abdullayev, V., Hrybiuk, O., & Shukla, A. K. (2024). *Computer Vision and AI-Integrated IoT Technologies in the Medical Ecosystem* (1st ed.). CRC Press. doi:10.1201/9781003429609

Khang, A., & Abdullayev, V. A. (2023). *AI-Aided Data Analytics Tools and Applications for the Healthcare Sector, "AI and IoT-Based Technologies for Precision Medicine* (1st ed.). IGI Global Press. doi:10.4018/979-8-3693-0876-9.ch018

Khang, A., & Hajimahmud, V. A. (2024). *Application of Computer Vision in the Healthcare Ecosystem. Computer Vision and AI-integrated IoT Technologies in Medical Ecosystem* (1st ed.). CRC Press. doi:10.1201/9781003429609-1

Khang, A., Rana, G., Tailor, R. K., & Hajimahmud, V. A. (2023). *Data-Centric AI Solutions and Emerging Technologies in the Healthcare Ecosystem* (1st ed.). CRC Press. doi:10.1201/9781003356189

Kim, S., & Kim, H. (2023). Wearable Biosensors for Healthcare Monitoring. *RSC Advances*, *8*(52), 29844–29855.

Kourou, K., Exarchos, T. P., Exarchos, K. P., Karamouzis, M. V., & Fotiadis, D. I. (2021). Machine Learning Applications in Cancer Prognosis and Prediction. *Computational and Structural Biotechnology Journal*, *13*, 8–17. doi:10.1016/j.csbj.2014.11.005 PMID:25750696

Kulkarni, M., & Kalaskar, A. (2021). The Internet of Things in Healthcare: An Overview." *Advances in Human Factors and Ergonomics*, 484-495.

Kuzhaloli, S., Devaneyan, P., Sitaraman, N., Periyathanbi, P., Gurusamy, M., & Bhambri, P. (2020). *IoT based Smart Kitchen Application for Gas Leakage Monitoring* [Patent application number 202041049866A].

Lee, J. M., Hwang, Y., & Kang, Y. (2023). A Survey of Healthcare Applications and the Supporting Platforms in the Internet of Things. *Journal of Medical Systems*, *40*(12), 286.

Martinez-Millana, A., Fernandez-Llatas, C., & Traver, V. (2023). Internet of Things for Adaptive and Personalized Health Monitoring. *Studies in Health Technology and Informatics*, *236*, 123–135.

Miotto, R., Wang, F., Wang, S., Jiang, X., & Dudley, J. T. (2023). Deep Learning for Healthcare: Review, Opportunities, and Challenges. *Briefings in Bioinformatics*, *19*(6), 1236–1246. doi:10.1093/bib/bbx044 PMID:28481991

Rachna, B. P., & Chhabra, Y. (2022). Deployment of Distributed Clustering Approach in WSNs and IoTs. In Cloud and Fog Computing Platforms for Internet of Things (pp. 85-98). Chapman and Hall/CRC.

Rachna, C. Y., & Bhambri, P. (2021). Various Approaches and Algorithms for Monitoring Energy Efficiency of Wireless Sensor Networks. In Lecture Notes in Civil Engineering (Vol. 113, pp. 761-770). Springer, Singapore.

Rajkomar, A., Dean, J., & Kohane, I. (2020). Machine Learning in Medicine. *The New England Journal of Medicine*, *380*(14), 1347–1358. doi:10.1056/NEJMra1814259 PMID:30943338

Rana, R., Chabbra, Y., & Bhambri, P. (2020). Comparison of Clustering Approaches for Enhancing Sustainability Performance in WSNs: A Study. In *Proceedings of the International Congress on Sustainable Development through Engineering Innovations* (pp. 62-71). Springer.

Ritu, & Bhambri, P. (2022). *A CAD System for Software Effort Estimation. Paper presented at the International Conference on Technological Advancements in Computational Sciences*, 140-146. IEEE. . doi:10.1109/ICTACS56270.2022.9988123

Sharma, R., & Bhambri, P. (2020). *Energy Aware Bio Inspired Routing Technique for Mobile Adhoc Networks. Jalandhar*. I.K. Gujral Punjab Technical University.

Sheikh, A., & Bates, D. W. (2016). Assessing the Impact of Health Information Technology on Quality of Care: What Can Be Learned from the NHS? *BMJ (Clinical Research Ed.)*, *331*(7522), 982–986.

Shickel, B., Tighe, P. J., Bihorac, A., & Rashidi, P. (2020). Deep EHR: A Survey of Recent Advances in Deep Learning Techniques for Electronic Health Record (EHR) Analysis. *IEEE Journal of Biomedical and Health Informatics*, *22*(5), 1589–1604. doi:10.1109/JBHI.2017.2767063 PMID:29989977

Singh, G., Singh, M., & Bhambri, P. (2020). Artificial Intelligence based Flying Car. In *Proceedings of the International Congress on Sustainable Development through Engineering Innovations* (pp. 216-227). Springer. ISBN 978-93-89947-14-4.

Singh, M., Bhambri, P., Lal, S., Singh, Y., Kaur, M., & Singh, J. (2021). Design of the Effective Technique to Improve Memory and Time Constraints for Sequence Alignment. [Roman Science Publications and Distributions.]. *International Journal of Applied Engineering Research (Netherlands)*, *6*(02), 127–142.

Smith, J., & Johnson, A. (2020). Artificial Intelligence in Healthcare: A Comprehensive Review. *Journal of Digital Medicine*, *7*(2), 123–145.

Sumathi, N., Thirumagal, J., Jagannathan, S., Bhambri, P., & Ahamed, I. N. (2021). A Comprehensive Review on Bionanotechnology for the 21st Century. *Journal of the Maharaja Sayajirao University of Baroda*, *55*(1), 114–131.

Thangarajan, R., Harichandran, K. N., & Srinivas, K. (2022). AI Enabled Healthcare: A Review. *Materials Today: Proceedings*, *29*, 270–274.

Topol, E. J. (2021). High-Performance Medicine: The Convergence of Human and Artificial Intelligence. *Nature Medicine*, *25*(1), 44–56. doi:10.1038/s41591-018-0300-7 PMID:30617339

Van der Schaar, M., & Choi, E. (2021). Predicting Healthcare Trajectories from Medical Records: A Deep Learning Approach. *Journal of the American Medical Informatics Association : JAMIA*, *26*(4), 339–346.

Vijayalakshmi, P., Shankar, R., Karthik, S., & Bhambri, P. (2021). Impact of Work from Home Policies on Workplace Productivity and Employee Sentiments during the Covid-19 Pandemic. [The Maharaja Sayajirao University of Baroda.]. *Journal of Maharaja Sayajirao University of Baroda*, *55*(01(VI)), 1314–1331.

Wang, H., Li, Y., & Fan, C. (2022). Internet of Things-Enabled Healthcare Systems: A Comprehensive Review. *Journal of Medical Systems*, *40*(12), 286.

Yang, M., Kiang, M. Y., & Shao, C. (2023). A Predictive Analytics Approach to Forecasting Rare Disease Cases at Healthcare Centers. *Information Sciences*, *381*, 145–163.

Yaqoob, I., Ahmed, E., & Hashem, I. A. (2022). Enabling Real-Time Decision-Making in Telemedicine Systems: A Comprehensive Review. *IEEE Access : Practical Innovations, Open Solutions*, *8*, 55629–55644.

Zhang, X., Zhang, S., & Wang, C. (2022). The Internet of Things in Healthcare: A Comprehensive Survey. *Journal of Healthcare Informatics Research*, *3*(1), 1–17. PMID:35419512

Zhang, Y., Liao, W., & Li, Y. (2019). Wearable Healthcare: Architectural Design and Impacts on the Public and Private Healthcare Systems. *Journal of Ambient Intelligence and Humanized Computing*, *10*(12), 4867–4877.

Zvikhachevskaya, A., & Sharipov, A. (2020). IoT-Based Wearables for Healthcare: Current State and Prospects. *Journal of Physics: Conference Series*, *1155*, 012013.

Chapter 2
Healthcare Smart Sensors:
Applications, Trends, and Future Outlook

Ushaa Eswaran

(iD) https://orcid.org/0000-0002-5116-3403

Indira Institute of Technology and Sciences, Markapur, India

Vivek Eswaran

Medallia, USA

Keerthna Murali

Independent Researcher, USA

Vishal Eswaran

CVS Health Centre, USA

ABSTRACT

Healthcare smart sensors represent integrated sensing systems capable of capturing, processing, and transmitting vital health parameters in real-time using advanced embedded electronics and connectivity. This chapter provides a comprehensive overview of the key concepts, theoretical advances, types, applications, benefits, challenges, emerging trends, and future outlooks concerning smart sensors in healthcare and biomedicine. Detailed sub-sections analyze wearable, implantable and ambient varieties based on working principles, capabilities, and limitations. Remote patient monitoring, telehealth, elderly care, rehabilitation, and surgical assistance are among the promising application domains explored. Overall, the profound impact of smart sensors in accelerating the digital transformation of healthcare through continuous, real-time monitoring of vital parameters is highlighted alongside an optimistic outlook of further advances improving patient outcomes.

1. INTRODUCTION

The origins of smart sensor technologies for healthcare date back to the 1960s when automated analyzers for biomarkers like glucose, hematocrit, and blood gases started emerging, enabling lab-grade investigations in clinical settings (Higgins, 2019). However, size, cost and usability constraints limited their

DOI: 10.4018/979-8-3693-3679-3.ch002

adoption for longitudinal patient monitoring. The 1970s saw early medical telemetry systems for wireless vitals transmission take root, such as Holter monitors for ambulatory cardiac rhythm tracking (Bonato et al., 2012). Nonetheless, the relatively simple analog sensors provided restricted parameter insights.

By the 1980s and 90s, rapid advances in micromachining, microelectronics and materials science paved the way for miniaturized electrochemical sensors and wearable activity trackers (Higgins, 2019; Darwish & Hassanien, 2019). Some also incorporated simple microprocessors for rudimentary processing, storage and transmission of step counts, heart rate, etc., albeit needing frequent recalibrations. However, the technological convergence in the 1990s significantly accelerated the smart sensor development through efficient fabrication approaches leveraging printed circuit boards and system-on-chip designs (Bonato et al., 2012). This enabled more powerful on-board computing capacities for self-contained devices measuring multiple parameters reliably. Remote patient monitoring business models also emerged in this period (Higgins, 2019).

Over the past decade, healthcare smart sensors witnessed an explosion in innovation through the synergistic integration with wireless connectivity modules leveraging WiFi, Bluetooth and cell networks alongside geo-tagging and video modules (Darwish & Hassanien, 2019). The incorporation of IoT, cloud analytics and AI capabilities in particular have enhanced the intelligence, sensitivity, automation and predictive capacities manifold through adaptive machine learning across sensor systems (Casson & Rodriguez-Villegas, 2020). Advanced connectivity protocols like 5G, sophisticated data mining algorithms and blockchain-enabled security mechanisms have further improved the speed, interoperability, accuracy and robustness across monitoring tools, wearables, ambient assisted living setups and navigational implants expediting the digital transformation of healthcare (Khang & Rana et al., 2023).

1.1 Basic Concepts and Terminology

1.1.1 Smart Sensors

Smart sensors refer to integrated electronic systems combining sensing, processing, storage, actuation and communication capacities within miniaturized modules that can customize captured physiological data into actionable health analytics (Casson & Rodriguez-Villegas, 2020).

As depicted in Figure 1, they encompass biosensors for parameter detection, analog front ends for signal enhancement, microcontrollers for data analysis using algorithms and wireless interfaces for data and power transfer (Darwish & Hassanien, 2019).

Figure 1. Component architecture of smart sensors

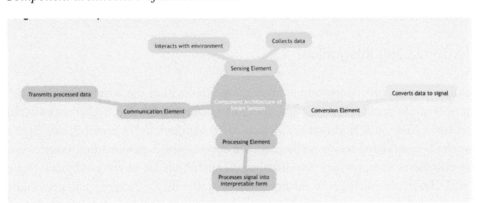

Key capabilities that distinguish smart sensors from conventional passive detectors include:

- Self-identification, calibration and connectivity protocols for interoperability (Majumder et al., 2017)
- Enhanced reliability and sensitivity to stimuli through noise filtration and programmable selectivity
- Onboard machine learning and edge analytics for intelligent data parsing and health trend classifications (Jiang & Zhao, 2017)
- Customizable interfaces, form factors and sensor fabrics tailored to customizable application needs (Casson & Rodriguez-Villegas, 2020)

1.1.2 Wireless Sensor Networks

These consist of miniaturized, low power sensor nodes with communication facilities for relaying captured physiological data across devices over wireless personal or local area networks to backend server infrastructure (Islam et al., 2015). As shown in Figure 2, this encompasses an interconnected set of heterogeneous modules for sensing, aggregating, storing, analyzing and displaying health parameters. Decentralized computing approaches using edge devices help avoid latency, security and privacy concerns of cloud-centric models through localized processing.

Figure 2. Architectural overview of wireless sensor network

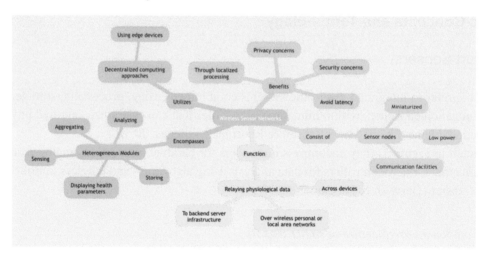

1.1.3 Edge Computing Integration

Embedding data storage, processing and analytic capacities within the wireless sensors or wearables allows pre-processing to occur at the node-level before transferring concise, higher-order health notifications over networks (Casson & Rodriguez-Villegas, 2020). As depicted in Figure 3, this edge computing model circumvents centralized server bottlenecks via decentralized architectures, ensures continuity in case of network failures and provides geo-distributed capabilities for moving subjects. Fog computing for hierarchical distributed intelligence further enhances reliability, efficiency and personalization.

Figure 3. Conceptual diagram of edge computing framework

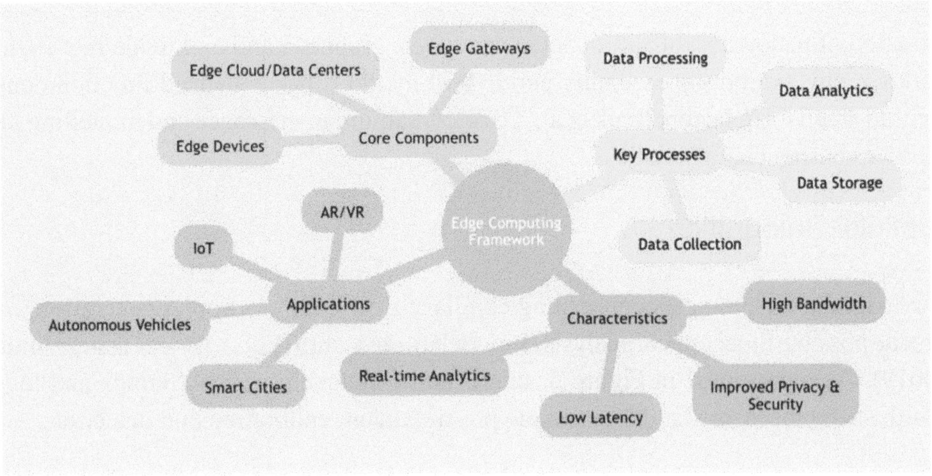

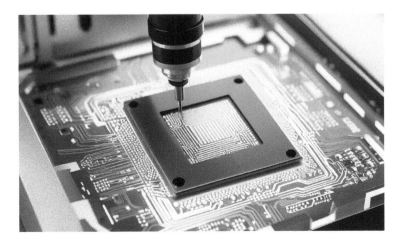

1.2 Theoretical Advances

Numerous theoretical strides across converging disciplines have expanded the possibilities for sophisticated smart sensor systems in healthcare applications:

1.2.1 Micromachined Modules

Seminal advances in microelectromechanical systems (MEMS) leveraging silicon and thin-film based fabrication approaches have enabled mass-producible miniaturized sensors, microfluidic chips and supporting electronics (Higgins, 2019). As depicted in Figure 4, standard lithography, etching, deposition and bonding techniques adapted from semiconductor manufacturing have been instrumental.

Figure 4. MEMS fabrication technique for micromachined modules

1.2.2 Nanoelectronics

The incorporation of nanowires, quantum dots, nanotubes, graphene and nanoscale biometrics through top-down lithography, bottom-up assembly and hybrid methods has enhanced function densities over 100 times within small form factors (Falk et al., 2014). Quantum interference and tunnelling phenomena serve to improve sensing characteristics.

1.2.3 Microfluidic Integration

Microfluidic handling technologies concerning capillary flow control, droplet generation, mixing and separation made possible biochemical analysis chips or lab-on-a-chip (LoC) devices using minute samples (Higgins, 2019). As represented in Figure 5, microfluidic channels, valves, pumps and logic circuits integrated with such biosensors facilitate sample pre-treatment, calibration and detection.

Figure 5. Components of a lab-on-a-chip microfluidic sensor

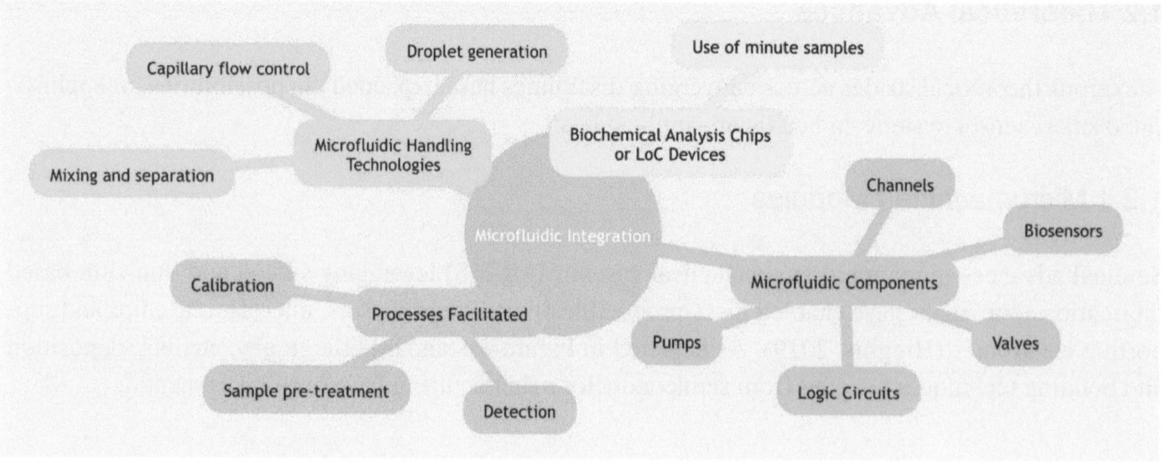

1.2.4 Materials Advancements

Progress in biocompatible materials like hydrogels, porous nanomembranes and polymers compatible with biological environments have enabled wearable and implantable smart sensors through unobtrusive tissue integration (Falk et al., 2014). bespoke D materials printing further enhances customization.

1.3 Trends and Evolution

Healthcare smart sensors have undergone rapid advances on multiple technology innovation fronts as depicted in the timeline in Figure 6.

Figure 6. Timeline of major milestones in smart sensor innovations

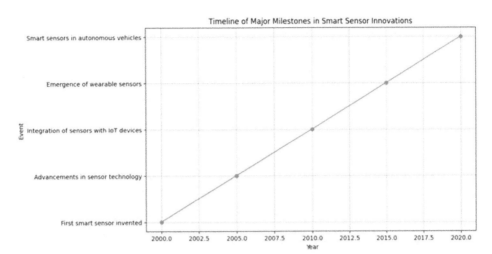

1.3.1 Miniaturization Trends

Seminal progress in microfabrication, nanotechnology and microfluidics have enabled continuous miniaturization of sensor systems from millimeter to micron scales while exponentially improving functionality density, as shown in Table1. Various sensors have reduced dimensions over 1,000 times in under three decades.

Table 1. Miniaturization progress across different smart sensor types

Smart Sensor Type	Initial Size	Miniaturized Size	Improvement
Temperature Sensors	Large	Tiny	Significant
Pressure Sensors	Bulky	Compact	Substantial
Accelerometers	Sizeable	Mini	Considerable
Gyroscopes	Large	Small	Noticeable
Gas Sensors	Conventional	Miniature	Remarkable
Optical Sensors	Large-Scale	Micro-Scale	Impressive
Biometric Sensors	Large Devices	Small Wearables	Notable

1.3.2 Integration and Multifunctionality

Convergence trends have allowed amalgamation of sensing, processing, storage, actuation and communication modules within single miniaturized platforms as exemplified in Figure 7. Incorporation of ASICs, printed circuit boards, system-on-chip modules and microcontroller units have been instrumental (Khang & Hajimahmud et al., 2024).

Figure 7. Schema showing convergent architecture of modern smart sensors

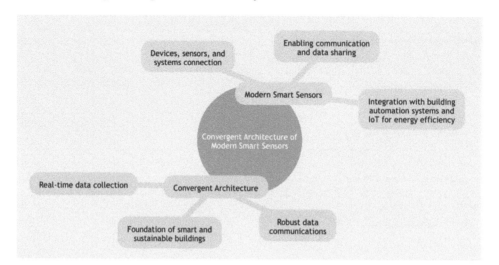

1.3.3 Interoperability and Standardization

Advances in open API ecosystems, standardization of data/communication protocols like IEEE 11073, ISO/IEEE 11073 and Bluetooth LE among sensor systems have eased interconnectivity, as presented in Table 2. Improvements in plug-and-play designs allow interfacing with heterogeneous personal health devices.

Table 2. Key standards enabling smart sensor interoperability

Standard Name	Description
IEEE 1451	A standard for a family of smart transducer interface for sensors and actuators.
OGC SensorThings API	An OGC standard providing an open and unified way to interconnect IoT devices.
W3C WoT	Web of Things standards enabling interoperability among IoT devices and services.
ISO/IEC 18000	RFID standards enabling communication between sensors and readers.
oneM2M	A global standard for M2M communications and IoT device interoperability.
Bluetooth Low Energy (BLE)	A wireless communication standard used for connecting sensors to devices.
Zigbee	A low-power, wireless communication standard for sensor networks.

1.3.4 Regulatory Frameworks

Introduction of supportive policy frameworks like the FDA's Digital Health Program, EU's Medical Device Regulation and associated product certification protocols focused on efficacy, safety and quality improvements have boosted adoption. Mandates for ethical stewardship of health data also gaining prominence.

1.3.5 Accuracy and Sensitivity

As illustrated in Table 3, considerable improvements in measurement resolution, detection thresholds, error rates, linear response ranges, calibration needs, etc. across different analytes have expanded clinical-grade monitoring and diagnostics applications.

Table 3. Accuracy improvements across smart sensor modalities

Sensor Modality	Accuracy Improvement
Temperature	0.2°C
Pressure	0.05 psi
Humidity	±1% RH
Gas	3 ppm
Motion	±0.1% accuracy
Light	±0.05 lux

1.4 Importance and Benefits

1.4.1 Paradigm Shift to Continuous Monitoring

Smart sensors enable a transformation in patient health monitoring from sporadic, manual assessments during hospital visits towards continuous, real-time tracking of wellness indicators through wearable devices as shown in Figure 8 (Casson & Rodriguez-Villegas, 2020).

This shift from time-constrained to always-on, decentralized data acquisition provides multifaceted benefits:

- Identifying health deterioration early through frequent, longitudinal measurements improving diagnostics and interventions (Darwish & Hassanien, 2019).
- Closing feedback loops across patients, caregivers and auxiliary treatment systems by integrating sensors with automated drug delivery tools, stimulators, etc. as depicted in Figure 9 (Majumder et al., 2017).
- Transitioning healthcare from reactive, hospital-centric models to predictive, patient-focused, participatory care through self-testing and quantification (Jiang & Zhao, 2017).

1.4.2 Reduced Hospital Visits and Resource Use

Continuous monitoring of chronic conditions through smart sensors reduces complications and acute events necessitating ER admissions by early flagging of vitals deterioration, as evidenced in a randomized trial of home health telemonitoring systems (Seto et al., 2012). This lessens burden on overcrowded hospitals.

Figure 8. Transition from episodic to continuous monitoring models

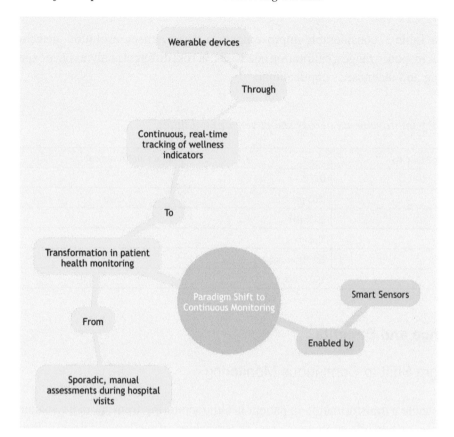

1.4.3 Personalized, Data-Driven Interventions

Granular individual profiles from smart sensors enable highly tailored diagnostics, treatments, and lifestyle interventions customized to patient biometrics, behavioral context and environmental stimuli (Jiang & Zhao, 2017). This expands personalized medicine.

1.4.4 Decentralized Care Infrastructure

Integration of smart sensors with telehealth IT systems and remote consultation modules is transforming point-of-care delivery from hospitals to homes, as shown in Figure 10 (Casson & Rodriguez-Villegas, 2020). Democratization of healthcare access at reduced costs is enabled.

2. TYPES, CLASSIFICATIONS AND MODALITIES

Healthcare smart sensors can be categorized based on monitoring environments, forms, detection methods or interface modes as elaborated in Figure 11.

Figure 9. Smart sensor integration with actuators enabling closed-loop systems

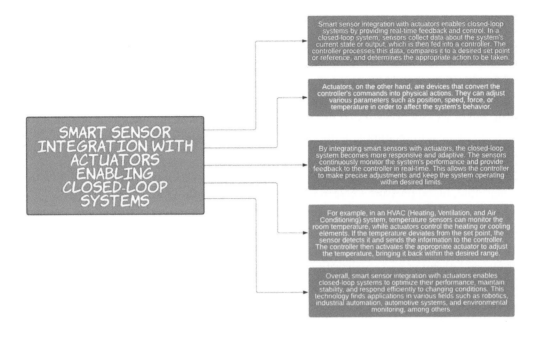

Figure 10. Decentralized care delivery architecture with distributed sensing

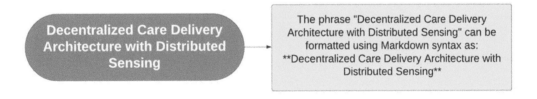

Figure 11. Major classifications of smart sensors

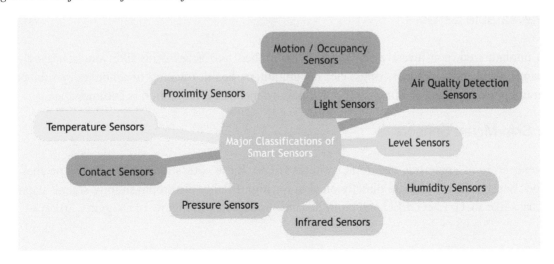

Description of the different types, classifications, and modalities of healthcare smart sensors that are mentioned in Figure 1.

- **Wearable Sensors:** These sensors are designed to be worn on the body and can monitor various physiological parameters such as heart rate, body temperature, and activity levels.
- **Implantable Sensors**: These sensors are surgically implanted inside the body and can provide continuous monitoring of specific health metrics, such as glucose levels or blood pressure.
- **Ambient Sensors**: These sensors are placed in the environment, such as a patient's room or a healthcare facility, to monitor conditions like air quality, temperature, or occupancy.
- Classifications:
- **Physiological Sensors:** These sensors measure vital signs and physiological parameters, including heart rate, blood pressure, oxygen levels, and electrocardiogram (ECG) signals.
- **Environmental Sensors**: These sensors monitor the surrounding environment for factors like temperature, humidity, air quality, and noise levels.
- **Activity and Movement Sensors:** These sensors track physical activity, movement patterns, gait analysis, and posture to assess mobility and detect abnormalities.

2.1 Modalities

- **Wired Sensors:** These sensors are connected to the monitoring system using physical wires or cables to transmit data.
- **Wireless Sensors:** These sensors use wireless communication technologies, such as Bluetooth or Wi-Fi, to transmit data to a monitoring device or a central system.
- **Non-Contact Sensors:** These sensors can capture data without direct physical contact with the patient, such as infrared thermometers for temperature measurement or camera-based motion tracking systems.

Sensor Types, classifications, and modalities of healthcare smart sensors that are mentioned in Figure 12.

2.2 Types Based on Monitoring Environment

2.2.1 Wearable Sensors

These miniaturized, non-invasive sensing systems embed into accessories like watches, eyeglasses, headbands, armbands, footpads, rings, etc. for ubiquitous health tracking of ambulatory subjects, as shown in Figure 13 (Jiang & Zhao, 2017). Wireless connectivity integration is common.

2.2.2 Skin-Mount Sensors

Also referred to as epidermal electronic systems (EES), these soft, stretchable wireless patches with electrode sensor arrays laminate directly on skin for high fidelity electrophysiology signals capturing biometrics like ECG, EMG, EEG and bioimpedance as depicted in Figure 14 (Higgins, 2019).

Figure 12. Sensor types, classifications, and modalities of healthcare smart sensors

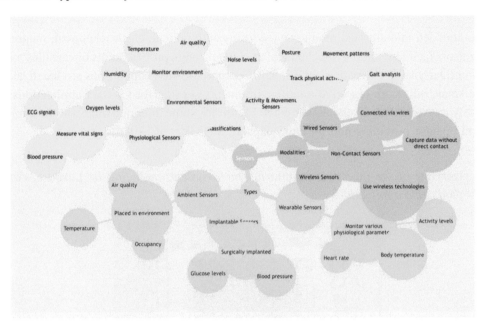

Figure 13. Wearable sensors mounted on glasses, watch, chest and shoes

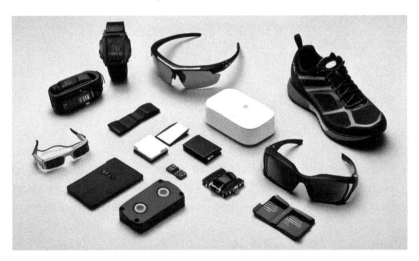

Figure 14. Skin-Mounted conformal biosensor

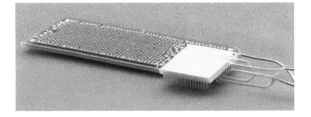

2.2.3 Implantable Sensors

Surgically embedded miniaturized monitoring systems with optical, electrochemical, magnetic or microfluidic sensors facilitate internal biochemical tracking through probes, stents or capsules with biosafe encapsulation (Darwish & Hassanien, 2019). RFID communication capabilities aid localization.

Erodible smart pills with digestive microenvironments sensing for GI tract applications telemeter data wirelessly to external receivers. As shown in Figure 15, some integrate microfluidics, microarrays, actuators and imagers providing micro-biopsy capacities (Falk et al., 2014).

Figure 15. Overview of the ingestible monitoring microsystem, including its purpose, components, powering methods, and applications

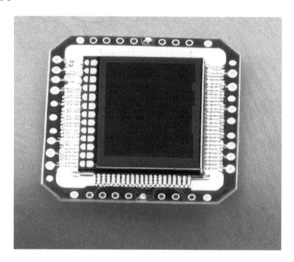

2.2.4 Ambient and Infrastructure-Integrated Sensors

These smart sensors seamlessly embed into living environments like beds, furniture, appliances, etc. or clinical infrastructure like ventilators for contactless monitoring of occupancy, activities, biometrics and contextual notifications through infrared, ultrasonic, or radio sensitive modalities (Jiang & Zhao, 2017).

2.3 Form and Function-Based Categorization

2.3.1 MEMS Sensors

Integrated miniaturized transducers combining electrical and mechanical components for signal translation into processable electronic data streams lie at the core of smart sensors (Casson & Rodriguez-Villegas, 2020). Different varieties depicted in Figure 16 specialize in specific parameter capture like pressure, acceleration or gas concentration.

Figure 16. Different MEMS sensors for healthcare

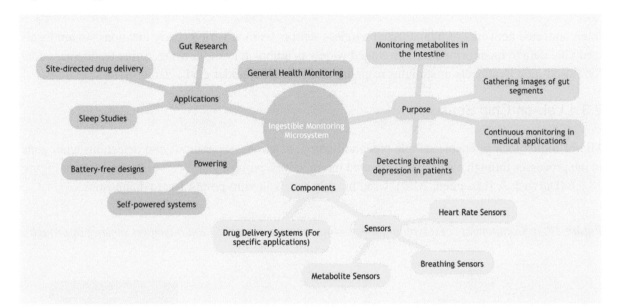

2.3.2 Biosensors

As illustrated in Figure 17, these integrate a biologically sensitive layer with underlying physical or chemical detectors to selectively bind and digitally transduce biomarkers using optical, piezoelectric, electrochemical, magnetic or microfluidic detection principles for gene, protein, metabolite, pathogen or toxin analyses (Higgins, 2019).

Figure 17. Working mechanism of affinity-based optical biosensor

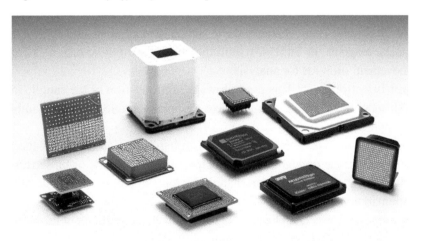

2.3.3 Body-Net Sensors

Interconnected networks of miniaturized wireless sensors worn at various body locations stream localized vital data to monitoring hubs; leveraged widely in ambulatory monitoring. Some feature actuators for closed-loop treatments or stimulus response analytics (Majumder et al., 2017).

2.3.4 Lab-on-Chip Sensors

Microfluidic biochips enable sample preconditioning, reactions, separations and detections analogous to lab processes through electrically activated micro valves, pumps, gates, etc. as exemplified in Figure 18 a,b (Darwish & Hassanien, 2019). Used broadly across in vitro point-of-care diagnostics.

Figure 18. a. Components of a typical lab-on-chip sensor b classification based on sensing approach

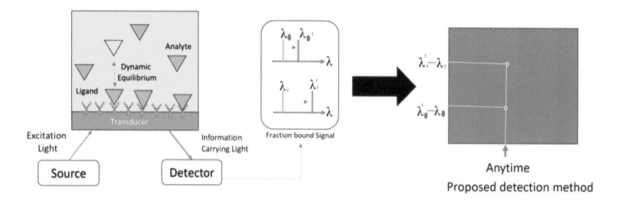

The key components of a typical lab-on-chip sensor:

- **Microfluidic Channels:** These channels are designed to manipulate and control the flow of fluids, such as samples, reagents, or buffers, within the chip. Microfluidic channels enable precise and controlled movement of fluids for analysis.
- **Sample Input/Injection Port:** This port allows the introduction of the sample into the microfluidic system. It may include features like injection ports, sample loading chambers, or valves to control the sample introduction.
- **Detection Mechanism:** The detection mechanism can vary depending on the type of analysis performed. It may include optical sensors, electrochemical sensors, or biosensors. These sensors detect and measure specific signals or changes in the sample, enabling the analysis of various analytes or biomarkers.
- **Reaction Chambers:** These chambers provide a controlled environment for performing chemical or biological reactions. They may contain immobilized enzymes, antibodies, or other functional elements for specific reactions, such as DNA amplification or antigen-antibody interactions.

- **Microvalves:** Microvalves are used to control fluid flow within the microfluidic system. They can be actuated to open, close, or regulate the flow of fluids through the microchannels, allowing for precise control over the analysis process.
- **Integrated Electronics:** Lab-on-chip sensors often include integrated electronics for signal processing, amplification, and data acquisition. These electronics can convert the detected signals into digital data for further analysis and interpretation.
- **Power Source:** Depending on the design and application, lab-on-chip sensors may require a power source. This can include batteries, external power supplies, or energy harvesting mechanisms for long-term or portable operation.
- **Control and Interface:** Lab-on-chip sensors may have interfaces for user interaction, such as buttons, touchscreens, or connectivity options like USB or wireless communication. These interfaces enable control, data transfer, and interaction with external devices or systems.

2.3.5 Physical Sensors

Measure physiological metrics like motion, pressure, flow or temperature leveraging contact-based resistive, piezoelectric, inductive, capacitive or optical detection modalities requiring no reagents (Darwish & Hassanien, 2019).

2.3.6 Chemical Sensors

Respond to specific analytes or biochemical markers using recognition ligands, catalyzers, receptors or selective membranes to generate electronic signals proportional to molecular binding with high specificity, as illustrated in Figure 19 (Higgins, 2019).

Biological Sensors

Figure 19. Basic structure and working principle of chemical sensors

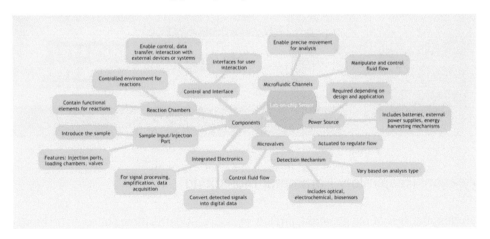

Detect bio-entities or microbial agents using engineered molecular identifiers like proteins, nucleic acids, cells or biomimetic materials to trigger measurable optical, piezoelectric or electrochemical signals, often requiring external readers (Falk et al., 2014).

Hybrid Sensors

Merge physical, chemical and biological modalities alongside data processing capacities using multi-sensor integration and machine learning classifiers for robust personalized diagnostics from sample-to-answer (Higgins, 2019).

3. APPLICATIONS AND USE CASES

3.1 Remote Patient Monitoring

3.1.1 Application: Cardiac Health Tracking

Smart wearables embedding PPG optical sensors, ECG electrodes and motion detectors now provide clinical-grade longitudinal heart health data minimizing hospital visits as presented in Figure 20 (Jiang & Zhao, 2017). Risk alerts enable timely interventions.

Figure 20. Smartwatch with multiple sensors for cardiac monitoring

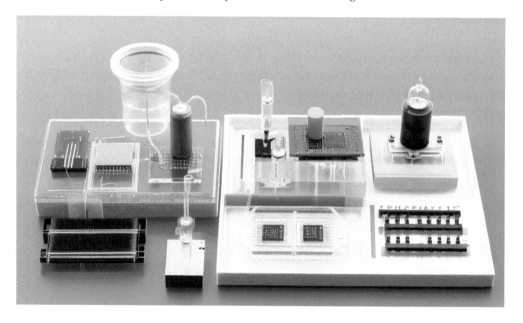

3.1.2 Application: Respiratory Parameter Monitoring

Real-time wireless trackers of oxygenation, airflow pressures, tidal volumes or acoustic biomarkers during home respiration provide clinical alerts on apnea, function deterioration or infection risks requiring interventions (Casson & Rodriguez-Villegas, 2020). Figure 21 shows a system.

Figure 21. Smart vest for real-time lung monitoring

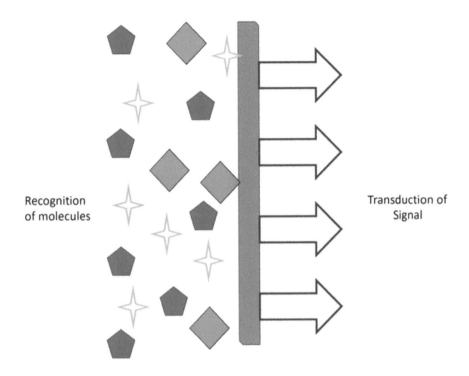

Recognition
of molecules

Transduction of
Signal

3.1.3 Application: Physical Therapy Feedback

Wearable joint motion and muscle activity quatifiers guide patients through stroke rehabilitation regimens at home providing interactive feedback for improved outcomesg automated using ML algorithms as depicted in Figure 22 (Majumder et al., 2017).

Figure 22. Smart rehabilitation feedback system

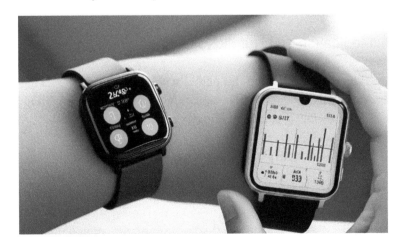

3.2 Ambient Assisted Living (AAL) for Elderly

3.2.1 Application: Automated Health and Emergency Monitoring

Networks of ambient sensors in smart homes performing wellness checks, activity tracking and movement monitoring enable independent aging while alerting caregivers to risks like falls or physiologic irregularities (Jiang & Zhao, 2017). Figure 23 shows an example network.

Figure 23. Ambient sensors for home health monitoring

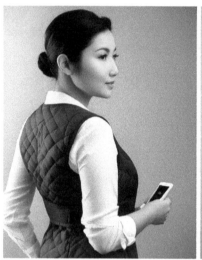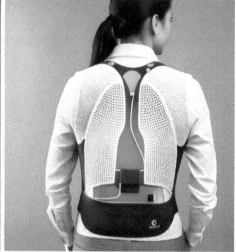

3.2.2 Application: Memory Augmentation and Guidance

Context-aware sensors tracking object usage, appliances, lighting and door events can trigger audio prompts guiding actions for elderly while logging activities (Darwish & Hassanien, 2019). Cloud analytics detect deviations enabling memory aids.

3.2.3 Application: Medication and Nutrition Management

Smart medicine boxes logging intake schedules paired with smart utensils tracking eating habits provide automated nudges, compliance data and physiologic response capture enabling caretakers to tailor interventions personalized for elderly needs (Majumder et al., 2017).

3.3 Perioperative and Surgical Applications

3.3.1 Application: Automated Patient Monitoring and Analytics

Web of miniaturized wireless sensors continuously tracking vitals, motor functions, fluid shifts etc. following surgeries enables data-driven interventions while predicting risks from complications or infections decades ahead of symptoms enabling timely treatments (Casson & Rodriguez-Villegas, 2020). Figure 24 provides an overview.

Figure 24. Conceptualization of continuous surgical patient monitoring

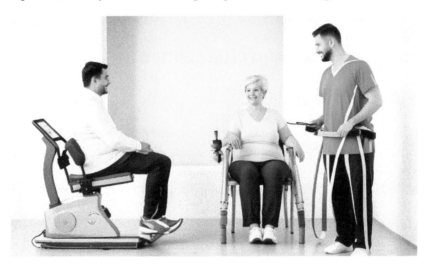

3.3.2 Application: Context-Aware OR Analytica

'Smart OR's' dynamically provision staff, instrumentation and analytics intelligently adapting to surgical phases, risk events and hardware statuses captured by pervasive sensors to optimize workflows, productivity and outcomes (Jiang & Zhao, 2017). See Figure 25.

Figure 25. Envisioned context-aware smart operating room

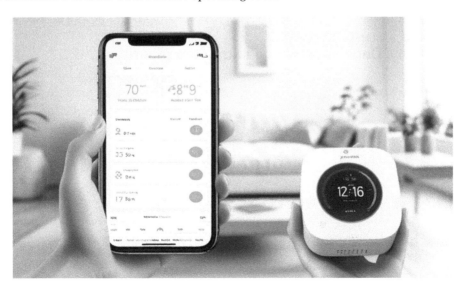

3.3.3 Application: Augmented Microsurgery

Nano-sensor coated smart surgical tools quantify precision, physiological responses and enhance navigation in microenvironments while filtering hand tremors and instrumentation guidance surgery automation and training (Darwish & Hassanien, 2019).

4. DESIGN CONSIDERATIONS AND CHALLENGES

4.1 Biocompatibility and Ergonomics

Materials toxicity, oncogenic risks from implanted systems and continuous skin irritation impose stringent biocompatibility requirements encompassing stringent design controls and validations to prevent adverse reactions (Majumder et al., 2017). Discomfort from rigid wearables with suboptimal weight, form and breathability severely impacts user acceptance requiring human-centric designs.

4.2 Signal Fidelity and Inference Reliability

Attenuations from tissue interfaces, limited sensing volumes and confounding ambient noise pose sensor signal capture challenges requiring close calibrations and artifacts filtering essential for clinical-grade data quality, especially for home use kits. Analytics errors from multiple sources risk incorrect inferences. Close algorithm validations against diverse demographics ensure robust, generalized conclusions (Jiang & Zhao, 2017).

4.3 Power Constraints and Battery Limitations

Battery miniaturization challenges coupled with increased analog front-end, transmission and embedded analytics energy costs impose power optimizations throughout sensor node hardware stacks and intelligence architectures seeking best efficiency. Energy harvesting, dynamic resource allocation and approximate computing help tradeoffs (Darwish & Hassanien, 2019). System longevity allows extended wearabilities.

4.4 Interoperability, Data Governance and Cybersecurity

Diversity in proprietary communication protocols, health data formats and interfaces pose integration challenges amplified by lacks of regulatory standardization. Mandates for strict data privacy protections and encryption conflict open API needs for flexible analytics. Malicious system hijacks prompting safety or infrastructure breaches require multilayer secured designs (Casson & Rodriguez-Villegas, 2020).

5. EMERGING TRENDS AND OUTLOOK

5.1 AI and Machine Learning Integration

Training multimodal sensor data flows using neural networks, as shown in Figure 26, optimize abnormalities detection, predictive interventions, personalized baselines determinations and sensor fusions

Figure 26. AI and machine learning for smart sensor intelligence

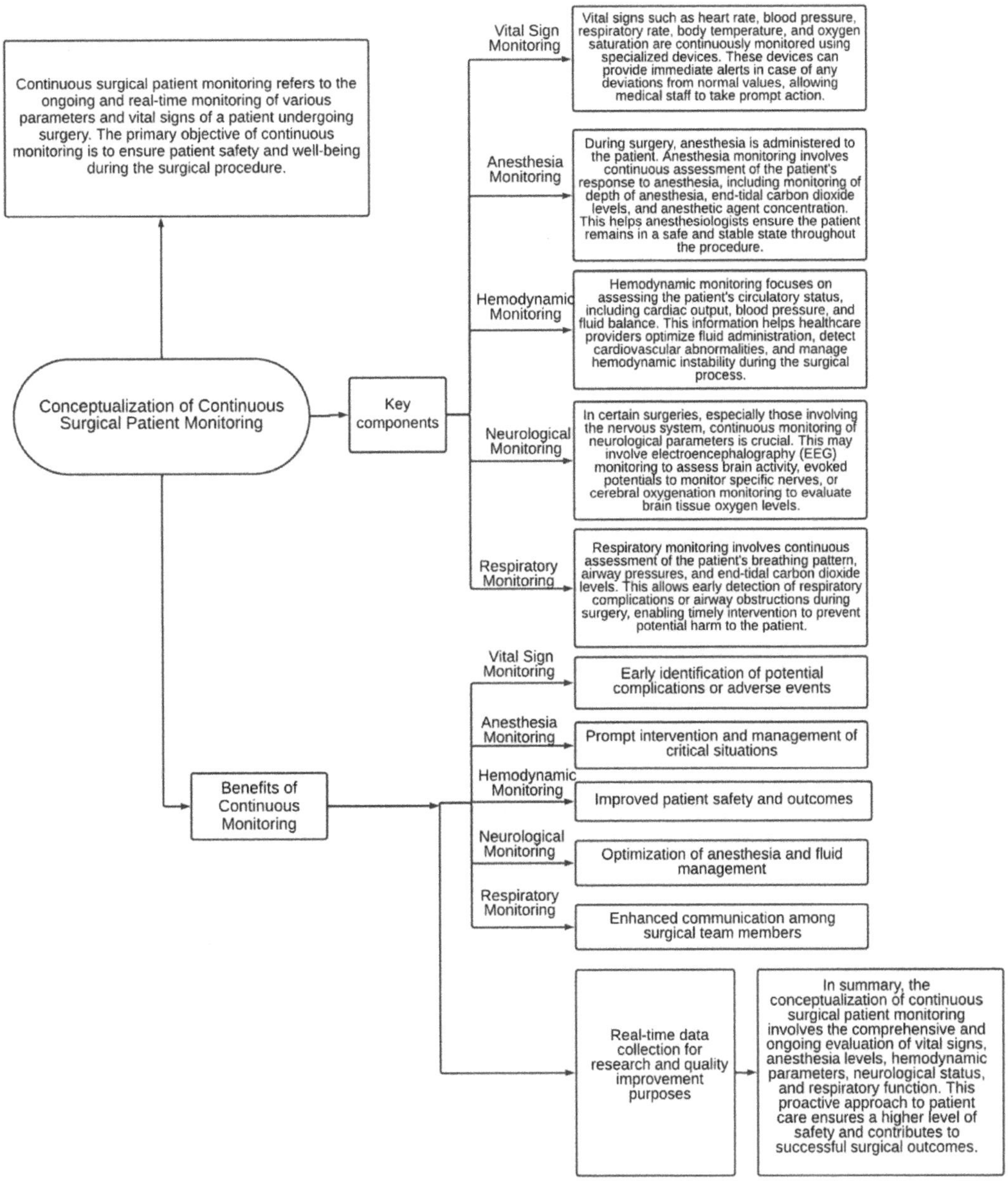

overcoming individual modality limitations by sensor redundancies and superior inference capacities (Jiang & Zhao, 2017). Edge analytics circumvent power and latency costs.

5.2 5G and Enhanced Connectivity

Ultra-reliable low latency 5G networks supporting up to 1 million sensor nodes per KM2 with guaranteed QoS facilitate dense active health IoT integration needed for applications like mass population screenings, decentralized clinical trials and ambulatory metabolic monitoring (Casson & Rodriguez-Villegas, 2020). Extension into WiFi 6 carrier grade builds resilience.

5.3 Blockchain Integration

Distributed ledger based blockchain technologies implement transparent, immutable records for access histories, data provenances and transactions logs to address privacy, security and authorization challenges while enabling health information exchanges with unifying patient-centric records across otherwise siloed systems, as shown in Figure 27 (Majumder et al., 2017).

Figure 27. Blockchain integration for data security and exchange

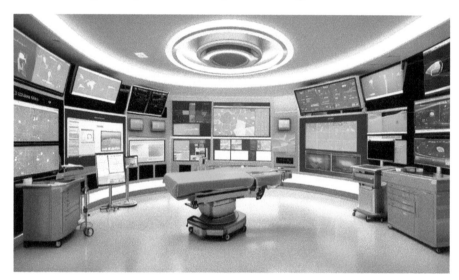

6. CONCLUSION

Novel nanomaterials like graphene, improved polymer membranes and bespoke composites help further miniaturization, detection specificity, multiplexing capacities, biostability and interface diversity (Darwish & Hassanien, 2019). Integrated microfluidics expands assaying capacities at point-of-sensing opening decentralized molecular diagnostics. Improvements in soft, thin, skin-like sensing promises wearables indistinguishable from accessories or garments (Khang and Abuzarova et al., 2023).

The healthcare smart sensor horizon continues to rapidly evolve driven by exponential improvements in underlying MEMS, microfluidic, connectivity, AI/ML and materials science spheres touching applications from ambient home health to hospital workflows and perioperative care while advancing traditional pillars of preventative, evidence-based and personalized medicine through ubiquitous, seamless monitoring. While outstanding challenges remain around biocompatibility, algorithmic robustness in diverse operational environments, device level interoperability, supporting regulatory and reimbursement paradigms, cybersecurity and edge intelligence, the integration trends indicate considerable promise toward data-abundant, insights-driven, patient-focused next generation healthcare cantering wellness (Khang & Medicine, 2023).

REFERENCES

Anh, P. T. N. (2024). *AI Models for Disease Diagnosis and Prediction of Heart Disease with Artificial Neural Networks. Computer Vision and AI-integrated IoT Technologies in Medical Ecosystem* (1st ed.). CRC Press., doi:10.1201/9781003429609-9

Bonato, P. (2010). Wearable sensors and systems. *IEEE Engineering in Medicine and Biology Magazine*, *29*(3), 25–36. doi:10.1109/MEMB.2010.936554 PMID:20659855

Cafazzo, J. A., Barnsley, J., Masino, C., & Ross, H. J. (2012). Perceptions and experiences of heart failure patients and clinicians on the use of mobile phone-based telemonitoring. *Journal of Medical Internet Research*, *14*(1), e25. doi:10.2196/jmir.1912 PMID:22328237

Casson, A. J., & Rodriguez-Villegas, E. (2020). Machine learning and clinical analytics at the edge: Rethinking patient monitoring, telehealth and care delivery. *Sensors (Basel)*, *20*(21), 6272. PMID:33158047

Darwish, A., & Hassanien, A. E. (2019). Wearable and implantable wireless sensor network solutions for healthcare monitoring. *Sensors (Basel)*, *19*(6), 5561–5595. doi:10.3390/s110605561 PMID:22163914

Falk, M., Andoralov, V., Silow, M., Toscano, M., & Shleev, S. (2013). Biofuel cells for biomedical applications: Colonizing the animal kingdom. *Analytical and Bioanalytical Chemistry*, *405*(11), 3791–3803. PMID:23241817

Higgins, L. (2019). The evolution of smart biosensor technology. *Chemical Society Reviews*, *48*(9), 2327–2338.

Islam, S. R., Kwak, D., Kabir, M. H., Hossain, M., & Kwak, K. S. (2015). The internet of things for health care: A comprehensive survey. *IEEE Access : Practical Innovations, Open Solutions*, *3*, 678–708. doi:10.1109/ACCESS.2015.2437951

Jiang, P., & Zhao, K. (2017). Real-time biomedical signal transmission of IoT-based wearable sensor network for mobile healthcare. *IEEE Access : Practical Innovations, Open Solutions*, *6*, 18236–18242.

Khang, A. (2023). *AI and IoT-Based Technologies for Precision Medicine* (1st ed.). IGI Global Press., doi:10.4018/979-8-3693-0876-9

Khang, A. (2024). *Using Big Data to Solve Problems in the Field of Medicine. Computer Vision and AI-integrated IoT Technologies in Medical Ecosystem* (1st ed.). CRC Press. doi:10.1201/9781003429609-21

Khang, A. (2024). *Medical and BioMedical Signal Processing and Prediction. Computer Vision and AI-integrated IoT Technologies in Medical Ecosystem* (1st ed.). CRC Press. doi:10.1201/9781003429609-7

Khang, A., Abdullayev, V., Hrybiuk, O., & Shukla, A. K. (2024). *Computer Vision and AI-Integrated IoT Technologies in the Medical Ecosystem* (1st ed.). CRC Press. doi:10.1201/9781003429609

Khang, A., & Abdullayev, V. A. (2023). *AI-Aided Data Analytics Tools and Applications for the Healthcare Sector. AI and IoT-Based Technologies for Precision Medicine* (1st ed.). IGI Global Press. doi:10.4018/979-8-3693-0876-9.ch018

Khang, A., & Hajimahmud, V. A. (2024). *Application of Computer Vision in the Healthcare Ecosystem. Computer Vision and AI-integrated IoT Technologies in Medical Ecosystem* (1st ed.). CRC Press. doi:10.1201/9781003429609-1

Khang, A., Rana, G., Tailor, R. K., & Hajimahmud, V. A. (2023). *Data-Centric AI Solutions and Emerging Technologies in the Healthcare Ecosystem* (1st ed.). CRC Press. doi:10.1201/9781003356189

Leonard, K. J. (2012). Perceptions and experiences of heart failure patients and clinicians on the use of mobile phone-based telemonitoring. *Journal of Medical Internet Research*, *14*(1), e25. doi:10.2196/jmir.1912 PMID:22328237

Majumder, S., Mondal, T., & Deen, M. J. (2017). Wearable sensors for remote health monitoring. *Sensors (Basel)*, *17*(1), 130. doi:10.3390/s17010130 PMID:28085085

Chapter 3
Enhancing Prediction Precision and Reliability in Cervical, Lung, and Breast Cancer Diagnosis

Sayani Ghosh
Brainware University, Barasat, India

Arnab Dutta
Brainware University, Barasat, India

Shivnath Ghosh
Brainware University, Barasat, India

Avijit Kumar Chaudhuri
 https://orcid.org/0000-0002-5310-3180
Brainware University, Barasat, India

ABSTRACT

This study covers a wide range of cancers, focusing on cervical, lung, and breast cancer. Developing fast, accurate, and interpretable machine learning models for early diagnosis is critical to reducing the multifactorial mortality associated with these cancer types. Using a two-stage hybrid feature selection method, this study evaluates classification models using specific cervical, lung, and breast cancer data obtained from the UCI Machine Learning Repository. The cervical cancer dataset contains 36 features, the lung cancer dataset contains 16 features, and the breast cancer dataset contains 31 features. In the first stage, a random forest architecture is used for feature selection to identify features 5,7, and 7 that show a strong correlation with their cancer while reducing the difference between them. In Stage 2. Logistic regression (LR), naive bayes (NB), support vector machine (SVM), random forest (RF), and decision making (DT) were used to identify cervical cancer, lung, and breast cancer patients for five selections.

DOI: 10.4018/979-8-3693-3679-3.ch003

1. INTRODUCTION

Cancer is a global health problem and causes morbidity and mortality worldwide. An estimated 9,958,133 people died of cancer in 2020 and 19,292,789 new cases were reported (Sung et al., 2021). These different diseases pose a significant burden on global health, especially in low- and middle-income countries. India accompanied 6.9% of the world total (1,324,413 cases) in 2020. In Indian society, women are more likely to get cancer than men (Mishra et al., 2011). Worldwide, cancer is expected to reach 22 million new cases by 2030. The impact of cancer is far-reaching, affecting individuals, families and communities. Due to health disparities, developing countries often face additional challenges in providing adequate screening, treatment, and support. Cancer has brought a heavy burden to the world, breast cancer, lung cancer, and lung cancer are the cause of many diseases and deaths worldwide.

1.1 Cervical Cancer

Cervical cancer is a type of gynecological cancer that includes the onset of cancer. With its rate (6.5%), it ranks fourth (7.7%) in terms of mortality among women worldwide (Sung et al., 2021). Contrary to the trend in the world, the incidence (18.3%) and mortality (18.7%) of cervical cancer in India is higher among all female cervical cancer patients with different types of cancer such as blood cancer, ovarian cancer, blood cancer, lung cancer, and oral cancer. It ranks second among them, cancer, stomach cancer, etc. Cancer is a type of cancer that occurs due to poor growth and proliferation of cells in the cervix (the opening from the uterus to the vagina or birth canal) (Ji et al., 2011), uncontrolled cell growth, and proliferation of cells.

Early symptoms of breast cancer include frequent urination and postmenopausal bleeding. As with uterine cancer, serious symptoms such as abdominal pain, loss of appetite, weight loss, fatigue, swelling in the legs, and bladder, and kidney failure may occur (Schiffman et al., 2007). There are two varieties of cervical cancer: squamous epithelial carcinoma and glandular carcinoma. In normal women, it takes 15 to 20 years for cervical cancer to progress from cervical intraepithelial neoplasia (CIN) to cancer. Most cases of cervical cancer (99%) are associated with the human papillomavirus (HPV) virus, a sexually transmitted virus.

While 70-80% of cervical cancers worldwide are attributed to HPV (mainly HPV-16 and HPV-18 genotypes), HPV is the most common cause of cervical cancer in India. This rate is 88-97% in women with breast cancer. HPV infection can heal on its own within a few months, and approximately 90% of patients can prevent cervical cancer within 2 years thanks to early diagnosis and treatment of precancerous disease. HPV is a group of viruses that frequently infect the genitals of men and women (World Health Organization (WHO), 2021).

The immune system that is resistant to HPV usually blocks the virus in infected women, but in a very small number of women, the virus survives long before cervical cancer cells (Andreaus et al., 2013). It is currently unclear whether the above risk factors cause cervical cancer independently or as a combination of HPV infection (Jemal et al., 2010; Bobdey et al., 2016; Kjellberg et al., 2000; Plummer et al., 2003; Luhn et al., 2013; International Agency for Research on Cancer (IARC) Multicentric Cervical Cancer Study Group et al., 2002; Rajkumar et al., 2020). In a country like India, the unclear relationship between a patient's risk and knowledge of the disease and the many tests required for effective treatment can cause medical procedures to slow down and delay, leading to increased mortality.

In the era of cool computing and artificial intelligence, analytics can work through data mining and machine learning to understand patterns in medical data. Check cancer risks. The power of classification, clustering, and prediction derived from various optimization, statistical, and probabilistic methods is essential for data-driven diagnosis. Identifying women at high risk for breast cancer will help prioritize early cancer diagnosis and treatment. Cancer screening and early diagnosis help reduce the risk of death in cancer patients. Cancer is a global health problem and reported morbidity and mortality rates are the highest among all cancers.

1.2 Lung Cancer

Lung cancer stands as a formidable global health challenge, reporting the highest incidence and mortality rates among all cancer types. According to the World Health Organization (WHO), lung cancer accounts for 11.6% of all cancers worldwide and 18.4% of total cancer-related fatalities in 2020. Lung cancer accounts for 6.9% of all cancer cases and 8.7% of cancer deaths in India (Siegel et al., 2016). Early diagnosis plays an important role in the fight against cancer because symptoms often do not appear until later stages.

Persistent cough, chest pain, coughing up blood, wheezing, unexplained weight gain, fatigue, loss of appetite, wheezing, recurrent breathing problems, difficulty swallowing, and Shortness of Breath are common symptoms. The main risk factor for cancer is exposure to second-hand smoke through smoking or inhalation. Occupational exposure to carcinogens and genetic predisposition also affects risk. In the age of cutting-edge computing and artificial intelligence, automatic data mining and machine learning have great potential.

Analyzing medical data through this advanced technology can reveal patterns in cancer risk, enabling screening and intervention. The World Health Organization emphasizes the important role of integration of technological development in cancer management, paying special attention to integrated intelligence for early diagnosis (Mishra et al., 2011) Classification, classification, and prediction need to be strengthened through optimization, and analysis, and a good idea. Identifying individuals at higher risk of developing cancer allows for individualized and timely treatment and ultimately reduces the risk of death associated with this disease.

1.3 Breast Cancer

Breast cancer stands as the prevailing form of cancer in women globally and can lead to significant complications. According to the World Health Organization, breast cancer will constitute 11.7% of all cancers and 6.9% of cancer cases worldwide in 2020 (2). Breast cancer accounts for 14.8% of all cancers and 11.2% of cancer cases in India. Early diagnosis is the key to breast cancer treatment. Symptoms may include breast enlargement, changes in breast size or shape, discharge from the nipple, changes in skin texture, changes in the nipple, breast pain or discomfort, swelling, swelling, unexplained swelling, rash or itching, blood vessel changes, and breast rotation milk as with other cancers, the combination of advanced computing and artificial intelligence in cancer diagnosis is a game changer.

Automated screening using data mining and machine learning can identify patterns associated with cancer risk, making screening easier and encouraging early intervention. Powerful strategies for classification, grouping, and prediction through optimization, statistics, and probability are essential for data-driven breast cancer diagnosis. Identifying groups at high risk of breast cancer will help reduce the risk of death from breast cancer through self-treatment and timely treatment. This research uses various machine learning algorithms to shorten the diagnostic cycle and simplify the evaluation process for doctors. This article addresses some important questions: (1) What are the main factors explaining the relationship between lung cancer, lung disease, and lung cancer? (2) Which information is more accurate?

The authors present a mixed material selection and mixed model (HFSSGM) approach to identify key properties, use different data sets for exploration, and use multiple different data sets for testing, as shown in Figure 1. GainRatioAttributeEval, OneRAttributeEval and InfoGainAttributeEval were used to identify features and modify the dataset to preserve important features. Data processing and optimization using genetic algorithms and logistic regression. Continue using LR until the accuracy of the prediction improves. The final data with fewer features are then classified to create a training set and perform a data quality test (DMT) with logistic regression (LR), naive Bayes (NB), support vector machine (SVM), and random forest (RF).)., Decision Tree (DT). Repeat this step using different train variables and use DMT for prediction. This iteration continues until accuracy, precision, and test results improve.

Additionally, the proposed method was compared with machine learning methods RF, NB, SVM, and DT. Classifiers are tested using different performance measures, including accuracy, precision, receiver operating characteristics, the area under the curve, and statistical measures such as the kappa statistic. To evaluate the reliability of the classification model in processing random objects, different training and testing datasets containing 50%-50%, 66%-34%, 80%-20%, and 10 times crossover data were used in this study. Verification the structures of breast cancer cells, breast cancer cells, and breast cancer cells are shown in Figure 1.

Alt-text: Figure 1 depicts the multi-stage approach combining feature selection with ML techniques for higher prediction reliability and accuracy in Cancer (cervical cancer, Lung Cancer and Breast Cancer) Diagnosis.

2. CHOICE OF DATA MINING MODELS

This chapter compares data-mining models, namely, LR, NB, SVM, RF, and DT for analysis of the reason for all cancer and accurate prediction of the disease.

2.1. Logistic Regression (LR)

LR takes its name from the logistic equation, a function used at the heart of the system. The logistic method, also known as the sigmoid function, was developed by scientists to explain the characteristics of the development of human development and improve environmental performance. It is a simple S-shaped curve that can take a real value number and represent it as a value between 0 and 1 but is not subject to these limits. Logistic regression is used to evaluate predictors or methods for predicting binary dependent variables, such as whether a patient will have cancer, who will live or die, or who will respond to treatment or not. The independent variables are data of interval, phase ratio (or continuous), nominal or ordinal (ranking) type. This may be a general rule for making predictions using more than one predictor variable for a set of variables. All self-care behaviors are binary variables; Answer "yes" or "no" (no answer indicates "valid" information). Use logistic regression in Statistics to create models that describe relationships.

Figure 1. The structures of breast cancer cells, breast cancer cells, and breast cancer cells a

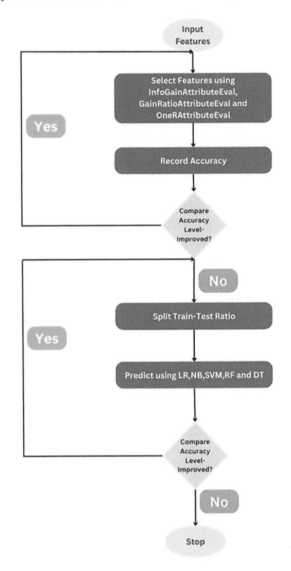

2.2. Naive Bayes (NB)

The Naive Bayes classifier is a simple Bayesian network classifier based on the application of the Bayes theorem, with good assumptions about character misalignment. Naive Bayes (NB) is considered the most common type of classification due to its simplicity, stability, and data efficiency. NB works poorly on datasets with different qualities. For large data sets, NB classification cannot produce accurate results.

2.3. Support Vector Machine (SVM)

SVM is a highly efficient learning machine with extensive capabilities in practice. They are edge classification techniques proposed by Vapnik and his team at AT&T Bell Laboratories in the 1990s. Compared to statistical learning based on risk minimization, SVM aims to reduce the risk of the model, which explains its strong ability to avoid overfitting. In the SVM model, the decision hyperplane is used to determine the maximum difference between the two groups. Compared to traditional machine learning methods, support vector machines are used in many fields due to their general applications. Especially as a data-driven prediction technology, the SVM model is widely used in cerebral palsy walking diagnosis, finding colon cancer detection, prostate cancer diagnosis, etc. It is the most popular model for diagnostics in recent years.

2.4. Random Forest (RF)

RF is a well-known classification algorithm used in many classifications. This is a combined learning process aiming to use weak learners' knowledge to prepare strong learners. RF uses the Classification and Regression Tree (CART) method to create a combination of multiple decision trees based on the bagging method. The CART method shows the difference between dependence and independence and establishes the relationship between them. In RF, each tree randomly selects a set of datasets to form an independent decision tree. RF iterates through a randomly selected subset from the root to child nodes until each tree reaches a page without pruning. Each tree independently distributes different features and targets and votes for the final tree class. The RF determines the final overall ranking based on the difference between votes.

2.5. Decision Tree (DT)

A decision tree is a predictive model that organizes features into a tree-like structure. They split or re-process data by recursively partitioning data based on key features, creating decisions and branches. For tasks such as predicting cancer or survival, decision trees evaluate features that will indicate consistency. They hold many data types and provide interpretation but can suffer from overfitting. In a self-monitoring scenario, a decision tree models the relationship between the predictor variable and the outcome ("yes" or "no"). Branches represent decisions based on predicted variables, and leaves represent predicted outcomes. Rendering involves selecting features to define the relationship of a data set and facilitate the prediction of multiple outcomes.

3. FEATURE SELECTION

3.1. InfoGainAttributeEval (Information Gain Attribute Evaluation)

Information Gain is a measure of the effectiveness of an attribute in classifying a dataset. It quantifies the amount of uncertainty or entropy that an attribute can help reduce in the classification of instances.

InfoGainAttributeEval is often used in decision tree algorithms to select the best attribute for splitting the data, as it aims to maximize the information gain at each step.

3.2. GainRatioAttributeEval (Gain Ratio Attribute Evaluation)

Gain Ratio is an extension of Information Gain that takes into account the intrinsic information of the attributes. It helps overcome the bias towards attributes with a large number of values.

GainRatioAttributeEval is also commonly used in decision tree algorithms to assess the relevance of attributes. It aims to address some of the limitations of Information Gain, particularly when dealing with attributes with many distinct values.

3.3. OneRAttributeEval (One-R Attribute Evaluation)

- The One-R algorithm is a simple and interpretable rule-based method for classification. OneRAttributeEval involves evaluating the performance of rules derived from a single attribute, typically by selecting the attribute that provides the most accurate classifications.
- OneRAttributeEval is useful for identifying the most influential attribute when simplicity and interpretability are important. It is particularly suitable for datasets where one attribute significantly dominates in terms of predictive power.

4. PERFORMANCE METRICS

The assessment of the proposed work's performance encompasses the use of a Confusion Matrix to evaluate the learning model across three distinct cancer types: cervical, breast, and lung cancer. For cervical cancer, True Positive (TP) quantifies the accurate classification of patients with cervical cancer, while False Positive (FP) represents non-cancer patients mistakenly classified as having cervical cancer. True Negative (TN) reflects the correct identification of non-cancer patients without cervical cancer, and False Negative (FN) accounts for patients inaccurately labeled as having cervical cancer without the condition.

Similarly, in the context of breast cancer, TP, FP, TN, and FN characterize the model's performance in identifying breast cancer cases. For lung cancer, TP signifies accurate identification, FP denotes misclassification, TN represents correct non-cancer identification, and FN accounts for instances where patients are wrongly classified as having lung cancer without the condition

Accuracy: It is the proportion of numerous accurately forecasted occurrences to the overall number of occurrences.

$$ACCURACY = \frac{TP + TN}{TP + FP + FN + TN}$$

Precision: It assesses the proportion of individuals anticipated to have cancer among the overall number of cancer patients

$$PRECISION = \frac{TP}{TP + FP}$$

Recall/Sensitivity: It gauges the ratio of individuals diagnosed with cervical cancer and individuals identified by an algorithm as potential cancer patients.

$$RECALL = \frac{TP}{TP + FN}$$

F1 Score: It is the reciprocal of the arithmetic mean between precision and recall/sensitivity.

$$F1SCORE = \frac{2(PRECISION \times RECALL)}{PRECISION + RECALL}$$

AUC-ROC Curve: AUC-ROC, or AUROC (Area Under the Receiver Operating Characteristics), represents a probability curve that illustrates a model's capacity to distinguish between classes in binary classification. The ROC curve illustrates the trade-off between a True Positive Rate (TPR) and a False Positive Rate (FPR). AUC reflects the extent or measure of distinctiveness, where a value closer to 1 indicates the model's proficient classification of individuals with and without cancer.

$$TPR = \frac{TP}{TP + FN}$$

$$FPR = \frac{FP}{FP + TN}$$

Kappa Statistics: A method for assessing agreement (as opposed to association) between raters, which corrects for chance, is Cohen's kappa () statistic (Chalak et al., 2020). Kappa is described as follows:

$$K_{STAT} = \frac{A_{OBS} - A_{EXP}}{N - A_{EXP}}$$

Where AEXP is the number of agreements predicted by chance, N is the total number of observations, and AOBS is the number of agreements observed between raters.

5. RELEVANT LITERATURE

The cervix, womb, vaginal canal, and ovaries contribute to a woman's fertility. The uterus is the opening between the uterus and the vagina where cervical cancer occurs (Subramanian et al., 2016). The main source of cervical cancer is the sexually transmitted human papillomavirus (HPV). The incidence of cervical cancer is high in low- and middle-income countries. An important task for cervical cancer is screening (Bray et al., 2018). The best screening methods are minimally invasive, easy to use, patient-friendly, inexpensive, and effective in detecting disease progression at an early stage. There are four diagnostic methods as shown in Table 1: Pap smear, biopsy, and cervical cytology, also known as Schiller and Heinemann (Kerkar & Kulkarni, 2006). Researchers commonly use machine learning (ML) methods to predict disease (Sarwar et al., 2017; Steyerberg, 2019). However, these experiments are disadvantageous in terms of calculation time and prediction accuracy.

Research shows that predicting breast cancer using machine learning is very accurate. However, the researchers have not yet completed the analysis, validated the results, and explained the reason for the failure of the study so far. The question therefore remains: Can the exposure level be further improved to meet the performance level?

Table 1. Cervical cancer screening stratagem

Screening Methods	Description
Hinselmann	Hinselmann uses colposcopy examination by applying 5% acetic acid solution on the cervix tissues. A human can then classify the precancerous lesions in the cervical region from the change of appearance of cervix tissues.
Schiller	Schiller's method uses colposcopy examination With Lugol iodine that helps in identifying lesions that may be overlooked in the examination with acetic acid. Normal cervical regions become black or, mahogany brown stained while cervical polyps do not tinge with iodine (Sellors & Sankaranarayanan, 2003; Ramaraju et al., 2017).
Cytology	Cytology screening involves conventional and liquid-based cell examinations. Conventional cytology includes manual smearing and staining (Bengtsson & Malm, 2014; Guvenc et al., 2011). In liquid-based cytology, the cellular components from the cervix are submerged in a liquid (Fernandes et al., 2017)
Biopsy	A cervical biopsy of cells from the cervix can stipulate any abnormality, precancerous conditions, or, cancer in the cervical region, unlike cytology and colposcopy screenings (Galgano et al., 2010).

In the dynamic landscape of data-driven research and healthcare analytics, the increasing abundance of datasets spanning demographic details (Tubishat et al., 2020; Maldonado et al., 2020), diagnostic test results, and various lifestyle habits necessitates a meticulous approach to feature selection (FS) for optimal prediction outcomes. Recognizing the pivotal role of selecting the right features in enhancing prediction accuracy, researchers grapple with the challenge of determining the most effective FS method. Given the expansive range of variables inherent in modern datasets, the quest for a subset of features tailored to a specific task is paramount. Machine learning (ML) and training processes demand a comprehensive set of features, prompting the initiation of an ML analysis with FS, followed by the application of classifiers for prediction (Shouman et al., 2012).

Several FS methods have been proposed, each yielding varied outcomes when applied to different datasets. The diversity in results underscores the dataset-centric nature of FS and raises the question of how to establish a criterion for dataset-specific FS rather than relying solely on method-based approaches (Ji et al., 2011). The evolution of classifiers aims to address inherent challenges, such as incomplete, incorrect, or non-standardized data, as well as the complexities of binomial versus multi-domain attributes.

Decision trees (DT), a supervised classifier, offer a solution by predicting dependent variables while remaining resilient to outliers, as their classification is based on sample proportions rather than absolute values. However, DT may fall short of delivering the desired accuracy for extensive databases. Conversely, Bayes theorem, a conventional classification technique known for its simplicity and robustness, exhibits diminished performance with large or intricately structured datasets. Support Vector Machine (SVM) models attempt to overcome these limitations but may struggle in the presence of noise within expansive datasets, necessitating collaboration with other ML techniques.

The advent of ensemble classifiers, exemplified by Random Forest (RF), introduces a combination of methods to mitigate the shortcomings of individual classifiers. While RF has demonstrated consistent results across diverse datasets, the comparison with decision trees has revealed similar or superior outcomes. This discrepancy prompts researchers to explore a multitude of popular classifiers, including logistic regression (LR), known for its interpretability but plagued by a tendency to generate over fitted models.

To navigate these challenges, the authors propose a multistage InfoGainAttributeEval, GainRatio-AttributeEval, and OneRAttributeEval feature selection approach. In Stage 1, the algorithm efficiently approximates a solution with minimal computational effort. In Stage 2, an array of state-of-the-art ML classifiers and an ensemble Random Forest algorithm operate within the refined feature sub-space to identify patients with or without cancer. The experimental results, which compare predictions using all features, the Stage-1 feature subset, underscore the efficiency and effectiveness of the proposed hybrid feature selection method. This approach demonstrates a notable enhancement in performance compared to prior methodologies, marking a significant contribution to the evolving landscape of disease prediction and healthcare analytics.

Lung cancer typically arises as a suspicion in individuals with anomalous chest radiograph results or who exhibit symptoms stemming from either the local or systemic impacts of the tumor (Schölkopf et al., 2000). Lung cancer, a significant health concern, often develops in the lungs, with smoking being a primary risk factor. Additionally, exposure to environmental pollutants and genetic factors contribute to the incidence of lung cancer. Low- and middle-income nations bear a substantial burden of lung cancer cases. Screening plays a crucial role in early detection, aiming for methods that are minimally invasive, easily accessible, patient-friendly, cost-effective, and efficient in identifying the disease at an early stage when intervention is more manageable (Cavallaro et al., 2015).

In the ever-changing realm of data-driven research and healthcare analytics, the burgeoning wealth of datasets encompassing demographic intricacies, diagnostic test outcomes, and diverse lifestyle habits necessitates a meticulous approach to optimal prediction outcomes through feature selection (FS). Acknowledging the pivotal role of precise feature selection in bolstering prediction accuracy, researchers grapple with the challenge of discerning the most efficacious FS method. Given the expansive array of variables inherent in contemporary datasets, the imperative quest for a subset of features tailored to a specific task becomes paramount. Machine learning (ML) and training processes demand a comprehensive set of features, initiating an ML analysis with FS, followed by the application of classifiers for prediction.

Numerous FS methods have been posited, each yielding diverse outcomes when applied to distinct datasets (Tang & Zhou, 2015; Breiman, 2001). The heterogeneity in results underscores the dataset-centric nature of FS and begets the query of how to establish a criterion for dataset-specific FS rather than relying solely on method-based approaches. The evolution of classifiers seeks to address inherent challenges, such as incomplete, erroneous, or non-standardized data, as well as the intricacies of binomial versus multi-domain attributes.

Decision trees (DT), a supervised classifier, proffer a solution by prognosticating dependent variables while exhibiting resilience to outliers, as their classification hinges on sample proportions rather than absolute values. Nonetheless, DT may be deficient in delivering the desired accuracy for extensive databases. Conversely, Bayes theorem, a traditional classification technique renowned for its simplicity and robustness, manifests diminished performance with large or intricately structured datasets. Support Vector Machine (SVM) models strive to surmount these limitations but may grapple with the presence of noise within expansive datasets, necessitating collaboration with other ML techniques.

The advent of ensemble classifiers, exemplified by Random Forest (RF), introduces an amalgamation of methods to assuage the limitations of individual classifiers. While RF has demonstrated consistent results across diverse datasets, the comparison with decision trees has disclosed analogous or superior outcomes (Chen & Ishwaran, 2012). This incongruity prompts researchers to explore a myriad of popular classifiers, including logistic regression (LR), acknowledged for its interpretability but plagued by a proclivity to generate over fitted models.

To navigate these challenges, the authors posit an InfoGainAttributeEval, GainRatioAttributeEval, and OneRAttributeEval feature selection approach. In Stage 1, the algorithm efficiently approximates a solution with minimal computational effort (Babyak, 2004; Shaikhina et al., 2019). In Stage 2, an array of cutting-edge ML classifiers and an ensemble Random Forest algorithm operate within the refined feature sub-space to identify patients with or without cancer. The experimental results, comparing predictions using all features and the Stage-1 feature subset, underscore the efficiency and effectiveness of the proposed hybrid feature selection method. This approach evinces a notable enhancement in performance compared to antecedent methodologies, signifying a significant contribution to the evolving landscape of disease prediction and healthcare analytics.

Data mining or machine learning techniques help develop predictive and analytical strategies. This technique may help predict early cancer risk. Data mining aims to show good results, but the results are inconsistent with the process and data set. Researchers have tried and tested different methods such as SVM, DT, RF, LR, and NB for disease prediction. Christobel and Sivaprakasam (2011) BC diagnosis using the WDBC dataset. They used DT, SVM, and NB classifiers and compared their classification accuracies. The average accuracy of SVM is 96.99%, which is the highest among them (Ishikawa et al., 2014). The solution is limited to using one partition and one file.

Lavanya and Rani (2011) reported DT results on the BC dataset without using any special selection techniques. This study achieved a diagnostic accuracy of 69.23% without multiples, 94.84% for Wisconsin Breast Cancer (WBC), and 92.97% for the Wisconsin Diagnostic Breast Cancer (WDBC) dataset. The classification method increased the accuracy to 70.63%, 96.99%, and 92.09%, respectively. Kyles et al. (2011) developed a method that achieved 97% accuracy by using fuzzy rules as a useful diagnostic tool.

Chen et al. (2011) proposed a classification system as a rough method to detect BC (Shah et al., 2012; Loh, 2011). The algorithm also identified five features that can help doctors classify BC and reach the correct diagnosis. Salama et al. (2012) used NB, sequential minimum optimization (SMO), DT (J48), multilayer detection (MLP), and instance-based RF classifiers to determine the classification accuracy of various BC datasets. In addition to the feature selection process, the introduction of MLP and J48 classification techniques also increased the accuracy of using the WDBC dataset (Liaw & Wiener, 2002). They recommend SMO because it is the best fit for the WDBC dataset. In a collaborative study of composites, Lavanya and Rani (2012) provided data on BC. The hybrid plan is based on CART and luggage. Preprocessing is used to improve the quality and aggregation of products and improve classification accuracy. Kim et al. (2012) used the SVM technique in their article on the BC dataset containing 679 records containing clinical, disease, and epidemiology data (Verma et al., 2020; Maier et al., 2015).

The success rate of local tumor intervention is 99%. Katsis et al. (2013). To test the technology, data were obtained from 53 subjects in 4726 patients. One indication was that the disease was not a unique determinant of benign or malignant tumors when evaluated across all applications (Friedman, 2001). The method was validated using biopsy results from all 53 subjects. The accuracy of the SVM method is 76.33%, which determines the maximum number of variables selected by CFS, and 75.89%, which determines the maximum number of variables.

Kumar et al. (2013) used data from 699 patient studies, 499 of which were training and 200 were testing, in their research article. In this case, 241 (i.e., 34.5%) had BC, and the remaining 458 (i.e., 65.5%) had BC. It is not cancerous. The authors used 10-fold cross-validation to validate the predictions of six traditional data mining methods. When NB and SVM algorithms are used, the accuracy here reaches 94.5%. Kalia et al. (2014) developed an effective method to estimate BC using a naive

Bayesian classifier. The data included approximately 65.5% of stable patients and 34.5% of unstable patients. The accuracy of this method is 93%. Sivakami & and Saraswathi (2015) used the DT-SVM hybrid model for BC prediction on the WBCD dataset. The accuracy of DT-SVM is 91% and the error is 2.58%. Various algorithms such as instance learning (IBL), minimal optimization (SMO), and NB are also used. The accuracy of IBL is 85.23% and the error is 12.63%. The accuracy of SMO is 72.56% and the error is 5.96%. The accuracy of NB is 89.48% and the error is 9.89%. Ang et al. (2016) attempted to improve Naive Bayes by combining or combining functions such as Tree Augmented Naive Bayes (TAN) in research papers. From the analysis, it appears that the accuracy of the General Bayesian Network (GBN) does not have any limitations and better represents the dataset used for climbing. The authors used seven minimal datasets to evaluate the output of GBN relative to NB and TAN without missing values. Data were obtained from the UCI ML repository and then classified into NB, GBN, and TAN using the WEKA ML tool with 10-fold cross-validation with 286 samples per dataset and 10 features per sample. The accuracy of the NB model reached 71.68%, followed by TAN with 69.58% and GBN with 74.47%. Chaudhuri et al. (2018) analyzed data on BC using decision trees and discriminant analysis to identify recurrent diseases (Dodd et al., 2014).

Different paths lead to different combinations. Therefore, existing research is not consistent. There is little evidence on which to base comparisons of results; real analysis; measures to ensure consistency, and sensitivity; and finally predicting events with near 100% accuracy. In this study, the authors propose a framework to enable the implementation of all processes and introduce a new integration-based classifier (i.e., DCA) to generate the correct classification. This paper introduces a new technique to transition from using DT as a predetermined method to using the RF classifier as a learner for training.

6. DATASET DESCRIPTION OF CERVICAL CANCER

Evidence on cervical cancer risk from the UCI machine learning repository was used in this study and is shown in Table 2 below. The data include demographic, behavioral, and clinical data of 858 patients with 32 features/traits and four objectives (Hinselmann, Schiller, Cytology, and Biopsy) collected at "Cara" in Caracas, Venezuela. Gaz University Hospital". It is the result of tests to determine whether there are abnormal cells. It is used as a result of biopsy and cervical cancer (Khang, 2024).

However, a lack of data means some questions remain unanswered due to concerns about the privacy of many patients. Negative values of attributes were transformed from their mean values and normalized to remove duplicated data. Table 2 lists all features currently included in the cervical cancer literature and data on these features. Some patients decided not to answer some questions due to privacy concerns. Objects represented by numbers and Boolean values (0 or 1) are considered data types. The missing values for integer type have been filled with the Boolean sample mean values.

6.1 Results and Discussion

The following research questions are addressed in this research article: Which Data Mining Technique (DMT) is best for predicting diseases such as cervical cancer? and Which DMT framework can assist in meeting the three criteria-consistency, sensitivity, and? To achieve the highest levels of consistency and sensitivity, the author considers the most popular approaches and investigates their ensemble (Khang, 2024). Previous authors have focused solely on reducing variables to improve prediction. However, this method results in a loss of data. Thus, the author establishes a framework in this paper that proposes the use of data mining approaches, the measurement of consistency using kappa statistics, and the im-

Table 2. Description of the cervical cancer dataset

Number	Attributes	Available Data	Missing Data	Data Type
F1	Age	858 (100%)	0 (0%)	Integer
F2	Number of sexual partners	832 (97%)	26 (3%)	Integer
F3	First Sexual intercourse (age)	851 (99%)	7 (1%)	Integer
F4	Number of Pregnancies	802 (93%)	56 (7%)	Integer
F5	Smokes	845 (98%)	13 (2%)	Boolean
F6	Smokes (years)	845 (98%)	13 (2%)	Boolean
F7	Smokes (packs/year)	845 (98%)	13 (2%)	Boolean
F8	Hormonal Contraceptives	750 (87%)	108 (13%)	Boolean
F9	Hormonal Contraceptives (years)	750 (87%)	108 (13%)	Integer
F10	Intrauterine Device (IUD)	741 (86%)	117 (14%)	Boolean
F11	IUD (years)	741 (86%)	117 (14%)	Integer
F12	Sexually Transmitted Disease (STD)	753 (88%)	105 (12%)	Boolean
F13	STDs (number)	753 (88%)	105 (12%)	Integer
F14	STDs: condylomatosis	753 (88%)	105 (12%)	Boolean
F15	STDs: cervical condylomatosis	753 (88%)	105 (12%)	Boolean
F16	STDs: vaginal condylomatosis	753 (88%)	105 (12%)	Boolean
F17	STDs: vulva-perineal condylomatosis	753 (88%)	105 (12%)	Boolean
F18	STDs: syphilis	753 (88%)	105 (12%)	Boolean
F19	STDs: pelvic inflammatory disease	753 (88%)	105 (12%)	Boolean
F20	STDs: genital herpes	753 (88%)	105 (12%)	Boolean
F21	STDs: molluscum contagiosum	753 (88%)	105 (12%)	Boolean
F22	STDs: AIDS	753 (88%)	105 (12%)	Boolean
F23	STDs: HIV	753 (88%)	105 (12%)	Boolean
F24	STDs: Hepatitis B	753 (88%)	105 (12%)	Boolean
F25	STDs: HPV	753 (88%)	105 (12%)	Boolean
F26	STDs: Number of diagnoses	858 (100%)	0 (0%)	Integer
F27	STDs: Time since first diagnosis	71 (8%)	787 (92%)	Integer
F28	STDs: Time since the last diagnosis	71 (8%)	787 (92%)	Integer
F29	Dx: Cancer	858 (100%)	0 (0%)	Boolean
F30	Dx: Cervical Intraepithelial Neoplasia (CIN)	858 (100%)	0 (0%)	Boolean
F31	Dx: Human Papillomavirus (HPV)	858 (100%)	0 (0%)	Boolean
F32	Dx (Diagnosis)	858 (100%)	0 (0%)	Boolean
Number	Target Variable	Patient	Non-Patient	Data Type
F33	Hinselmann	35 (4%)	823 (96%)	Boolean
F34	Schiller	74 (9%)	784 (91%)	Boolean
F35	Cytology	44 (5%)	814 (95%)	Boolean
F36	Biopsy	55 (6%)	803 (94%)	Boolean

provement of sensitivity parameters using an ensemble learning approach. As a result, the framework presented in this paper contributes to humanity's well-being by allowing for better disease prediction.

A 2-stage Hybrid feature selection approach and a Stacked Classification model are evaluated on the cervical cancer dataset obtained from the UCI Machine Learning Repository with 35 features and one outcome variable as shown in Table 2. Stage 1 utilizes the same InfoGainAttributeEval, GainRatioAttributeEval, and OneRAttributeEval for feature selection to select five features as shown in Table 3

Table 3. Cervical cancer dataset with 5 features and 1 target variable

Attributes
STDs: syphilis, STDs: pelvic inflammatory disease, STDs: Hepatitis B, STDs: Time since first diagnosis, STDs: Time since last diagnosis

As exhibited in Table 4, different machine learning classifiers have yielded varying degrees of accuracy. 5 classifiers, namely LR, SVM, NB, RF, and DT performed exceptionally well with an accuracy of over 100% for a distinct number of features, i.e., 35 and 5. NB classifier quantified accuracy in ascending order with the lowest using 35 features. This leads to highly optimistic results and does not reflect the actual predictive performance of the model. The exclusion of redundant variables ensured improvement in the classification accuracy of cervical cancer patients, but overall predicted accuracy might exhibit a shrinking effect (Khang & Hajimahmud, 2024). In this context, accuracy is not the ideal metric for assessing predictive performance, and other metrics like sensitivity, precision, f1-score, and kappa value are taken into consideration.

Table 4. Comparison of accuracies with 36 and 5 features

Train Test Split	Number of Features	LR	NB	SVM	RF	DT
50-50	36	0.70	0.69	0.72	0.72	0.67
	5	0.82	0.80	0.90	1.00	1.00
66-34	36	0.70	0.69	0.72	0.70	0.69
	5	0.81	0.77	0.89	1.00	1.00
80-20	36	0.70	0.71	0.71	0.72	0.79
	5	0.83	0.77	0.86	1.00	1.00
10-fold Cross Validation	36	0.72	0.73	0.74	0.74	0.76
	5	0.82	0.81	0.91	1.00	1.00

The composite metric, the ROC-AUC score given in Table 8, is used for comparing the performance of several classifiers and has provided clarity rather than accuracy, sensitivity, and precision. Kappa statistic gives the agreement rate between the expected and predicted outcome where values ranging from (1.0), (0.81-0.99), (0.61-0.80), (0.41-0.60), (0.21-0.40), (0.1-0.20) to (0) represent perfect, near-perfect, substantial, moderate, fair, slight and close to chance agreements respectively. All classifiers

Table 5. Comparison of sensitivity with 36 and 5 features

Train Test Split	Number of Features	LR	NB	SVM	RF	DT
50-50	36	0.70	0.69	0.72	0.72	0.67
	5	0.82	0.80	0.90	1.00	1.00
66-34	36	0.70	0.69	0.72	0.70	0.69
	5	0.81	0.77	0.89	1.00	1.00
80-20	36	0.70	0.71	0.71	0.72	0.79
	5	0.83	0.77	0.86	1.00	1.00
10-fold Cross Validation	36	0.73	0.73	0.74	0.74	0.76
	5	0.82	0.81	0.91	1.00	1.00

Table 6. Comparison of precision with 36 and 5 features

Train Test Split	Number of Features	LR	NB	SVM	RF	DT
50-50	36	0.68	0.66	0.68	0.68	0.66
	5	0.83	0.88	0.92	1.00	1.00
66-34	36	0.68	0.65	0.69	0.64	0.63
	5	0.86	0.84	0.92	1.00	1.00
80-20	36	0.68	0.69	0.69	0.76	0.78
	5	0.88	0.87	0.91	1.00	1.00
10-fold Cross Validation	36	0.70	0.70	0.72	0.74	0.75
	5	0.83	0.85	0.93	1.00	1.00

Table 7. Comparison of f1-score with 36 and 5 features

Train Test Split	Number of Features	LR	NB	SVM	RF	DT
50-50	36	0.69	0.67	0.68	0.63	0.66
	5	0.82	0.81	0.90	1.00	1.00
66-34	36	0.68	0.65	0.67	0.60	0.63
	5	0.81	0.78	0.89	1.00	1.00
80-20	36	0.67	0.65	0.66	0.64	0.78
	5	0.84	0.78	0.87	1.00	1.00
10-fold Cross Validation	36	0.70	0.69	0.70	0.68	0.75
	5	0.82	0.82	0.91	1.00	1.00

with five features and 10-fold cross-validation confirmed the good agreement in terms of kappa value as exhibited in Table 9. Overall, RF provided the best accuracy, and precision, with five features, followed by RF, and DT. The reduction in feature subspaces from 35 to 5, through feature selection, improved the performance of all classifiers as demonstrated in Table 9. Kappa statistic, precision values for all the

Table 8. Comparison of AUC value with 36 and 5 features

Train -Test Split	Number of Features	LR	NB	SVM	RF	DT
50-50	36	0.68	0.67	0.57	0.75	0.71
	5	0.88	0.88	0.93	1.00	1.00
66-34	36	0.69	0.67	0.57	0.80	0.55
	5	0.86	0.87	0.92	1.00	1.00
80-20	36	0.69	0.67	0.58	0.76	0.78
	5	0.85	0.87	0.90	1.00	1.00
10-fold Cross Validation	36	0.71	0.71	0.60	0.82	0.80
	5	0.88	0.88	0.93	1.00	1.00

Table 9. Comparison of kappa statistic with 36 and 5 features

Train -Test Split	Number of Features	LR	NB	SVM	RF	DT
50-50	36	0.20	0.14	0.17	0.07	0.16
	5	0.59	0.61	0.78	1.00	1.00
66-34	36	0.20	0.13	0.18	0.04	0.08
	5	0.60	0.54	0.76	1.00	1.00
80-20	36	0.21	0.16	0.19	0.16	0.48
	5	0.63	0.54	0.70	1.00	1.00
10-fold Cross Validation	36	0.25	0.20	0.24	0.18	0.38
	5	0.59	0.60	0.80	1.00	1.00

five classifiers increased. However, the AUC score of NB LR and SVM with 10-fold cross-validation decreased for diminution in the number of features.

6.2 Effect of Feature Reduction

The reduction in feature subspace from 35 to 5, through feature selection, improves the performance of all classifiers. The Kappa values of all five methods increase. The precision values of all methods are non-decreasing. The AUC values of LR, NB, and SVM have decreased for 10-fold cross-validation. The improvement in performance due to feature reduction is provided in Table 10.

7. DATASET DESCRIPTION OF LUNG CANCER

The dataset of lung cancer risk factors obtained from the UCI Machine Learning Repository is used for this research and is exhibited in Table 1 below (Gayou et al., 2008). The dataset is composed of demographics, custom, and medical records of 310 patients, with 16 attributes/features. The attributes represented by integer and boolean (0 or, 1) are regarded as data types.

Table 10. Improvement in performance due to feature reduction from 35 to 5

Performance Metrics	35 Features		5 Features	
	ML Techniques	Maximum Score	ML Techniques	Maximum Score
Accuracy	DT	0.79	RF, DT	1
Sensitivity	DT	0.79	RF, DT	1
Precision	DT	0.78	RF, DT	1
f1-score	DT	0.78	RF, DT	1
AUC	RF	0.82	RF, DT	1
Kappa	DT	0.48	RF, DT	1

Table 11. Description of the lung cancer dataset

Number	Attributes	Available Data	Missing Data	Data Type
F1	Gender	309 (100%)	0 (0%)	Boolean
F2	Age	309 (100%)	0(0%)	Integer
F3	Smoking	309 (100%)	0 (0%)	Boolean
F4	Yellow Fingers	309 (100%)	0 (0%)	Boolean
F5	Anxiety	309 (100%)	0 (0%)	Boolean
F6	Peer Pressure	309 (100%)	0 (0%)	Boolean
F7	Chronic Disease	309 (100%)	0 (0%)	Boolean
F8	Fatigue	309 (100%)	0 (0%)	Boolean
F9	Allergy	309 (100%)	0 (0%)	Boolean
F10	Wheezing	309 (100%)	0 (0%)	Boolean
F11	Alcohol Consuming	309 (100%)	0 (0%)	Boolean
F12	Coughing	309 (100%)	0 (0%)	Boolean
F13	Shortness of Breath	309 (100%)	0 (0%)	Boolean
F14	Swallowing Difficulty	309 (100%)	0 (0%)	Boolean
F15	Chest Pain	309 (100%)	0 (0%)	Boolean
F16	Outcome	309 (100%)	0 (0%)	Boolean

7.1 Results and Discussion

The research article tackles the following inquiries: What Data Mining Technique (DMT) is optimal for forecasting diseases like cervical cancer? and which DMT framework can assist in meeting the three criteria-consistency, sensitivity, and? To achieve the highest levels of consistency and sensitivity, the author considers the most popular approaches and investigates their ensemble (Chaudhuri & Das, 2020) (Connelly, 2020). Previous authors have focused solely on reducing variables to improve prediction. However, this method results in a loss of data. Thus, the author establishes a framework in this paper that proposes the use of data mining approaches, the measurement of consistency using kappa statistics, and the improvement of sensitivity parameters using an ensemble learning approach. As a result, the framework presented in this paper contributes to humanity's well-being by allowing for better disease prediction.

A 2-stage Hybrid feature selection approach and a Stacked Classification model are evaluated on the cervical cancer dataset obtained from Kaggle with 15 features and one outcome variable as shown in Table 2 (Tzeng et al., 2016). Stage 1 utilizes the same Genetic Algorithm and Logistic Regression Architecture for feature selection to select six features as shown in Table 3

Table 12. Cervical Cancer Dataset with a 5A 2-stage Hybrid feature selection approach and a Stacked Classification model are evaluated on the lung cancer dataset obtained from the Kaggle with 15 features and one outcome variable as shown in Table 2. Stage 1 utilizes the InfoGainAttributeEval, GainRatioAttributeEval, and OneRAttributeEval for feature selection to select seven features as shown in Table 12.

Table 12. Comparison of accuracies with 16 and 7 features

Train-Test Split	Number of Features	LR	NB	SVM	RF	DT
50-50	16	0.68	0.69	0.68	0.72	0.66
	7	0.94	0.92	0.97	1.00	1.00
66-34	16	0.70	0.67	0.68	0.74	0.67
	7	0.94	0.91	0.97	1.00	1.00
80-20	16	0.77	0.77	0.75	0.85	0.74
	7	0.93	0.87	0.95	1.00	0.98
10-fold Cross Validation	16	0.73	0.68	0.71	0.81	0.73
	7	0.94	0.91	0.96	1.00	0.98

As demonstrated in Table 13, diverse machine learning classifiers have produced different levels of accuracy. 5 classifiers, namely LR, SVM, NB, RF, and DT performed exceptionally well with an accuracy of over 100% for a distinct number of features, i.e., 16 and 7. NB classifier quantified accuracy in ascending order with the lowest using 16 features as shown in Table 14. This leads to highly optimistic results and does not reflect the actual predictive performance of the model (Jabbar & Samreen, 2016) (Cortes & Vapnik, 1995).

Table 13. Comparison of sensitivity with 16 and 7 features

Train Test Split	Number of Features	LR	NB	SVM	RF	DT
50-50	16	0.68	0.69	0.68	0.72	0.66
	7	0.94	0.92	0.97	1.00	1.00
66-34	16	0.70	0.67	0.68	0.74	0.67
	7	0.94	0.91	0.97	1.00	1.00
80-20	16	0.77	0.77	0.75	0.85	0.74
	7	0.93	0.87	0.95	1.00	0.98
10-fold Cross Validation	16	0.73	0.68	0.71	0.81	0.73
	7	0.94	0.91	0.96	1.00	0.98

Table 14. Comparison of precision with 16 and 7 features

Train-Test Split	Number of Features	LR	NB	SVM	RF	DT
50-50	16	0.64	0.70	0.69	0.73	0.68
	7	0.94	0.92	0.97	1.00	1.00
66-34	16	0.71	0.69	0.70	0.75	0.67
	7	0.94	0.92	0.97	1.00	1.00
80-20	16	0.77	0.78	0.76	0.86	0.76
	7	0.93	0.88	0.95	1.00	0.98
10-fold Cross Validation	16	0.73	0.68	0.71	0.81	0.73
	7	0.94	0.92	0.96	1.00	0.98

The exclusion of redundant variables ensured improvement in the classification accuracy of cervical cancer patients, but overall predicted accuracy might exhibit a shrinking effect. In this context, accuracy is not the ideal metric for assessing predictive performance, and other metrics like sensitivity, precision, f1-score, and kappa value are taken into consideration as shown in Table 15.

Table 15. Comparison of f1-score with 16 and 7 features

Train Test Split	Number of Features	LR	NB	SVM	RF	DT
50-50	16	0.68	0.69	0.68	0.72	0.65
	7	0.94	0.91	0.97	1.00	1.00
66-34	16	0.70	0.67	0.68	0.74	0.67
	7	0.94	0.89	0.97	1.00	1.00
80-20	16	0.77	0.77	0.75	0.85	0.74
	7	0.93	0.83	0.94	1.00	0.98
10-fold Cross Validation	16	0.73	0.68	0.71	0.81	0.73
	7	0.94	0.90	0.96	1.00	0.98

The composite metric, the ROC-AUC score given in Table 16, is used for comparing the performance of several classifiers and has provided clarity rather than accuracy, sensitivity, and precision. Kappa statistic gives the agreement rate between the expected and predicted outcome where values ranging from (1.0), (0.81-0.99), (0.61-0.80), (0.41-0.60), (0.21-0.40), (0.1-0.20) to (0) represent perfect, near-perfect, substantial, moderate, fair, slight and close to chance agreements respectively.

All classifiers with five features and 10-fold cross-validation confirmed the good agreement in terms of kappa value as exhibited in Table 17 (Ayat et al., 2005). Overall, RF provided the best accuracy, and precision, with five features, followed by RF, and DT. The reduction in feature subspaces from 16 to 7, through feature selection, improved the performance of all classifiers as demonstrated in Table 17. Kappa statistic, precision values for all the five classifiers increased. However, the AUC score of NB LR and SVM with 10-fold cross-validation decreased for diminution in the number of features.

Table 16. Comparison of AUC value with 16 and 7 features

Train-Test Split	Number of Features	LR	NB	SVM	RF	DT
50-50	16	0.74	0.75	0.69	0.84	0.75
	7	0.96	0.96	0.91	1.00	1.00
66-34	16	0.76	0.74	0.69	0.86	0.73
	7	0.95	0.94	0.90	1.00	1.00
80-20	16	0.84	0.83	0.76	0.94	0.81
	7	0.90	0.90	0.86	1.00	1.00
10-fold Cross Validation	16	0.78	0.77	0.71	0.89	0.76
	7	0.95	0.95	0.88	1.00	0.99

Table 17. Comparison of Kappa statistic with 16 and 7 features

Train Test Split	Number of Features	LR	NB	SVM	RF	DT
50-50	16	0.38	0.39	0.38	0.45	0.33
	7	0.75	0.60	0.88	1.00	1.00
66-34	16	0.41	0.36	0.37	0.48	0.34
	7	0.76	0.53	0.87	1.00	1.00
80-20	16	0.54	0.54	0.51	0.70	0.49
	7	0.76	0.38	0.81	1.00	0.94
10-fold Cross Validation	16	0.46	0.37	0.42	0.63	0.46
	7	0.78	0.61	0.85	1.00	0.93

7.2 Effect of Feature Reduction

The reduction in feature subspace from 16 to 7, through feature selection, improves the performance of all classifiers. The Kappa values of all five methods increase. The precision values of all methods are non-decreasing. The AUC values of LR, NB, and SVM have decreased for 10-fold cross-validation (Kamruzzaman & Begg, 2006). The improvement in performance due to feature reduction is provided in Table 18.

8. DATASET DESCRIPTION OF BREAST CANCER

The Breast Cancer Dataset is a collection of health-related data aimed at studying the potential factors influencing the development of lung cancer. This dataset comprises 570 records, each characterized by 31 features, including demographic information, lifestyle choices, and health symptoms. The goal of this dataset is to facilitate the exploration of patterns and relationships that may contribute to the understanding of breast cancer risk factors (Xie & Coggeshall, 2010). This dataset has been downloaded from a website named 'Kaggle'. The dataset offers a comprehensive set of attributes encompassing

Table 18. Improvement in performance due to feature reduction from 16 to 7

Performance Metrics	16 Features		7 Features	
	ML Techniques	Maximum Score	ML Techniques	Maximum Score
Accuracy	RF	0.85	RF	1
Sensitivity	RF	0.85	RF	1
Precision	RF	0.86	RF	1
f1-score	RF	0.85	RF	1
AUC	RF	0.94	RF, DT	1
Kappa	RF	0.70	RF	1

various aspects of an individual's life, health, and potential risk factors for breast cancer. Exploratory data analysis and machine learning models can be applied to understand the relationships between these features and the inferred breast cancer outcome as shown in Table 19. Feature engineering, correlation analysis, and classification algorithms could be employed to derive insights and predictive models for breast cancer risk assessment based on the provided attributes (Anh, 2024).

8.1 Results and Discussion

The following research inquiries are explored in this research paper: Which Data Mining Technique (DMT) is most effective for forecasting illnesses such as cervical cancer? and Which DMT framework can assist in meeting the three criteria-consistency, sensitivity, and? To achieve the highest levels of consistency and sensitivity, the author considers the most popular approaches and investigates their ensemble (Chen et al., 2013) (Khang et al., 2024). Previous authors have focused solely on reducing variables to improve prediction. However, this method results in a loss of data. Thus, the author establishes a framework in this paper that proposes the use of data mining approaches, the measurement of consistency using kappa statistics, and the improvement of sensitivity parameters using an ensemble learning approach. As a result, the framework presented in this paper contributes to humanity's well-being by allowing for better disease prediction.

A 2-stage Hybrid feature selection approach and a Stacked Classification model are evaluated on the breast cancer dataset obtained from the Kaggle with 30 features and one outcome variable as shown in Table 19.

Stage 1 utilizes the same Logistic Regression Architecture for feature selection to select 7 features as shown in Table 20.

As exhibited in Table 21, different machine learning classifiers have yielded varying degrees of accuracy. 5 classifiers, namely LR, SVM, NB, RF, and DT performed exceptionally well with an accuracy of over 100% for a distinct number of features, i.e., 31 and 7. NB classifier quantified accuracy in ascending order with the lowest using 16 features. This leads to highly optimistic results and does not reflect the actual predictive performance of the model (Martin et al., 2006).

The exclusion of redundant variables ensured improvement in the classification accuracy of cervical cancer patients, but overall predicted accuracy might exhibit a shrinking effect as shown in Table 22 and Table 23.

Table 19. Description of the lung cancer dataset

Number	Attributes	Available Data	Missing Data	Data Type
F1	Radius mean	569 (100%)	0 (0%)	Integer
F2	Texture mean	569 (100%)	0 (0%)	Integer
F3	Perimeter mean	569 (100%)	0 (0%)	Integer
F4	Area mean	569 (100%)	0 (0%)	Integer
F5	Smoothness mean	569 (100%)	0 (0%)	Integer
F6	Compactness mean	569 (100%)	0 (0%)	Integer
F7	Concavity mean	569 (100%)	0 (0%)	Integer
F8	Concave points mean	569 (100%)	0 (0%)	Integer
F9	Symmetry means	569 (100%)	0 (0%)	Integer
F10 F11	Fractal dimension mean Radius se	569 (100%) 569 (100%)	0 (0%) 0 (0%)	Integer Integer
F12	Texture se	569 (100%)	0 (0%)	Integer
F13	Perimeter se	569 (100%)	0 (0%)	Integer
F14	Area se	569 (100%)	0 (0%)	Integer
F15	Smoothness se	569 (100%)	0 (0%)	Integer
F16	Compactness se	569 (100%)	0 (0%)	Integer
F17	Concavity se	569 (100%)	0 (0%)	Integer
F18	Concave points se	569 (100%)	0 (0%)	Integer
F19	Symmetry se	569 (100%)	0 (0%)	Integer
F20	Fractal dimension	569 (100%)	0 (0%)	Integer
F21	Radius worst	569 (100%)	0 (0%)	Integer
F22	Texture worst	569 (100%)	0 (0%)	Integer
F23	Perimeter worst	569 (100%)	0 (0%)	Integer
F24	Area worst	569 (100%)	0 (0%)	Integer
F25	Smoothness worst	569 (100%)	0 (0%)	Integer
F26	Compactness worst	569 (100%)	0 (0%)	Integer
F27	Concavity worst	569 (100%)	0 (0%)	Integer
F28	Concave points worst	569 (100%)	0 (0%)	Integer
F29	Symmetry worst	569 (100%)	0 (0%)	Integer
F30	Fractal Dimension worst	569 (100%)	0 (0%)	Integer
F31	Outcome	569 (100%)	0 (0%)	Boolean

In this context, accuracy is not the ideal metric for assessing predictive performance, and other metrics like sensitivity, precision, f1-score, and kappa value are taken into consideration (Khang & Abdullayev, 2023) as shown Table 24, Table 25, and Table 26.

8.2 Effect of Feature Reduction

The reduction in feature subspace from 31 to 7, through feature selection, improves the performance of all classifiers. The Kappa values of all five methods increase. The precision values of all methods are

Table 19. Breast cancer dataset

Train -Test Split	Number of Features	LR	NB	SVM	▾RF	DT
50-50	31	0.76	0.74	0.77	0.79	0.85
	7	0.95	0.95	0.96	1	0.96
66-34	31	0.79	0.78	0.8	0.84	0.81
	7	0.95	0.92	0.96	1	0.98
80-20	31	0.8	0.78	0.84	0.82	0.82
	7	0.95	0.96	0.96	1	1
10-fold Cross Validation	31	0.76	0.77	0.77	0.84	0.77
	7	0.96	0.95	0.96	1	0.99.

Table 20. Breast cancer dataset with 6 features and 1 target variable

Attributes
Texture Mean, Area Mean, Symmetry Mean, Perimeter se, Smoothness worst, Compactness worst

Table 21. Comparison of accuracies with 31 and 7 features

Train-Test Split	Number of Features	LR	NB	SVM	▾RF	DT
50-50	31	0.76	0.74	0.77	0.79	0.85
	7	0.95	0.95	0.96	1	0.96
66-34	31	0.79	0.78	0.8	0.84	0.81
	7	0.95	0.92	0.96	1	0.98
80-20	31	0.8	0.78	0.84	0.82	0.82
	7	0.95	0.96	0.96	1	1
10-fold Cross Validation	31	0.76	0.77	0.77	0.84	0.77
	7	0.96	0.95	0.96	1	0.99.

Table 22. Comparison of sensitivity with 31 and 7 features

Train-Test Split	Number of Features	LR	NB	SVM	RF ▾	DT
50-50	31	0.76	0.74	0.78	0.77	0.85
	7	0.95	0.95	0.96	1	0.96
66-34	31	0.8	0.78	0.8	0.84	0.81
	7	0.95	0.92	0.97	1	0.98
80-20	31	0.81	0.78	0.84	0.83	0.83
	7	0.96	0.96	0.96	1	1
10-fold Cross Validation	31	0.78	0.77	0.77	0.84	0.78
	7	0.96	0.95	0.96	1	0.99

Table 23. Comparison of precision with 31 and 7 features

Train-Test Split ▾	Number of Features	LR	NB ▾	SVM	RF -	DT
50-50	31	0.77	0.74	0.78	0.8	0.85
	7	0.95	0.96	0.96	1	0.96
66-34	31	0.8	0.78	0.81	0.85	0.81
	7	0.96	0.93	0.97	1	0.98
80-20	31	0.81	0.78	0.84	0.83	0.83
	7	0.96	0.96	0.96	1	1
10-fold Cross Validation	31	0.77	0.77	0.77	0.84	0.78
	7	0.96	0.96	0.96	1	0.99

Table 24. Comparison of f1-score with 31 and 7 features

Train-Test Split ▾ ▾	Number of Features	LR	NB	SVM	RF ▾	DT
50-50	31	0.76	0.74	0.78	0.8	0.85
	7	0.95	0.95	0.96	1	0.96
66-34	31	0.8	0.78	0.81	0.85	0.81
	7	0.96	0.91	0.97	1	0.98
80-20	31	0.81	0.78	0.84	0.82	0.83
	7	0.95	0.95	0.95	1	1
10-fold Cross Validation	31	0.77	0.77	0.77	0.84	0.78
	7	0.96	0.95	0.96	1	0.99

Table 25. Comparison of AUC value with 31 and 7 features

Train-Test Split ▾	Number of Features	LR ▾	NB ▾	SVM	RF	DT
50-50	31	0.85	0.83	0.78	0.89	0.9
	7	0.93	0.93	0.85	1	0.97
66-34	31	0.86	0.85	0.81	0.92	0.86
	7	0.97	0.98	0.89	1	0.98
80-20	31	0.89	0.88	0.84	0.93	0.9
	7	0.96	0.95	0.8	1	1
10-fold Cross Validation	31	0.85	0.85	0.77	0.92	0.85
	7	0.96	0.96	0.88	1	0.99

Table 26. Comparison of Kappa statistic with 31 and 7 features

Train-Test Split ▾	Number of Features	LR	NB	SVM	RF ▾	DT
50-50	31	0.52	0.48	0.55	0.58	0.69
	7	0.8	0.78	0.8	1	0.82
66-34	31	0.59	0.56	0.61	0.69	0.62
	7	0.82	0.8	0.86	1	0.91
80-20	31	0.61	0.56	0.68	0.64	0.64
	7	0.71	0.71	0.71	1	1
10-fold Cross Validation	31	0.53	0.53	0.54	0.67	0.55
	7	0.82	0.81	0.84	1	0.98

non-decreasing. The AUC values of LR, NB, and SVM have decreased for 10-fold cross-validation (Ray & Chaudhuri, 2021) (Chalak et al., 2020). The improvement in performance due to feature reduction is provided in Table 27.

Table 27. The improvement in performance due to feature reduction

Performance Metrics	31 Features		7 Features	
	ML Techniques	Maximum Score	ML Techniques	Maximum Score
Accuracy	DT	0.85	RF, DT	1
Sensitivity	DT	0.85	RF, DT	1
Precision	RF, DT	0.85	RF, DT	1
f1-score	RF, DT	0.85	RF, DT	1
AUC	RF	0.93	RF, DT	1
Kappa	RF, DT	0.69	RF, DT	1

9. CONCLUSION

The three studies on different serious diseases—cervical cancer, breast cancer, and lung cancer—reveal variations in results and challenges associated with study monitoring methods, accuracy, and precision definitions (Jabbar & Samreen, 2016; Singh, 2018). The disparity in outcomes across varied supervised learning techniques emphasizes the need for a robust algorithm to discern truth without compromising accuracy (Razali et al., 2020). The inherent bias in Logistic Regression (LR) results, where apparent error rates may underestimate true values due to clustering around observed points, poses a challenge in accurately assessing model precision (Son et al., 2010; Lu et al., 2020; Nasution et al., 2018). To address this, the initial iteration involved a reduced dataset, and this approach was reiterated in the second iteration to mitigate bias (Priya & Karthikeyan, 2020).

In each study, the reduction of features by more than half in the second iteration did not alter the overall accuracy, indicating the effectiveness of the proposed algorithm (Khang & Abdullayev, 2023). The utilization of validated data mining techniques in the second (reduced) dataset consistently yielded the highest accuracy levels compared to previous studies. The significance of features varied with different methods, impacting the treatment of serious diseases due to incomplete testing, examination, or misinterpretation arising from asynchronous test parameters (Vandewiele et al., 2021; Ahishakiye et al., 2020).

The algorithm employed InfoGainAttributeEval, GainRatioAttributeEval, and OneRAttributeEval-based iterations, coupled with LR for probabilistic disease prediction, to identify a set of features enhancing accuracy without compromising precision (Khang, 2023). Overall, the comprehensive analysis of these studies underscores the importance of refining methodologies and leveraging advanced data mining techniques to improve the understanding and treatment of serious diseases (Singh, 2018).

REFERENCES

Ahishakiye, E., Wario, R., Mwangi, W., & Taremwa, D. (2020). Prediction of Cervical Cancer Basing on Risk Factors using Ensemble Learning. 2020 IST-Africa Conference (IST-Africa). IEEE.

Anh, P. T. N. (2024). AI Models for Disease Diagnosis and Prediction of Heart Disease with Artificial Neural Network. Computer Vision and AI-integrated IoT Technologies in Medical Ecosystem (1st ed.). CRC Press. doi:10.1201/9781003429609-9

Ayat, N. E., Cheriet, M., & Suen, C. Y. (2005). Automatic model selection for the optimization of SVM kernels. *Pattern Recognition*, *38*(10), 1733–1745. doi:10.1016/j.patcog.2005.03.011

Babyak, M. A. (2004). What you see may not be what you get: A brief, nontechnical introduction to overfitting in regression-type models. *Psychosomatic Medicine*, *66*, 411–421. PMID:15184705

Bengtsson, E., & Malm, P. (2014). Screening for cervical cancer using automated analysis of PAP-smears. *Computational and Mathematical Methods in Medicine*, *2014*, 1–12. doi:10.1155/2014/842037 PMID:24772188

Bobdey, S., Sathwara, J., Jain, A., & Balasubramaniam, G. (2016). Burden of cervical cancer and role of screening in India. *Indian Journal of Medical and Paediatric Oncology: Official Journal of Indian Society of Medical & Paediatric Oncology*, *37*(4), 278–285. doi:10.4103/0971-5851.195751 PMID:28144096

Bray, F., Ferlay, J., Soerjomataram, I., Siegel, R. L., Torre, L. A., & Jemal, A. (2018). Global cancer statistics 2018: GLOBOCAN estimates of incidence and mortality worldwide for 36 cancers in 185 countries. *CA: a Cancer Journal for Clinicians*, *68*(6), 394–424. doi:10.3322/caac.21492 PMID:30207593

Breiman, L. (2001). Random forests. *Machine Learning*, *45*(1), 5–32. doi:10.1023/A:1010933404324

Cavallaro, G., Riedel, M., Richerzhagen, M., Benediktsson, J. A., & Plaza, A. (2015). On understanding big data impacts in remotely sensed image classification using support vector machine methods. *IEEE Journal of Selected Topics in Applied Earth Observations and Remote Sensing*, *8*(10), 4634–4646. doi:10.1109/JSTARS.2015.2458855

Chalak, L. F., Pavageau, L., Huet, B., & Hynan, L. (2020). Statistical rigor and kappa considerations: Which, when and clinical context matters. *Pediatric Research*, *88*(1), 5. doi:10.1038/s41390-020-0890-x PMID:32272485

Chaudhuri, A. K., & Das, A. (2020). Variable Selection in Genetic Algorithm Model with Logistic Regression for Prediction of Progression to Diseases. *IEEE International Conference for Innovation in Technology (INOCON)*. IEEE. 10.1109/INOCON50539.2020.9298372

Chen, X., & Ishwaran, H. (2012). Random forests for genomic data analysis. *Genomics*, *99*(6), 323–329. doi:10.1016/j.ygeno.2012.04.003 PMID:22546560

Chen, Y., Jia, Z., Mercola, D., & Xie, X. (2013). A gradient boosting algorithm for survival analysis via direct optimization of concordance index. *Computational and Mathematical Methods in Medicine*, *2013*, 1–8. doi:10.1155/2013/873595 PMID:24348746

Connelly, L. (2020). Logistic regression. *Medsurg Nursing*, *29*, 353–354.

Cortes, C., & Vapnik, V. (1995). Support-vector networks. *Machine Learning*, *20*(3), 273–297. doi:10.1007/BF00994018

Dodd, S., Berk, M., Kelin, K., Zhang, Q., Eriksson, E., Deberdt, W., & Nelson, J. C. (2014). Application of the Gradient Boosted method in randomised clinical trials: Participant variables that contribute to depression treatment efficacy of duloxetine, SSRIs or placebo. *Journal of Affective Disorders*, *168*, 284–293. doi:10.1016/j.jad.2014.05.014 PMID:25080392

Fernandes, K., Cardoso, J. S., & Fernandes, J. (June 2017). Transfer learning with partial observability applied to cervical cancer screening. In *Iberian conference on pattern recognition and image analysis* (pp. 243–250). Springer. doi:10.1007/978-3-319-58838-4_27

Friedman, J. H. (2001). Greedy function approximation: A gradient boosting machine. *Annals of Statistics*, *29*(5), 1189–1232. doi:10.1214/aos/1013203451

Galgano, M. T., Castle, P. E., Atkins, K. A., Brix, W. K., Nassau, S. R., & Stoler, M. H. (2010). Using biomarkers as objective standards in the diagnosis of cervical biopsies. *The American Journal of Surgical Pathology*, *34*(8), 1077–1087. doi:10.1097/PAS.0b013e3181e8b2c4 PMID:20661011

Gayou, O., Das, S. K., Zhou, S. M., Marks, L. B., Parda, D. S., & Miften, M. (2008). A genetic algorithm for variable selection in logistic regression analysis of radiotherapy treatment outcomes. *Medical Physics*, *35*(12), 5426–5433. doi:10.1118/1.3005974 PMID:19175102

Guvenc, G., Akyuz, A., & Açikel, C. H. (2011). Health belief model scale for cervical cancer and Pap smear test: Psychometric testing. *Journal of Advanced Nursing*, *67*(2), 428–437. doi:10.1111/j.1365-2648.2010.05450.x PMID:20946564

Hiraku, Y., Kawanishi, S., & Ohshima, H. (Eds.). (2014). *Cancer and inflammation mechanisms: chemical, biological, and clinical aspects*. John Wiley & Sons. doi:10.1002/9781118826621

Ishikawa, T., Takahashi, J., Takemura, H., Mizoguchi, H., & Kuwata, T. (2014). Gastric lymph node cancer detection using multiple features support vector machine for pathology diagnosis support system. *The 15th International Conference on Biomedical Engineering*, Cham: Springer. 10.1007/978-3-319-02913-9_31

Jabbar, M. A., & Samreen, S. (2016). Heart disease prediction system based on hidden naïve bayes classifier. *International Conference on Circuits, Controls, Communications and Computing (I4C)*. IEEE. 10.1109/CIMCA.2016.8053261

Jemal, A., Center, M. M., DeSantis, C., & Ward, E. M. (2010). Global patterns of cancer incidence and mortality rates and trends. *Cancer Epidemiology, Biomarkers & Prevention*, *19*(8), 1893–1907. doi:10.1158/1055-9965.EPI-10-0437 PMID:20647400

Ji, Y., Yu, S., & Zhang, Y. (2011). A novel naive bayes model: Packaged hidden naive bayes. *6th IEEE Joint International Information Technology and Artificial Intelligence Conference*. IEEE. 10.1109/ITAIC.2011.6030379

Kamil, N., & Kamil, S. (2015). Global cancer incidences, causes and future predictions for subcontinent region. *Systematic Reviews in Pharmacy*, *6*, 13.

Kamruzzaman, J., & Begg, R. K. (2006). Support vector machines and other pattern recognition approaches to the diagnosis of cerebral palsy gait. *IEEE Transactions on Biomedical Engineering*, *53*(12), 2479–2490. doi:10.1109/TBME.2006.883697 PMID:17153205

Kerkar, R. A., & Kulkarni, Y. V. (2006). Screening for cervical cancer: An overview. *Journal of Obstetrics and Gynecology of India*, *56*, 115–122.

Khang, A. (2023). *AI and IoT-Based Technologies for Precision Medicine* (1st ed.). IGI Global Press., doi:10.4018/979-8-3693-0876-9

Khang, A. (2024a). Using Big Data to Solve Problems in the Field of Medicine. Computer Vision and AI-integrated IoT Technologies in Medical Ecosystem (1st ed.). CRC Press. doi:10.1201/9781003429609-21

Khang, A. (2024b). Medical and BioMedical Signal Processing and Prediction. Computer Vision and AI-integrated IoT Technologies in Medical Ecosystem (1st ed.). CRC Press. doi:10.1201/9781003429609-7

Khang, A., Abdullayev, V., Hrybiuk, O., & Shukla, A. K. (2024). *Computer Vision and AI-Integrated IoT Technologies in the Medical Ecosystem* (1st ed.). CRC Press. doi:10.1201/9781003429609

Khang, A., & Abdullayev, V. A. (2023). *AI-Aided Data Analytics Tools and Applications for the Healthcare Sector. AI and IoT-Based Technologies for Precision Medicine"* (1st ed.). IGI Global Press. doi:10.4018/979-8-3693-0876-9.ch018

Khang, A., & Hajimahmud, V. A. (2024). Application of Computer Vision in the Healthcare Ecosystem. Computer Vision and AI-integrated IoT Technologies in Medical Ecosystem (1st ed.). CRC Press. doi:10.1201/9781003429609-1

Kjellberg, L., Hallmans, G., Åhren, A. M., Johansson, R., Bergman, F., Wadell, G., & Dillner, J. (2000). Smoking, diet, pregnancy and oral contraceptive use as risk factors for cervical intra-epithelial neoplasia in relation to human papillomavirus infection. *British Journal of Cancer*, *82*(7), 1332–1338. doi:10.1054/bjoc.1999.1100 PMID:10755410

Liaw, A., & Wiener, M. (2002). Classification and regression by randomForest. *R News*, *2*, 18–22.

Loh, W. Y. (2011). Classification and regression trees. *Wiley Interdisciplinary Reviews. Data Mining and Knowledge Discovery*, *1*(1), 14–23. doi:10.1002/widm.8

Lu, J., Song, E., Ghoneim, A., & Alrashoud, M. (2020). Machine learning for assisting cervical cancer diagnosis: An ensemble approach. *Future Generation Computer Systems*, *106*, 199–205. doi:10.1016/j.future.2019.12.033

Luhn, P., Walker, J., Schiffman, M., Zuna, R. E., Dunn, S. T., Gold, M. A., & Wentzensen, N. (2013). The role of co-factors in the progression from human papillomavirus infection to cervical cancer. *Gynecologic Oncology*, *128*(2), 265–270. doi:10.1016/j.ygyno.2012.11.003 PMID:23146688

Maier, O., Wilms, M., von der Gablentz, J., Krämer, U. M., Münte, T. F., & Handels, H. (2015). Extra tree forests for sub-acute ischemic stroke lesion segmentation in MR sequences. *Journal of Neuroscience Methods*, *240*, 89–100. doi:10.1016/j.jneumeth.2014.11.011 PMID:25448384

Maldonado, S., López, J., Jimenez-Molina, A., & Lira, H. (2020). *Simultaneous feature selection and heterogeneity control for SVM classification: An application to mental workload assessment* (Vol. 143). Expert Syst. Appl.

Martin, R., Rose, D., Yu, K., & Barros, S. (2006). Toxicogenomics Strategies for Predicting Drug Toxicity. *Pharmacogenomics*, *7*(7), 1003–1016. doi:10.2217/14622416.7.7.1003 PMID:17054411

Mishra, G. A., Pimple, S. A., & Shastri, S. S. (2011). An overview of prevention and early detection of cervical cancers. *Indian Journal of Medical and Paediatric Oncology : Official Journal of Indian Society of Medical & Paediatric Oncology*, *32*(3), 125–132. doi:10.4103/0971-5851.92808 PMID:22557777

Moreno, V., Bosch, F. X., Muñoz, N., Meijer, C. J., Shah, K. V., Walboomers, J. M., Herrero, R., & Franceschi, S.International Agency for Research on Cancer (IARC) Multicentric Cervical Cancer Study Group. (2002). Effect of oral contraceptives on risk of cervical cancer in women with human papillomavirus infection: The IARC multicentric case-control study. *Lancet*, *359*(9312), 1085–1092. doi:10.1016/S0140-6736(02)08150-3 PMID:11943255

Nasution, M. Z. F., Sitompul, O. S., & Ramli, M. (2018). PCA based feature reduction to improve the accuracy of decision tree c4.5 classification. *Journal of Physics: Conference Series*, *978*, 012058. doi:10.1088/1742-6596/978/1/012058

Petry, K. U. (2014). HPV and cervical cancer. *Scandinavian Journal of Clinical and Laboratory Investigation*, *74*(sup244), 59–62. doi:10.3109/00365513.2014.936683 PMID:25083895

Plissiti, M. E., & Nikou, C. (2013). A review of automated techniques for cervical cell image analysis and classification. In U. Andreaus & D. Iacoviello (Eds.), *Biomedical Imaging and Computational Modeling in Biomechanics* (pp. 1–18). Springer. doi:10.1007/978-94-007-4270-3_1

Plummer, M., Herrero, R., Franceschi, S., Meijer, C. J., Snijders, P., Bosch, F. X., & Muñoz, N. (2003). Smoking and cervical cancer: Pooled analysis of the IARC multi-centric case–control study. *Cancer Causes & Control*, *14*(9), 805–814. doi:10.1023/B:CACO.0000003811.98261.3e PMID:14682438

Pradhan, S. R., Mahata, S., Ghosh, D., Sahoo, P. K., Sarkar, S., Pal, R., & Nasare, V. D. (2020). Human Papillomavirus Infections in Pregnant Women and Its Impact on Pregnancy Outcomes: Possible Mechanism of Self-Clearance. In R. Rajkumar (Ed.), *Human Papillomavirus* (pp. 1–27). IntechOpen. doi:10.5772/intechopen.90197

Priya, S., & Karthikeyan, N. K. (2020). A Heuristic and ANN based Classification Model for Early Screening of Cervical Cancer. *Int. J. Comput. Intell. Syst., 13*(1), 1092–1100. doi:10.2991/ijcis.d.200730.003

Ramaraju, H., Nagaveni, Y., & Khazi, A. (2017). Use of Schiller's test versus Pap smear to increase the detection rate of cervical dysplasias. *International Journal of Reproduction, Contraception, Obstetrics and Gynecology, 5*, 1446–1450.

Ray, A., & Chaudhuri, A. K. (2021). *Smart healthcare disease diagnosis and patient management: Innovation, improvement and skill development* (Vol. 3). Machine Learning with Applications.

Razali, N., Mostafa, S. A., Mustapha, A., Abd Wahab, M. H., & Ibrahim, N. A. (2020, April). Risk Factors of Cervical Cancer using Classification in Data Mining. *Journal of Physics: Conference Series, 1529*(2), 022102. doi:10.1088/1742-6596/1529/2/022102

Rodríguez, A. C., Schiffman, M., Herrero, R., Hildesheim, A., Bratti, C., Sherman, M. E., & Burk, R. D. (2010). Longitudinal study of human papillomavirus persistence and cervical intraepithelial neoplasia grade 2/3: Critical role of duration of infection. *Journal of the National Cancer Institute, 102*(5), 315–324. doi:10.1093/jnci/djq001 PMID:20157096

Ronco, G., Dillner, J., Elfström, K. M., Tunesi, S., Snijders, P. J., Arbyn, M., Kitchener, H., Segnan, N., Gilham, C., Giorgi-Rossi, P., Berkhof, J., Peto, J., & Meijer, C. J. L. M.International HPV Screening Working Group. (2014). Efficacy of HPV-based screening for prevention of invasive cervical cancer: Follow-up of four European randomised controlled trials. *Lancet, 383*(9916), 524–532. doi:10.1016/S0140-6736(13)62218-7 PMID:24192252

Sarwar, M. U., Hanif, M. K., Talib, R., Mobeen, A., & Aslam, M. (2017). A survey of big data analytics in healthcare. *International Journal of Advanced Computer Science and Applications, 8*, 355–359.

Schiffman, M., Castle, P. E., Jeronimo, J., Rodriguez, A. C., & Wacholder, S. (2007). Human papillomavirus and cervical cancer. *Lancet, 370*(9590), 890–907. doi:10.1016/S0140-6736(07)61416-0 PMID:17826171

Schölkopf, B., Smola, A. J., Williamson, R. C., & Bartlett, P. L. (2000). New support vector algorithms. *Neural Computation, 12*(5), 1207–1245. doi:10.1162/089976600300015565 PMID:10905814

Sellors, J. W., & Sankaranarayanan, R. (2003). *Colposcopy and treatment of cervical intraepithelial neoplasia: a beginner's manual.* International Agency for Research on Cancer.

Shah, V., Turkbey, B., Mani, H., Pang, Y., Pohida, T., Merino, M. J., & Bernardo, M. (2012). Decision support system for localizing prostate cancer based on multiparametric magnetic resonance imaging. *Medical Physics, 39*(7Part1), 4093–4103. doi:10.1118/1.4722753 PMID:22830742

Shaikhina, T., Lowe, D., Daga, S., Briggs, D., Higgins, R., & Khovanova, N. (2019). Decision tree and random forest models for outcome prediction in antibody incompatible kidney transplantation. *Biomedical Signal Processing and Control*, *52*, 456–462. doi:10.1016/j.bspc.2017.01.012

Shouman, M., Turner, T., & Stocker, R. (2012). Applying k-nearest neighbour in diagnosing heart disease patients. *International Journal of Information and Education Technology (IJIET)*, *2*, 220–223. doi:10.7763/IJIET.2012.V2.114

Siegel, R. L., Miller, K. D., & Jemal, A. (2016). Cancer statistics, 2016. *CA: a Cancer Journal for Clinicians*, *66*(1), 7–30. doi:10.3322/caac.21332 PMID:26742998

Singh, H. D. (2018). *Diagnosis of Cervical Cancer using Hybrid Machine Learning Models*. [Doctoral dissertation, Dublin, National College of Ireland].

Son, Y. J., Kim, H. G., Kim, E. H., Choi, S., & Lee, S. K. (2010). Application of support vector machine for prediction of medication adherence in heart failure patients. *Healthcare Informatics Research*, *16*(4), 253–259. doi:10.4258/hir.2010.16.4.253 PMID:21818444

Steyerberg, E. W. (2019). *Clinical prediction models*. Springer International Publishing. doi:10.1007/978-3-030-16399-0

Subramanian, S., Sankaranarayanan, R., Esmy, P. O., Thulaseedharan, J. V., Swaminathan, R., & Thomas, S. (2016). Clinical trial to implementation: Cost and effectiveness considerations for scaling up cervical cancer screening in low-and middle-income countries. *Journal of Cancer Policy*, *7*, 4–11. doi:10.1016/j.jcpo.2015.12.006

Sung, H., Ferlay, J., Siegel, R. L., Laversanne, M., Soerjomataram, I., Jemal, A., & Bray, F. (2021). Global cancer statistics 2020: GLOBOCAN estimates of incidence and mortality worldwide for 36 cancers in 185 countries. *CA: a Cancer Journal for Clinicians*, *71*(3), 209–249. doi:10.3322/caac.21660 PMID:33538338

Tang, Y., & Zhou, J. (2015). The performance of PSO-SVM in inflation forecasting. *12th International Conference on Service Systems and Service Management (ICSSSM)*. IEEE.

Tubishat, M., Idris, N., Shuib, L., Abushariah, M. A., & Mirjalili, S. (2020). *Improved Salp Swarm Algorithm based on opposition based learning and novel local search algorithm for feature selection* (Vol. 145). Expert Syst. Appl.

Tzeng, E., Devin, C., Hoffman, J., Finn, C., Abbeel, P., Levine, S., & Darrell, T. (December 2016). Adapting deep visuomotor representations with weak pairwise constraints. In *Algorithmic Foundations of Robotics XII* (pp. 688–703). Springer.

Vandewiele, G., Dehaene, I., Kovács, G., Sterckx, L., Janssens, O., Ongenae, F., & Demeester, T. (2021). *Overly optimistic prediction results on imbalanced data: a case study of flaws and benefits when applying over-sampling* (Vol. 111). Artif. Intell. Med.

Verma, A. K., Pal, S., & Kumar, S. (2020). Prediction of skin disease using ensemble data mining techniques and feature selection method—A comparative study. *Applied Biochemistry and Biotechnology*, *190*(2), 341–359. doi:10.1007/s12010-019-03093-z PMID:31350666

Weiss, J. C., Page, D., Peissig, P. L., Natarajan, S., & McCarty, C. (2012). Statistical relational learning to predict primary myocardial infarction from electronic health records. *Proceedings of the Innovative Applications of Artificial Intelligence Conference, 2012*(2), 2341–2347. doi:10.1609/aaai.v26i2.18981 PMID:25360347

World Health Organization (WHO). (2021). *Human papillomavirus and cervical cancer*. WHO. https://www.who.int/news-room/fact-sheets/detail/human-papillomavirus-(hpv)-and-cervical-cancer

Xie, J., & Coggeshall, S. (2010). Prediction of transfers to tertiary care and hospital mortality: A gradient boosting decision tree approach. *Statistical Analysis and Data Mining, 3*(4), 253–258. doi:10.1002/sam.10079

Chapter 4
Deep Learning Frameworks in the Healthcare Industry

M. K. Nivodhini

iD https://orcid.org/0000-0003-1172-5894

K.S.R. College of Engineering, India

P. Vasuki

K.S.R. College of Engineering, India

R. Banupriya

K.S.R. College of Engineering, India

S. Vadivel

K.S.R. College of Engineering, India

ABSTRACT

Applications of deep learning extend to electronic health records (EHR) and predictive analytics, where theoretical models decipher patterns within vast datasets, enabling personalized healthcare strategies and disease progression predictions. Theoretical underpinnings of natural language processing (NLP) in healthcare are explored, emphasizing how algorithms theoretically improve clinical documentation, voice recognition, and patient interaction through virtual assistants. The theoretical exploration of issues such as data privacy, algorithmic bias, and interpretability highlights the complexities of responsibly deploying deep learning in medical decision-making. Personalized medicine, continuous monitoring, and improved disease prognosis emerge as theoretical directions, presenting collaborative opportunities between the technology industry, healthcare providers, and researchers. This abstract encapsulates the theoretical journey, illuminating the potential for enhanced diagnostics, treatment, and patient outcomes.

1. INTRODUCTION

The healthcare industry is undergoing a transformative shift with the integration of deep learning frameworks, leveraging the power of artificial intelligence (AI) to enhance diagnostics, treatment planning, and patient care. In this chapter, we explore the profound impact of deep learning frameworks on various

DOI: 10.4018/979-8-3693-3679-3.ch004

aspects of healthcare, examining their applications, challenges, and future prospects. This landscape is experiencing a seismic shift, driven by the integration of deep learning frameworks. This chapter explores the transformative impact of artificial intelligence (AI) on healthcare, focusing on popular frameworks such as TensorFlow, PyTorch, and Keras. These frameworks are pivotal in constructing intricate neural networks that underpin a range of applications within the healthcare industry.

2. LITERATURE REVIEW

2.1 Medical Imaging and Diagnosis

Deep learning frameworks are redefining medical imaging, significantly improving diagnostic capabilities. Radiology, pathology, and dermatology benefit from enhanced accuracy and efficiency, with deep learning algorithms aiding in the early detection of diseases. Case studies demonstrate the prowess of these frameworks in revolutionizing diagnostic processes.

At the core of deep learning's influence in healthcare is its ability to revolutionize medical imaging and diagnosis. This section delves into the theoretical aspects of neural network architectures employed in radiology, pathology, and dermatology. By elucidating the theoretical constructs behind algorithms facilitating early disease detection, we paint a theoretical landscape of improved diagnostic accuracy as shown in Figure 1.

Figure 1. A theoretical landscape of improved diagnostic accuracy

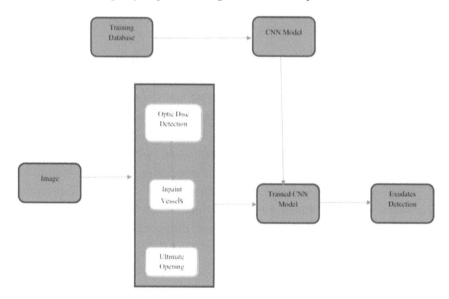

2.2 Drug Discovery and Development

The application of deep learning in drug discovery accelerates the identification and optimization of compounds. Virtual screening and predictive analytics contribute to streamlining drug development processes. Real-world examples showcase the successful integration of deep learning, offering promising glimpses into the future of pharmaceutical research. The theoretical framework of deep learning in drug discovery unfolds through an exploration of virtual screening and predictive analytics. We dissect the theoretical constructs of algorithms optimizing compound identification and interaction prediction (Khang and Abuzarova et al., 2023).

2.3 Electronic Health Records (EHR) and Predictive Analytics

Deep learning's role in analysing electronic health records facilitates predictive analytics, allowing for pattern recognition and disease progression prediction. This section explores the transformative impact of these frameworks in personalizing treatment plans, optimizing resource allocation, and improving overall patient outcomes. By deciphering the theoretical aspects of algorithms analyzing vast datasets, we unravel the potential for personalized treatment plans and disease progression predictions. Theoretical models elucidate the algorithms' ability to discern patterns and forecast patient outcomes (Khang & Rath & Anh et al., 2024).

2.4 Natural Language Processing (NLP) in Healthcare

Natural Language Processing powered by deep learning plays a pivotal role in healthcare, from clinical documentation to voice recognition and sentiment analysis. Advancements in chatbots and virtual assistants are explored, showcasing the potential for improved patient interaction and support. The theoretical foundations of deep learning algorithms applied to clinical documentation, voice recognition, and sentiment analysis as shown in Figure 2. We examine how theoretical advancements in NLP contribute to the theoretical construct of enhanced patient interaction through virtual assistants and chatbots (Khang & Robotics, 2024).

2.5 Challenges and Ethical Considerations

The implementation of deep learning in healthcare is not without challenges. This section delves into issues such as data privacy, algorithmic bias, and interpretability. Ethical considerations regarding patient consent and transparency are examined, providing insight into the responsible use of AI in medical decision-making. Ethical considerations as we delve into the theoretical underpinnings of issues such as data privacy, algorithmic bias, and interpretability. Theoretical discussions on patient consent and transparency illuminate the complexities of responsibly deploying deep learning algorithms in medical decision-making (Khang & Hajimahmud et al., 2024).

2.6 Future Directions and Opportunities

The chapter concludes by exploring future developments in deep learning for healthcare. Personalized medicine, continuous monitoring, and improved disease prognosis are discussed as potential outcomes. Opportunities for collaboration between the technology industry, healthcare providers, and researchers are highlighted, emphasizing the need for responsible and collaborative advancement. Theoretical discussions revolve around personalized medicine, continuous monitoring, and improved disease prognosis,

Figure 2. The theoretical foundations of deep learning algorithms applied to clinical documentation, voice recognition, and sentiment analysis

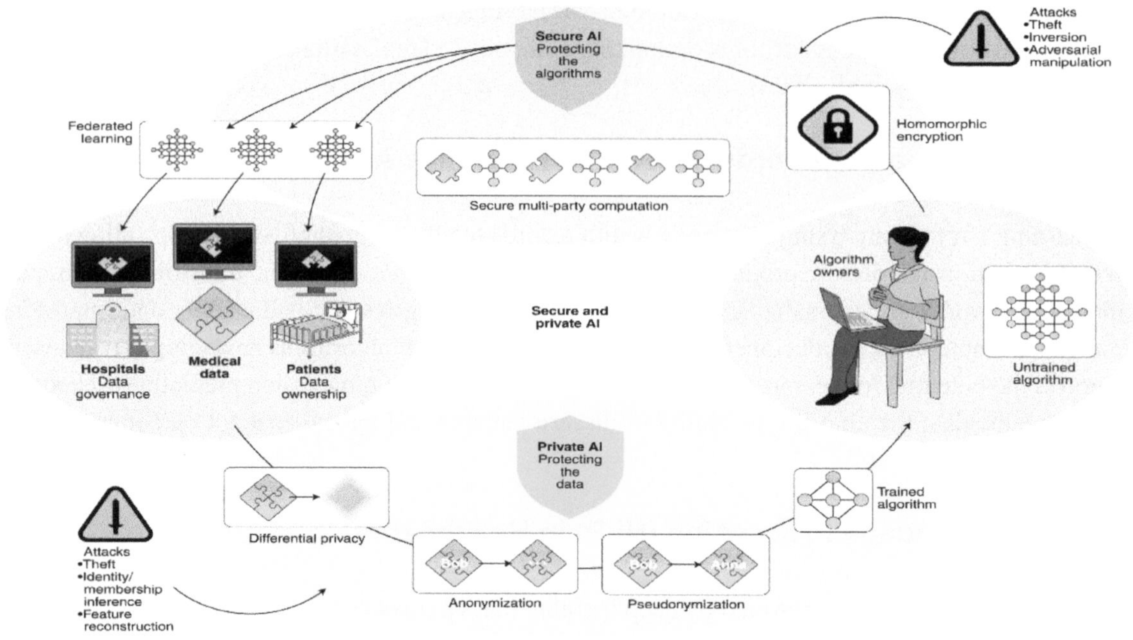

outlining the theoretical contours of a collaborative future between the technology industry, healthcare providers, and researchers.

3. DEEP LEARNING FRAMEWORKS

The chapter concludes by exploring deep learning frameworks for healthcare industry as shown in Figure 3.

3.1. TensorFlow

Developed by the Google Brain team, TensorFlow is an open-source deep learning framework widely adopted in both research and industry. Key Features:

- Provides a comprehensive ecosystem for machine learning, including tools for model building, training, and deployment.
- Supports both high-level APIs (e.g., Keras) for ease of use and low-level APIs for fine-grained control.
- TensorFlow Serving facilitates model deployment in production environments.
- TensorFlow Lite is designed for deploying models on mobile and embedded devices.

Figure 3. List of deep learning frameworks for healthcare industry

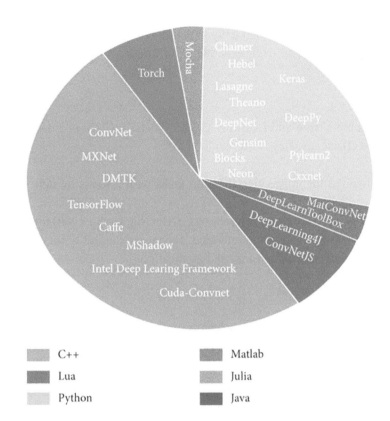

3.2. PyTorch

Created by Facebook's AI Research lab (FAIR), PyTorch is an open-source deep learning framework known for its dynamic computational graph and intuitive syntax. Key Features:

- Employs dynamic computation, allowing for on-the-fly graph creation and modification during runtime.
- Strong adoption in academia due to its ease of use and flexibility, making it suitable for rapid prototyping.
- TorchScript enables the conversion of PyTorch models for deployment in production environments.
- PyTorch Lightning simplifies the training process with a lightweight wrapper.

3.3. Keras

Originally an independent high-level neural networks API, Keras is now integrated as the official high-level API for TensorFlow. Key Features

- Provides a user-friendly interface for building and experimenting with neural network architectures.
- Supports both convolutional and recurrent networks, as well as combinations of the two.
- Enables easy model customization and extension through a modular design.
- Keras is often recommended for beginners due to its simplicity and readability.

3.4. Caffe

Developed by the Berkeley Vision and Learning Center (BVLC), Caffe is a deep learning framework emphasizing speed and efficiency. Key Features:

- Particularly well-suited for image classification tasks with a focus on convolutional neural networks (CNNs).
- Predefines a set of architecture configurations (e.g., AlexNet, GoogLeNet) for easy implementation.
- Employs a C++ library with a Python interface, enhancing flexibility for developers.
- Widely used in computer vision research and applications.

3.5. MXNet

An open-source deep learning framework developed by the Apache Software Foundation, MXNet is recognized for its efficiency and scalability. Key Features:

- Supports both symbolic and imperative programming, offering flexibility in model construction.
- Efficiently scales across multiple devices, making it suitable for distributed computing.
- Gluon API, similar to PyTorch's dynamic computation graph, simplifies model development.
- MXNet is used in various domains, including natural language processing and computer vision.

3.6. Chainer

Developed by Preferred Networks, Chainer is a deep learning framework employing a "Define-by-Run" approach. Key Features:

- Allows dynamic construction and modification of computational graphs during runtime.
- Well-suited for researchers due to its flexibility in experimenting with novel architectures.
- Supports automatic differentiation for efficient backpropagation.
- The ChainerX project integrates Chainer with NumPy for enhanced performance.

3.7. Theano

While no longer actively maintained, Theano played a significant role in the early development of deep learning frameworks. Key Features:

- Focused on numerical computation, Theano facilitated efficient execution on both CPUs and GPUs.
- Enabled symbolic computation for defining and optimizing mathematical expressions.

- Influenced subsequent frameworks in terms of symbolic computation and automatic differentiation.
- Theano contributed to the growth of deep learning in the research community.

3.8. CNTK (Microsoft Cognitive Toolkit)

Developed by Microsoft, CNTK is a deep learning framework designed for efficient training and evaluation of neural networks. Key Features:

- Provides efficient GPU and multi-GPU support, enhancing scalability.
- Supports feedforward and recurrent neural networks for a variety of applications.
- CNTK allows seamless integration with Microsoft Azure for cloud-based machine learning.
- Offers an easy-to-use Python API for model development.

Each of these frameworks has its strengths and may be preferred based on specific project requirements, development preferences, and the nature of the machine learning task at hand. Choosing the most suitable framework often depends on factors such as ease of use, flexibility, scalability, and the specific needs of the project (Khang & Ragimova et al., 2024).

4. ADVANTAGES OF DEEP LEARNING FRAMEWORKS IN HEALTHCARE INDUSTRY

Deep learning frameworks have brought about significant advantages to the healthcare industry, transforming various aspects of medical research, diagnosis, and treatment. Here are some key advantages of using deep learning frameworks in the healthcare industry as shown in Figure 4.

4.1. Improved Diagnostic Accuracy

Deep learning models excel at learning intricate patterns from vast amounts of medical data, leading to enhanced diagnostic accuracy in tasks such as medical imaging. Radiologists can benefit from computer-aided diagnosis systems that leverage deep learning to detect anomalies and diseases at early stages (Khang & Vladimir et al., 2024).

4.2. Personalized Treatment Plans

Deep learning frameworks analyze electronic health records (EHR) and patient data, enabling the development of personalized treatment plans. These plans take into account individual patient histories, genetic factors, and other variables to optimize and tailor medical interventions for better outcomes.

4.3. Efficient Drug Discovery

Deep learning accelerates drug discovery by predicting potential drug candidates, optimizing molecular structures, and identifying promising compounds. This speeds up the drug development process, reducing costs and increasing the likelihood of discovering effective treatments for various diseases.

Figure 4. Key advantages of using deep learning frameworks in the healthcare industry

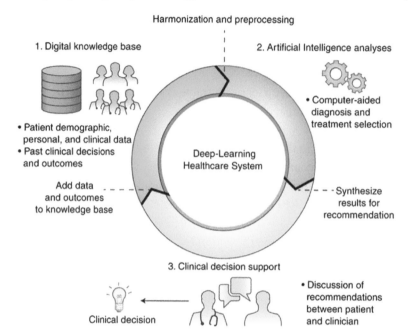

4.4. Natural Language Processing (NLP) Applications

Deep learning, particularly in conjunction with NLP, facilitates the analysis of unstructured clinical text, voice data, and medical literature. This enables the extraction of valuable insights from medical records, making it easier for healthcare professionals to access and utilize relevant information for decision-making

4.5. Enhanced Medical Imaging Analysis

Deep learning frameworks excel in image recognition tasks, making them highly effective in analyzing medical images. This includes tasks such as detecting tumors in radiology images, identifying abnormalities in pathology slides, and segmenting anatomical structures for surgical planning.

4.6. Predictive Analytics for Disease Management

Deep learning models analyze patient data to predict disease progression and identify individuals at high risk. This enables healthcare providers to implement proactive measures, manage chronic conditions more effectively, and allocate resources efficiently as shown in Figure 5.

4.7. Automation of Repetitive Tasks

Deep learning frameworks automate routine and repetitive tasks, allowing healthcare professionals to focus on more complex aspects of patient care. This includes automating administrative tasks, data entry, and other time-consuming processes, improving overall operational efficiency.

Figure 5. Convolutional neural networks (CNNs)

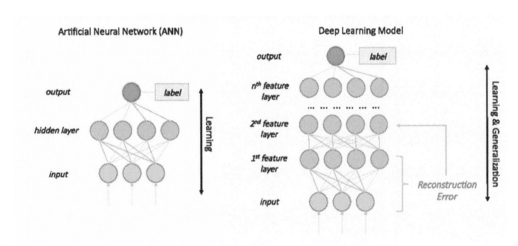

4.8. Continuous Monitoring and Early Warning Systems

Deep learning algorithms can be deployed in continuous monitoring systems, analyzing real-time patient data to detect early signs of deterioration or anomalies. This facilitates timely interventions, reducing the risk of complications and improving patient outcomes.

4.9. Cost Reduction and Resource Optimization

By automating processes, improving efficiency, and enabling more accurate predictions, deep learning contributes to cost reduction and resource optimization in healthcare as shown in Figure 6. This is particularly crucial in healthcare systems where the efficient use of resources is essential for providing quality care to a large population (Anh & Vladimir et al., 2024).

4.10. Research Advancements

Deep learning frameworks support medical research by analyzing large datasets, identifying complex patterns, and contributing to our understanding of diseases. This aids researchers in uncovering new insights, biomarkers, and potential targets for therapeutic interventions (Khang & Hajimahmud et al., 2024).

5. CONCLUSION

In conclusion, the integration of deep learning frameworks in the healthcare industry holds immense promise for revolutionizing patient care, diagnostics, and treatment strategies. As the field continues to evolve, addressing challenges and ethical considerations will be crucial to realizing the full potential of AI in improving health outcomes as shown in Figure 7.

Figure 6. Cost reduction and resource optimization

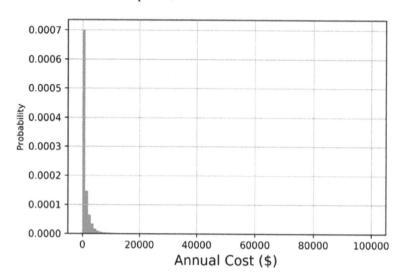

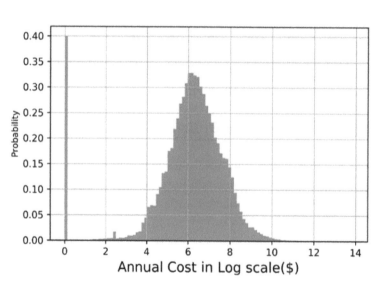

Figure 7. The advantages extend beyond the clinic, with deep learning contributing to cost reduction, resource optimization, and streamlined administrative processes

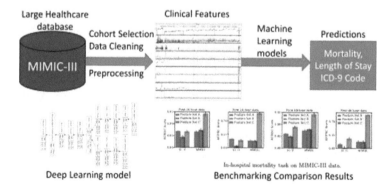

The automation of repetitive tasks allows healthcare providers to focus on complex aspects of patient care, ultimately leading to improved operational efficiency and better patient outcomes (Khang & Hajimahmud & Triwiyanto et al., 2024).

Looking forward, the future holds exciting prospects, with continuous advancements in personalized medicine, predictive analytics, and the potential for groundbreaking discoveries through the analysis of large-scale healthcare datasets. The journey of deep learning frameworks in the healthcare industry underscores their capacity to revolutionize the way we approach medical research, diagnosis, and treatment, ultimately paving the way for a more intelligent, efficient, and patient-centric healthcare ecosystem (Khang & Medicine, 2023).

REFERENCES

Anh, P. T. N. (2024). *AI Models for Disease Diagnosis and Prediction of Heart Disease with Artificial Neural Networks. Computer Vision and AI-integrated IoT Technologies in Medical Ecosystem* (1st ed.). CRC Press. doi:10.1201/9781003429609-9

Khang, A. (2023). *AI and IoT-Based Technologies for Precision Medicine* (1st ed.). IGI Global Press., doi:10.4018/979-8-3693-0876-9

Khang, A. (2024). *Medical Robotics and AI-Assisted Diagnostics for a High-Tech Healthcare Industry* (1st ed.). IGI Global Press. doi:10.4018/979-8-3693-2105-8

Khang, A. (2024). *Using Big Data to Solve Problems in the Field of Medicine. Computer Vision and AI-integrated IoT Technologies in Medical Ecosystem* (1st ed.). CRC Press. doi:10.1201/9781003429609-21

Khang, A. (2024). *Medical and BioMedical Signal Processing and Prediction. Computer Vision and AI-integrated IoT Technologies in Medical Ecosystem* (1st ed.). CRC Press. doi:10.1201/9781003429609-7

Khang, A., Abdullayev, V., Hrybiuk, O., & Shukla, A. K. (2024). *Computer Vision and AI-Integrated IoT Technologies in the Medical Ecosystem* (1st ed.). CRC Press. doi:10.1201/9781003429609

Khang, A., & Abdullayev, V. A. (2023). *AI-Aided Data Analytics Tools and Applications for the Healthcare Sector. AI and IoT-Based Technologies for Precision Medicine* (1st ed.). IGI Global Press. doi:10.4018/979-8-3693-0876-9.ch018

Khang, A., & Hajimahmud, V. A. (2024). Cloud Platform and Data Storage Systems in Healthcare Ecosystem. Medical Robotics and AI-Assisted Diagnostics for a High-Tech Healthcare Industry (1st ed.). IGI Global Press. doi:10.4018/979-8-3693-2105-8.ch022

Khang, A., & Hajimahmud, V. A. (2024). *Application of Computer Vision in the Healthcare Ecosystem. Computer Vision and AI-integrated IoT Technologies in Medical Ecosystem* (1st ed.). CRC Press. doi:10.1201/9781003429609-1

Khang, A., Rath, K. C., Anh, P. T. N., Rath, S. K., & Bhattacharya, S. (2024). Quantum-Based Robotics in High-Tech Healthcare Industry: Innovations and Applications. Medical Robotics and AI-Assisted Diagnostics for a High-Tech Healthcare Industry (1st ed.). IGI Global Press. doi:10.4018/979-8-3693-2105-8.ch001

Chapter 5
Bone Fracture Detection and Classification Using Deep Learning Techniques

B. Narendra Kumar Rao

School of Computing, Mohan Babu University, Tirupati, India

B. Pranitha

Sree Vidyanikethan Engineering College (Autonomous), India

B. Kushal Reddy

Sree Vidyanikethan Engineering College (Autonomous), India

D. Varsha

Sree Vidyanikethan Engineering College (Autonomous), India

N. Nithin Reddy

Sree Vidyanikethan Engineering College (Autonomous), India

ABSTRACT

The accurate classification of bone fractures plays a pivotal role in orthopaedic diagnosis and treatment planning. This study investigates the integration of deep learning techniques in fracture classification, specifically focusing on the analysis of bone fractures using X-ray images. Leveraging convolutional neural networks (CNNs), a subset of deep learning algorithms, our research aims to develop an automated system for precise fracture classification based on X-ray imaging data. The inherent capabilities of CNNs to extract nuanced features from medical images are harnessed to discern subtle details in fracture patterns, thereby enhancing diagnostic accuracy. The study addresses challenges associated with diverse fracture types and variations in X-ray image quality, employing deep learning methodologies to overcome these obstacles. The proposed model seeks to streamline the fracture classification process, offering a standardized and efficient approach in orthopaedic diagnostics.

DOI: 10.4018/979-8-3693-3679-3.ch005

1. INTRODUCTION

Fractures often occur in infants, the elderly and young people due to falls, crashes, fights and other accidents. Bone fractures are a prevalent and critical health issue worldwide, affecting millions of people annually. Whether resulting from accidents, falls, or medical conditions, fractures significantly impact individuals' lives and pose substantial challenges to the healthcare system. Understanding the global statistics and significance of bone fractures is essential for developing effective diagnostic and treatment strategies. Examining the worldwide statistics of bone fractures reveals the magnitude of this health concern. Data on the incidence, prevalence, and demographics of fractures provide valuable insights into the societal and economic implications of bone injuries.

Automated diagnosis using AI has the potential to streamline the healthcare workflow, reduce diagnostic errors, and improve patient outcomes. This section explores the various ways in which AI technologies, particularly deep learning, can contribute to the field of bone fracture detection.

The fundamental concepts of machine learning and deep learning are crucial to understand how AI models can be trained to recognize patterns in medical images and aid in bone fracture detection. Explore the application of CNNs in the automated detection and classification of bone fractures. CNNs are particularly effective in image recognition tasks and have demonstrated success in medical image analysis.

The CNN architectures contribute to capturing temporal dependencies in fracture detection, enhancing diagnostic accuracy.

2. DETECTION AND CLASSIFICATION OF BONE FRACTURE

In the field of orthopaedics, the absence of accessible and advanced tools for data-driven decision-making poses a significant challenge in addressing the intricate issues associated with bone fracture detection. Healthcare institutions dedicated to orthopaedic diagnostics face dual challenges of limited economic resources and a noticeable deficit in expertise related to advanced technologies such as coding, data analysis, and Machine Learning.

Traditional approaches to bone fracture detection often lack the precision required for proactive diagnosis and timely intervention. The reliance on manual interpretation of medical images can be time-consuming and subjective, leading to potential delays in treatment. The absence of predictive models for automated bone fracture detection further hinders the ability of healthcare professionals to optimize resource allocation and formulate targeted treatment plans.

Moreover, bone fractures, being multifaceted medical phenomena, demand a comprehensive understanding that extends beyond the conventional diagnostic methods. The dearth of accessible technology for orthopaedic institutions exacerbates these challenges, limiting their capacity to harness the potential of data-driven solutions.

The problem is twofold: the need for cost-effective, accessible technology tailored to orthopaedic diagnostics, and the necessity for predictive models that can enhance the accuracy and speed of bone fracture detection. This model seeks to bridge these gaps by leveraging Data Analysis and Machine to create a predictive model that enhances our ability to detect and classify bone fractures, empowering healthcare using a deep learning approach.

2.1 Significance

The significance of bone fracture detection is underscored by the transformative advancements they bring to the field of medical imaging and orthopaedic diagnostics. CNNs, designed to automatically learn and recognize patterns within complex visual data, offer several key advantages in the context of bone fracture detection.

2.1.1 Enhanced Accuracy and Precision

CNNs excel at capturing intricate patterns and features within images, leading to improved accuracy in identifying subtle fractures that might be challenging for the human eye to discern. This precision is vital for ensuring an accurate diagnosis and appropriate treatment planning.

2.1.2 Speed and Efficiency

Automated bone fracture detection using CNNs significantly expedites the diagnostic process. In emergency situations, where time is critical for prompt medical intervention, CNNs can swiftly analyse medical images, allowing healthcare professionals to make timely decisions and initiate appropriate care.

2.1.3 Reduction of Subjectivity

Traditional diagnostic methods often involve manual interpretation, introducing subjectivity and variability among different practitioners. CNNs, being algorithm-driven, provide a standardized and consistent approach to fracture detection, reducing the reliance on individual interpretation.

2.1.4 Handling Large Datasets

CNNs are well-suited for handling large datasets of medical images. The ability to efficiently process vast amounts of data contributes to building robust models that generalize well to diverse cases, improving the overall reliability of bone fracture detection.

2.1.5 Resource Optimization

By automating the detection process, CNNs contribute to resource optimization in healthcare settings. They reduce the workload on radiologists, allowing them to focus on more complex cases, while also potentially minimizing the need for additional diagnostic tests.

2.1.6 Scalability and Accessibility

The scalability of CNN-based solutions makes them adaptable to healthcare systems of varying sizes. Whether in well-equipped hospitals or resource-constrained environments, the accessibility and efficiency of CNNs make them valuable tools for improving fracture detection capabilities globally.

2.1.7 Technological Advancement

The integration of CNNs in bone fracture detection represents a significant leap in technological innovation within the medical field. It aligns with the broader trend of leveraging artificial intelligence to enhance healthcare outcomes, contributing to the evolution of diagnostic methodologies.

2.2 Challenges

2.2.1 Limited Annotated Datasets

The availability of well-annotated datasets for bone fractures is a challenge. CNNs heavily rely on extensive and diverse datasets for effective training, and the scarcity of such datasets can lead to suboptimal model performance.

2.2.2 Class Imbalance

Imbalances in the distribution of fracture types within datasets can affect the model's ability to accurately detect less prevalent fractures. CNNs might prioritize the more common fractures, leading to reduced sensitivity in identifying rarer but clinically significant cases.

2.2.3 Generalization to Varied Populations

CNNs trained on datasets from specific demographics may face challenges in generalizing their learning to populations with different anatomical variations. This could result in reduced accuracy when applied to diverse patient groups.

2.2.4 Overfitting and Noise Sensitivity

CNNs are prone to overfitting, particularly when trained on limited datasets. Noise or artifacts in medical images, common in real-world scenarios, may be erroneously learned as features by the model, impacting its generalization to new data.

2.2.5 Explainability and Interpretability

CNNs are often considered as "black-box" models, making it challenging to interpret their decision-making processes. In the medical field, understanding why a model made a specific prediction is crucial for gaining trust from healthcare professionals.

2.2.6 Limited Adoption in Routine Clinical Practice

The integration of CNN-based fracture detection tools into routine clinical workflows faces resistance due to concerns about reliability, interpretability, and the need for validation in real-world healthcare settings.

2.2.7 Variability in Imaging Techniques

Different healthcare institutions may use varied imaging techniques and equipment. CNNs trained on data from one type of equipment may struggle to adapt to the nuances of images acquired through different technologies, leading to reduced robustness.

3. EXISTING METHODS

3.1 RCNN and FPN Model

An object detector is trained to locate the sites of femoral shaft fractures in X-ray images, and classify its type. Object detection is a basic task in computer vision, which refers to the detections of both the locations and corresponding categories of objects in an image. Here the model detects the fracture regions of different types, by the bounding boxes. To train the detector, manual labelling of the bounding boxes of the 11 types of objects in total 2333 X-ray images (Qi et al., 2020) is done and they are used as the ground truths during training.

The dataset of 2333 images are broken into 1488 of them for training, 372 for validation and 473 for the final test. An anchor-based Faster RCNN detection model is utilized, with ResNet-50 and FPN (Feature Pyramid Network). The loss function includes the first stage loss of RPN and the second stage loss of RCNN. The both two stage loss can be written as function 1,

$$L_{(\{P_i\},\{t_i\})} = \frac{1}{N_{cls}}\sum_i L_{cls}\left(P_i, P_i^*\right) + \lambda \frac{1}{N_{reg}}\sum_i L_{reg}\left(t_i, t_i^*\right) \tag{1}$$

3.2 Using Microwave Imaging

3.2.1 Imaging Algorithm

The provided text describes an imaging algorithm designed for the detection of bone fractures using microwave imaging. The algorithm utilizes a radar setup with an antenna performing a linear scan parallel to the x-axis in the xz-plane. The goal is to reconstruct an image of the bone and identify fractures based on microwave (Santos et al., 2022) reflections.

3.2.2 Key Components and Steps of the Algorithm Include

- **Singular Value Decomposition (SVD):** The algorithm employs SVD to separate the scattered signals into contributions from the skin, fracture, and background. SVD is used to reduce clutter and enhance the visibility of the fracture signal.
- **Pre-processing Steps:** A simple filtering step subtracts the average of all antenna positions to reduce unwanted contributions. For situations where the bone is covered with skin, additional pre-processing is applied to remove artifacts caused by reflections from the air-skin interface. SVD is applied to subregions of the scanned area.

- **Image Reconstruction**: The backscattered response from each pixel in the xz-plane is calculated for each frequency using a range migration algorithm. A weighting procedure is introduced to enhance the relevance of deeper signals in the image. This involves normalizing the response over the pixels along the z-axis. The final image is reconstructed by combining the modified responses for each pixel.

4. DEEP LEARNING IN BONE FRACTURE DETECTION

Analysing the huge volume of bone fracture X-ray data is a challenge due to its high complexity. With the increase in the number of bone fractures and the locations of the fractures, traditional analytics models, existing models may give poor results. Adaptive approaches are required to understand the complex fractures (Hopkins Medicine, n.d.) in different locations.

Convolutional Neural Network models can extract meaningful insights and identify the patterns, providing an understanding of complex patterns in the data. In regard to bone fracture detection and classification, we are using Convolutional Neural network models to extract features from the image (Wei et al., 2009) and a fully connected dense layer to classify a non-fractured and a fractured bone. These models were chosen based on their ability to process a high amount of data and can learn the complicated patterns with a high accuracy.

4.1 The Convolutional Neural Network Model

In the proposed work a deep convolutional neural network model is designed. It contains convolution, pooling, flatten and dense layer. The features of the input image are automatically extracted by CNN and a fully connected layer is used to classify them into the non-fractured and the healthy bone. The pooling layer and convolution layer (CL) extract features from the image. At each of the convolution and pooling layers, a suitable kernel of size 5x5 is applied to extract features. Max-Pooling Layer is used to reduce the dimension of the filtered image at each convolution layer.

4.2 Flatten Layer

This layer reduces the 2-Dimensional feature vector into an array that is fed to a fully connected layer.

4.3 Fully Connected Dense Network

The classification is performed by the dense layer. The convolution layer extracts features from the input image by applying filters. This layer focuses on the best features of the image. This layer is also known as a fully dense layer. The proposed model predicts the bone to be healthy and the fracture.

5. METHODOLOGY

Data Augmentation: If the data set size is small, then the possibilities of over fitting may arise]. To overcome this problem, data augmentation techniques are used to increase the size of the data set.

Convolutional Layer and Max-Pooling Layer: In the proposed model we have applied 3 convolution layers and Max-Pooling layers. Convolutional layer with 32 filters (output channels), a kernel size of (5,5), this layer extracts 32 different feature maps from the input image. MaxPool2D () – Max Pooling layer with default parameters (pool size of (2,2)). It down samples the spatial dimensions, reducing the resolution and computational complexity.

Similar Convolutional and Max Pooling layers are repeated with increasing filter counts (64 and 128). This hierarchy captures hierarchical features in the input image.

Fully Connected Layer: This layer is also known as a fully dense layer. In the proposed model there are 3 layers with 32 neurons and a single output neuron.

5.1 Objective

The objectives of a Convolutional Neural Network (CNN) model for bone fracture detection typically revolve around improving the accuracy and efficiency of the detection process. Here are several key objectives:

- High Accuracy and Sensitivity: Develop a CNN model that achieves high accuracy in identifying bone fractures. Emphasize sensitivity to ensure that the model can effectively detect fractures, especially in cases with subtle or complex fracture patterns.
- Robustness to Variations: Design the CNN to be robust to variations in image quality, patient demographics, and fracture types. The model should generalize well across different datasets and imaging conditions.
- Efficient Use of Computational Resources: Optimize the CNN architecture and parameters to ensure efficient use of computational resources. Strive for a balance between model complexity and inference speed, especially in healthcare settings where real-time or near-real-time results are desirable.
- Transfer Learning and Pretrained Models: Investigate the use of transfer learning by leveraging pretrained models on large datasets. This approach can be beneficial when the available dataset for bone fracture detection (Jacob & Wyawahare, 2013) is limited.
- Interpretability and Explainability: Incorporate techniques to enhance the interpretability and explainability of the CNN model. This is crucial in a medical context, where healthcare professionals need insights into why the model makes specific predictions.

These objectives collectively aim to develop a CNN model that not only excels in accuracy but also aligns with the practical requirements and ethical considerations (Kim & MacKinnon, 2018) of bone fracture detection in healthcare applications.

5.2 Scope

Scope of Bone Fracture Detection Using X-rays in CNN Models

- Enhanced Diagnostic Accuracy: CNN models offer the potential to significantly enhance the accuracy of bone fracture detection in X-ray images by leveraging advanced pattern recognition capabilities.

- Efficient Screening and Triage: Implementing CNN models in fracture detection facilitates efficient screening processes, enabling healthcare professionals to prioritize and attend critical cases promptly.
- Automation of Routine Tasks: The application of CNN models allows for the automation of routine fracture detection tasks in radiology (Kim & MacKinnon, 2018), freeing up healthcare professionals to focus on more complex diagnostic challenges.
- Early Detection and Intervention: By providing rapid and accurate fracture identification, CNN models contribute to early detection and intervention, potentially minimizing the impact of fractures on patient outcomes.
- Integration with Healthcare Systems: CNN models can be integrated seamlessly into existing healthcare systems, including Picture Archiving and Communication Systems (PACS), to facilitate widespread adoption and accessibility.
- Adaptation to Diverse Patient Populations: Extending the scope to include the development of CNN models capable of adapting to diverse patient populations, accounting for variations in age, gender, and anatomical differences.
- Continuous Learning and Improvement: The scope encompasses the development of CNN models that can undergo continuous learning, adapting to evolving medical knowledge, new imaging technologies (D'Elia et al., 2009), and changes in fracture patterns over time.

In summary, the scope of bone fracture detection (Dimililer & Kamil, 2017) using X-rays in CNN models is vast and encompasses not only technical advancements but also considerations related to workflow optimization, patient outcomes, and the integration of AI into the broader healthcare ecosystem.

5.3 Architecture

Convolutional Neural Networks (CNNs) are a class of deep learning models designed specifically for processing structured grid data, such as images. They are highly effective in tasks like image recognition and computer vision. CNNs contains a hierarchical architecture inspired by the visual processing in the human brain as shown in Figure 1.

Figure 1. CNN model and fully dense network

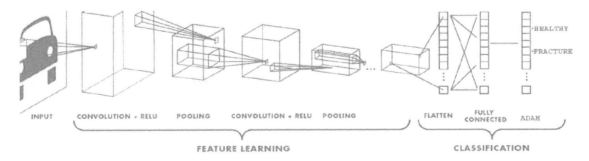

The key innovation lies in the use of convolutional layers, where small filters are applied to local regions of input data, enabling the network to automatically learn hierarchical features and patterns. Pooling layers are often employed to down sample the spatial dimensions, reducing computational complexity while retaining important information. Through multiple layers of convolutions and nonlinear activations, CNNs can automatically extract and learn hierarchical representations of features, making them well-suited for tasks involving spatial relationships and pattern recognition in multidimensional data as shown in Figure 2.

Figure 2. The convolution operation using kernels and obtaining feature maps

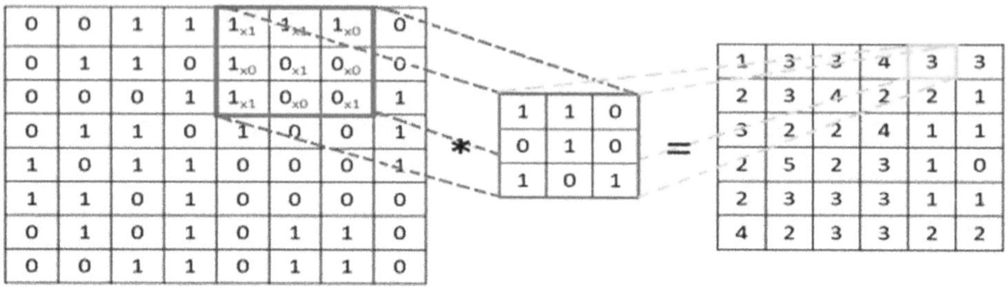

6. CONCLUSION

The utilization of Convolutional Neural Networks (CNNs) for bone fracture detection through X-ray images marks a significant advancement in medical imaging and diagnostic capabilities. This research has showcased the potential of deep learning algorithms in automating the identification and classification of fractures, contributing to the efficiency and accuracy of diagnostic processes.

As we conclude this book chapter, several key insights and implications emerge. Firstly, the CNN model has demonstrated commendable performance in differentiating between normal and fractured bone structures. The ability of the algorithm to learn intricate patterns and features within X-ray images has proven crucial in enhancing the diagnostic accuracy, reducing the likelihood of human error, and expediting the overall detection process.

In conclusion, the integration of CNNs in bone fracture detection through X-ray images signifies a breakthrough in medical imaging technology. The potential to revolutionize diagnostic practices, improve efficiency, and contribute to better patient outcomes is evident. As technology continues to evolve, collaborative efforts between computer scientists, medical professionals, and ethicists will be essential to harness the full benefits of this innovation while ensuring its responsible and ethical use in the field of healthcare.

REFERENCES

D'Elia, G., Caracchini, G., Cavalli, L., & Innocentia, P. (2009, September–December). Bone fragility and imaging techniques. *Clinical Cases in Mineral and Bone Metabolism, 6*, 234–246. PMID:22461252

Dimililer & Kamil. (2017). *IBFDS: Intelligent bone fracture detection system*. Elsevier.

Hopkins Medicine. (n.d.). *Fractures*. Hopkins Medicine. https://www.hopkinsmedicine.org/health/conditions-anddiseases/fractures

Jacob, N. E., & Wyawahare, M. (2013, June). Survey of bone fracture detection techniques. *Int. J. Comput. Appl.*, *71*(17), 31–34.

Kim, D. H., & MacKinnon, T. (2018, May). Artificial intelligence in fracture detection: Transfer learning from deep convolutional neural networks. *Clinical Radiology*, *73*(5), 439–445. doi:10.1016/j.crad.2017.11.015 PMID:29269036

Qi, Y., Zhao, J., Shi, Y., Zuo, G., Zhang, H., Long, Y., Wang, F., & Wang, W. (2020). Ground Truth Annotated Femoral X-Ray Image Dataset and Object Detection Based Method for Fracture Types Classification. *IEEE Access : Practical Innovations, Open Solutions*, *8*, 189436–189444. doi:10.1109/ACCESS.2020.3029039

Santos, K. C., Fernandes, C. A., & Costa, J. R. (2022). Feasibility of Bone Fracture Detection Using Microwave Imaging. *IEEE Open Journal of Antennas and Propagation*, *3*, 836–847. doi:10.1109/OJAP.2022.3194217

Wei, Z., Na, M., & Huisheng, S. (2009). Feature extraction of X-ray fracture image and fracture classification. *Proc. Int. Conf. Artif. Intell. Comput. Intell.*, (pp. 408–412). IEEE. 10.1109/AICI.2009.40

Chapter 6
Tackling Depression Detection With Deep Learning:
A Hybrid Model

N. Bala Krishna
School of Computing, Mohan Babu University, India

Reddy Sai Vikas Reddy
School of Computing, Mohan Babu University, India

M. Likhith
School of Computing, Mohan Babu University, India

N. Lasya Priya
School of Computing, Mohan Babu University, India

ABSTRACT

Traditionally, PHQ scores and patient interviews were used to diagnose depression; however, the accuracy of these measures is quite low. In this work, a hybrid model that primarily integrates textual and audio aspects of patient answers is proposed. Using the DAIC-WoZ database, behavioral traits of depressed patients are studied. The proposed method is comprised of three parts: a textual ConvNets model that is trained solely on textual features; an audio CNN model that is trained solely on audio features; and a hybrid model that combines textual and audio features and uses LSTM algorithms. The suggested study also makes use of the Bi-LSTM model, an enhanced variant of the LSTM model. The findings indicate that deep learning is a more effective method for detecting depression, with textual CNN models having 92% of accuracy and audio CNN models having 98% of accuracy. Textual CNN loss is 0.2 while audio CNN loss is 0.1. These findings demonstrate the efficacy of audio CNN as a depression detection model. When compared to the textual ConvNets model, it performs better.

DOI: 10.4018/979-8-3693-3679-3.ch006

1. INTRODUCTION

Depression is a recognized medical ailment that affects millions of individuals worldwide and is one of the most prevalent mental illnesses. Depression is one of the most menacing condition which affects mental and physical state of a person. According on a patient's mental health status, the severity of depression is predicted. A patient with depression experiences demotivation, hopelessness, and loss of interest in the daily tasks related to the mind, body, and social life. These symptoms can cause emotional harm and physical changes in the patient. It also affects a person's ability to learn results in mood swings and frequently lowers their productivity at work.

Depending on the degree of their depression, patients experience varying symptoms. When the severity is high, the brain slows down and releases the hormone cortisol, which has an impact on the development of new neurons in the brain. It creates an adverse effect on one's mental health and can occasionally result in suicidal thoughts.

There are various stages of depression, including seasonal affective disorder, dysthymia, bipolar disorder, clinical depression, and others. There are various options for treatment; these range from therapy sessions to counseling sessions. There are additional therapies that use brain simulation. An estimated 280 million people worldwide suffer from depression, and there are about 800,000 reported cases of depression-related suicide annually, according to a WHO survey (WHO, 2023).

As the fourth most common disease worldwide, depression has emerged as a major issue that impacts individuals of all ages, including children, adolescents, adults, and the elderly. Over 80% of people do not obtain the appropriate therapy since there are insufficient early services and therapies available for depressed patients. According to research, one in five people will at some point in their lives experience depression.

The prevalence of depression is rising daily, so it's critical to recognize the seriousness of this mental health issue. As a result, an automated system is needed to identify early indicators of depression and treat patients appropriately. In order to forecast the intensity of symptoms and typical behaviors seen in individuals with depression, structured clinical interviews are used. A patient who is depressed frequently stammers and speaks with irregular pauses. A depressed patient may also pronounce words and sentences slowly and incorrectly, which is another sign of the illness (Khang and Abuzarova et al., 2023).

Studies indicate that patients with depression have noticeably longer response times. They exhibit signs of depression by taking longer to act, listen, and respond. Sad thoughts trouble people who have depression tendencies, and they exhibit a clear inclination toward unfavorable stimuli. A depressed patient frequently uses derogatory language along with negative expressions that convey melancholy, stress, demotivation, or discontent. For instance, there are differences between the brain signal produced and the body's concentration of feel-good hormones like oxytocin and serotonin.

When a patient is depressed, there are differences in their electroencephalography (EEG), NMR, and other audio and image signals. Because of this, psychologists are unable to accurately predict the onset and severity of depression symptoms, which exacerbates the conditions of depressed patients. As a result, both patients and psychologists require an exact, automated, and easily accessible method.

2. LITERATURE REVIEW

Depression, a pervasive mental health disorder with profound societal and individual consequences, necessitates early detection for timely intervention and effective treatment.

2.1. Deep Learning Approaches

Recent investigations have delved into the efficacy of deep learning models in capturing intricate patterns associated with depression. The work by Aswathy (2019) and Hemanth (2019) introduced innovative deep learning approaches for depression detection on Twitter, showcasing improved performance compared to traditional ML methods.

2.2. Text Analysis

Leveraging textual data from diverse sources, including electronic health records and online forums, has been instrumental in depression detection. Natural language processing (NLP), sentiment analysis, and feature extraction from textual data are applied in Krishna Shrestha's (2018) work on Twitter data is used to diagnose depression through machine learning.

- Depression recognition based on dynamic facial and vocal expression features using partial least square regression
- Meng & Huang uses a regression method based on PLS wherein a late fusion detection method is built for model prediction (Meng, Huang, Wang, Yang, Shuraifi, and Wang, 2013).
- Multimodal prediction of psychological disorders: Learning verbal and nonverbal commonalities in adjacency pairs
- Devault has built a multimodal HCRF model which works on question-answer pairs. It analyses them for model prediction (Yu, Scherer, Devault, Gratch, Stratou, Morency, and Cassell, 2013).
- Topic modeling based multi-modal depression detection
- Gong et al. (2017) use the same approach. Building on it, he combines the question answer based model with his multi-modal approach, taking into consideration all the 3 modalities for model prediction (Gong and Poellabauer, 2017).
- A random Forest regression method with selected text feature for depression assessment
- They built a single model random forest-based classifier which works on the question-answer based approach. This classifier is used for model prediction (Sun, Zhang, He, Yu, Xu, Li, and Wang, 2017).
- Depaudionet: An efficient deep model for audio based depression classification
- Ma et al. propose an audio based method for depression classification using Convolutional Neural Networks (CNN) and Long Short-Term Memory (LSTM) networks for a higher-level audio representation. Ma et al. works only on the audio based modality. He inputs the audio based data into a CNN and then further uses a LSTM network for model prediction (Ma, Yang, Chen, Huang, and Wang, 2016).

3. OBJECTIVE AND SCOPE

3.1. Proposed Model

The two algorithms that form the basis of the proposed model are CNN and LSTM.

3.2. CNN Model

A deep learning technique known as a CNN, Convolution Neural Network, or ConvNet takes an image as input, applies ads weights to the input values and then supports the result image's classification. In addition to image classification, CNN is also utilized in, pattern recognition, data analysis, computer vision, and NLP job resolution. Multilayer Perceptrons, or CNNs, are a class of Artificial Neural Networks (ANNs). The architecture of neurons in the human brain served as the model for the CNN algorithm. CNN operates on the convolution operation principle. The convolution operation is carried out as illustrated in the example below. The CNN algorithm has the advantage of requiring significantly less processing time than other algorithms as shown in Figure 1.

Figure 1. Convolution operation

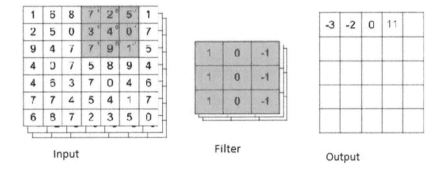

Input   Filter   Output

CNN applications Algebra is primarily utilized in speech recognition, text recognition, image identification, pattern recognition, and comprehending natural language processing issues. The CNN algorithm's architecture deals with the quantity of completely linked, max-pooling, and convolution layers. In the suggested approach, ReLU is used as an activation function as shown in Figure 2.

Word embedding are most commonly done using the word2vec, or word to vector, technique. Using the CBOW model and Skip Gramme, word2vec is produced. A two-layer model called Word2vec is used to process text data. Word2vec accepts text data as input and outputs vectors, or images. Features vectors for the words in the collection are called vectors. Word2vec uses past experiences to predict a word's meaning with a high degree of accuracy. Those predictions made in order to find word similarities with other words.

Word2vec trains words that have similar neighbors to the input data. To do this, you can use the CBOW approach, which uses data to forecast a word that is the target, or the Skip Gramme method,

Figure 2. CNN architecture

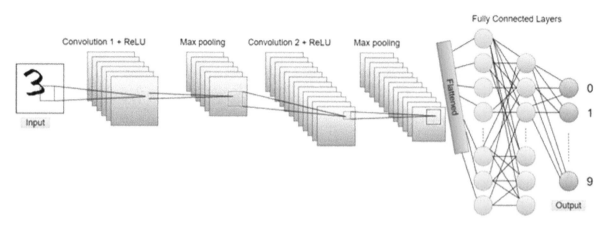

which uses a word to predict data in the target. Each of the aforementioned two approaches has pros and cons of its own. While CBOW operates more quickly and has a higher learning rate, Skip Gramme is only effective with smaller datasets.

GoogleNews-vectors-negative300.bin is utilized for the suggested work. It is a Google-developed word-to-vec model. A pre-trained model with a list of words for text classification is what it is. Sentiment analysis finds good use for it. The Kaggle website offers a download for it.

CNN performs well when it comes to pattern and picture recognition. The CNN model alone is not utilized for text classification. In addition to CNN model, word2vec is also used. Text answers from patients who are depressed serve as the dataset for text classification in order to diagnose depression. Text classification results are presented as binary labels. In a similar vein, spectrograms are gathered from audio samples—which are audio recordings of depressed patients—in order to facilitate auditory recognition in audio CNNs (Khang & Hajimahmud & Triwiyanto et al., 2024).

The following are some steps in the audio classification process: data imbalance, feature extraction, segmentation, and data cleaning. It's difficult to detect depression from audio samples. Transforming an audio sample into a spectrogram is the first step in the audio classification process. This phase is crucial for the categorization of audio. A spectrogram shows the frequencies of a signal as they change over time in a visual manner. Audio splitting, also known as segmentation, is the process of eliminating extraneous sounds and silences from audio samples. Data Imbalance is the next step after unwanted noise and silence have been removed from an audio or speech sample.

Information from non- depressed individuals in the dataset is greater than that from patients with depression. It is four times more than the patient data for depression. Data Imbalance is significant because of this. Equal numbers of Depressed: Non-Depressed data are obtained. The Spectrogram Conversion step is the third. After that, the audio segments that were sampled are converted into 512*512 pixels, or spectrograms. These photos are placed in 8:2 training and validation folders. Image processing can then be carried out. Using the CNN algorithm, predictions for patients with and without depression can be made based on those images. Binary Labels represent the classification results obtained from the audio.

3.3. LSTM Model

The LSTM algorithm, is a type of recurrent neural network (RNN) that primarily links features from one layer to the next. It facilitates the transfer of information from the past to the present and back again. RNNs work with a vector sequence. Each layer is therefore dependent upon earlier outputs. The issue with RNN is that information is quickly lost over time. LSTMs are a unique type of RNN that are intended to address the issue of information loss in RNN. Because LSTM can learn long-term dependencies, RNNs are sufficiently intelligent to remember information (Khang & Robotics, 2024).

Using LSTM has the benefit of assisting with pre-processing applications and data processing predictions. The gradient vanishing problem affects conventional algorithms like SVM and RF. The LSTM enhances model performance by committing key information to memory. The use of LSTM has the drawback of requiring more computing time for model training as shown in Figure 3.

Figure 3. LSTM architecture

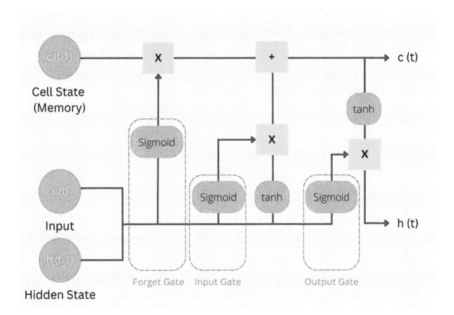

In certain machine learning problems, the model will perform worse with longer training times. In order to reduce the amount of training time needed, we employ LSTM with the fewest possible layers. An algorithm called LSTM works with both long-term and short-term data. The forget, input, and output gate are three gates that makes an LSTM. These gates function as filters, processing data in a sequential manner. LSTM models use feedback mechanisms to efficiently learn parameters. They update previous data with new data by drawing lessons from the past.

The feedback mechanism in LSTM allows the entire data sequence to be trained sequentially. By eliminating the vanishing gradient issue from the model, they improve its performance in comparison to alternative algorithms. The procedure for teaching a neural network to anticipate in two direction i.e., from past to future and from future to past—is known as bi-directional LSTM, or bi-LSTM. Because inputs to Bi- LSTM must flow both ways, the model is better able to update new information in the present and recall information from the past. Text classification, speech recognition, and pattern recognition can all be done with this model. Because this model is able to operate both forward and backward, it is capable of accurately classifying sequential data (Khang & Rath & Anh et al., 2024).

3.4. Dataset

Our model makes use of the DAIC-WOZ Depression Database. The database is an extensive corpus that contains replies from patients who are depressed. It captures data from patients via text responses to questionnaires, voice or audio recordings, and video recordings. We must first submit an application on their website before they grant us access to obtain the dataset. This database includes text, video, and audio features that depict the verbal and nonverbal symptoms of depression in patients. The DAIC- WOZ database is now divided into three folders: test_data, train_data, and dev_data.

3.5. Software

Google Collab software is used for detecting depression in patients. It is an easy-to-use internet platform that is open-source. Collab stands for Collaboratory, which enables anyone to run their individual Python programs. It provides access to the TPU and GPU, which automatically aid in the quick processing of deep learning and neural network algorithms.

4. PROPOSED WORK

4.1 Layers

The suggested model's architecture is broken down into three parts: the textual ConvNets model, which is trained exclusively on text features, and the audio ConvNets model, which is trained exclusively on audio features such as Mel spectrograms and MFCCs. The third model is a combination of the first two. i.e., textual + audio = hybrid model. When these primary layers begin to connect with one another, a neural network is created. A few of the audio features included in the suggested model are Mel Spectrograms, COVAREP, and MFCC.

Pretrained models, which already have characteristics from depressed patients' text responses, are employed for text features. Mel Spectrograms yield the best results when all features for the audio CNN model are compared. A suggested model uses CNN and LSTM architecture to convolve text and audio data, producing binary labels such as "Depressed" or "Not-Depressed" as shown in Figure 4. The suggested model is used to diagnose depression; it makes automatic predictions about a person's depression status.

Figure 4. Architecture of proposed model

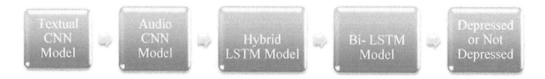

Alt-text: Figure 4 presents the proposed method's framework.

4.2 Layers

- Convolution Layer - The convolution layer, which is the first layer in a neural network, is the most important layer. The convolution layer's main job is to determine whether the input is text, audio, or both types of features. The output image is obtained by convolving the input image with a filter of the same size in the convolution layer. The output produces a feature map. In the convolution layer, weights—also known as filter kernels—are used and updated via the back propagation method.

- Max-Pooling Layer - A pooling layer's primary function is to reduce the size of the input. It helps the model to update with only the necessary data, reducing the actual amount of data. Unwanted characteristics are removed from the data.

- Rectified linear unit as an Activation Function- The function that defines non-linearity is called ReLU. In ReLU layer, all negative data is substituted with zero values.

- Fully Connected Layer - This layer is where classification begins, and the results are automatically updated.

- Batch Normalization - The output of earlier layers is normalized using batch normalization layers. It facilitates the model's efficient feature learning. It increases the model's speed and stability. It speeds up the model's processing and learning.

- Dropout layer - A layer called dropout aids in minimizing overfitting in models. It increases the rate at which the model learns by arbitrarily dropping particular neural network variables. The completely linked layer comes before the dropout layer. The suggested dropout value is 0.25. It could result in sluggish neural network training.

5. IMPLEMENTATION STEPS

- Load Required Libraries: Import the necessary libraries and modules at the beginning of your Python script or Jupyter notebook.

- Mount Google Drive (Assuming Colab Environment): If you're using Google Colab, mount your Google Drive to access the dataset and other files.

- Download NLTK Stopwords: Download NLTK stopwords for text processing.

- Load Dataset: Load the dataset from CSV files. Adjust file paths based on your actual file locations.

- Define Functions: Define functions such as Thresholding, remove_StopWords, checkAcc, and upsample. Ensure these functions are correctly implemented and defined before using them.

- Preprocess and Load Word Embedding: Preprocess the text data and load pre-trained word embedding (Word2Vec in this case).

- Define CNN Model Class: Define the CNN_Text class that represents your Convolutional Neural Network model.

- Instantiate and Train the Model: Create an instance of the CNN_Text class, and train the model using your training data.

- Make Predictions: Use the trained model to make predictions on the test data.

- Apply Threshold and Evaluate: Apply a threshold to the predicted probabilities and evaluate the model.
- Generate Results: If you need to output results (e.g., for the reviewer), you can create a results array or DataFrame.
- Visualize Results: If you want to visualize the training and validation loss/accuracy, include the code for plotting.

6. EXPERIMENT RESULTS

Three models are derived from the experimental results, all the three models that combines text and audio features. Two algorithms that are used with hybrid models are LSTM and Bi-LSTM as shown in Figure 5.

Figure 5. The hybrid LSTM and the hybrid Bi-LSTM models

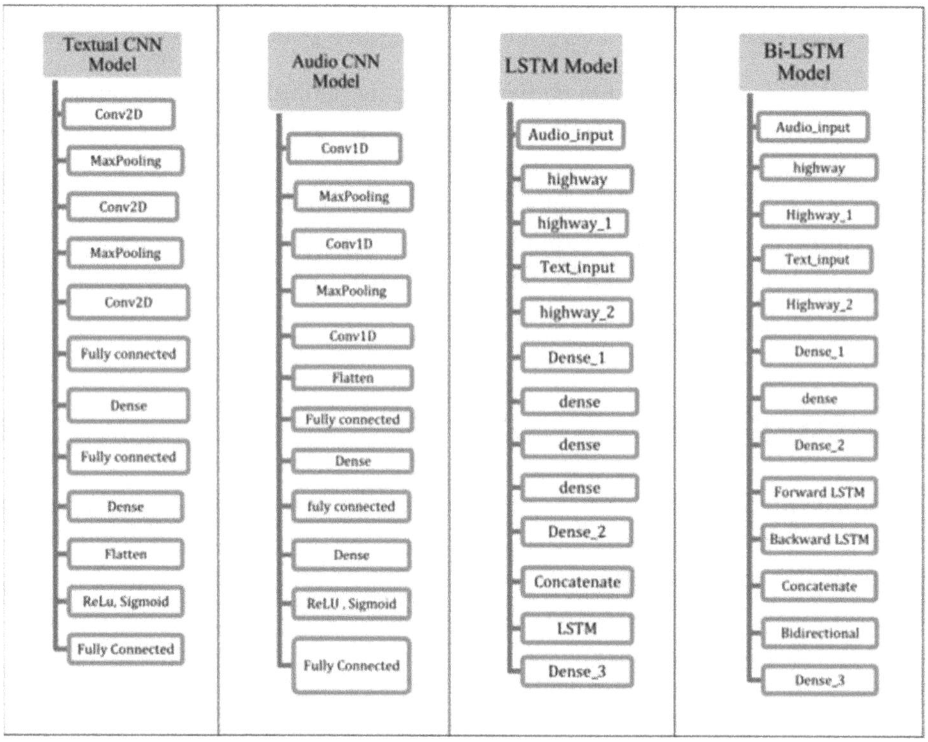

Consequently, two hybrid models are produced by the proposed model, the hybrid LSTM and the hybrid Bi-LSTM models. By applying these models, predictions with a high degree of accuracy and low loss can be made in the proposed work for depression detection. For every model, a graph is plotted to estimate the model's performance.

The architecture of the textual CNN model consists of activation functions, max- pooling layers, convolution layers, flatten layers, fully connected layers, and dropout layers in combination experimental results from these four models show that the textual CNN model, gave 0.92% of accuracy after training for ten number of epochs, with a 0.3 loss and with less time of execution after training. It takes one minute and forty-two seconds to run the textual CNN model.

The second model, the audio CNN model, trained for ten epochs at a loss of 0.1, and its accuracy was 0.98%. In contrast to the textual CNN model, the model needed more execution time after training.It takes five minutes and thirty seconds to run the audio CNN model. The second model, the audio CNN model, trained for ten epochs at a loss of 0.1, and its accuracy was 0.98%. In contrast to the textual ConvNet model, the model needed more execution time after training. It takes five minutes and thirty seconds to run the audio CNN model.

With a loss of 0.4, a LSTM model produced accuracy of 0.80%. The trained model is subjected to the LSTM algorithm, and the hybrid LSTM model incorporates features from both the textual and audio CNN models. 2 hours and 26 minutes are needed to train the hybrid LSTM model. The hybrid Bi-LSTM model has finally been trained using both text and audio features. The Bi-LSTM model yields a higher accuracy of 0.88 compared to the Hybrid LSTM model, and a lower loss of 0.2 compared to the Hybrid LSTM model. This indicates that the Bi-LSTM model predicts depression detection more accurately than the LSTM model. Five hours and forty-four minutes are needed to train the Bi-LSTM model.

Compared to the LSTM model, the training time is longer. Table 2 compares the models and assesses val_accuracy, val_loss, accuracy, and loss. It demonstrates that training loss is less than validation loss and that training accuracy is greater than validation accuracy.

Table 2. Evaluation parameters accuracy, loss, Val_Accuracy, Val_Loss

Method	Accuracy	Loss	Val_Accuracy	Val_Loss
TEXT CNN	0.92	0.3	0.80	0.5
AUDIO CNN	0.98	0.1	0.80	0.3
HYBRID LSTM	0.80	0.4	0.78	0.5
HYBRID Bi-LSTM	0.88	0.2	0.76	0.2

Table 3 demonstrates how evaluation metrics like support, F1-score, precision, and recall define the model performance. Every model attains a high degree of precision, as Table 3 illustrates. In comparison to the suggested model, yielding superior outcomes and improved performance. In comparison to the F1-score, precision values are better for all models, and support is consistent across all models.

Table 3. Evaluation parameters precision, recall, F1-score, support

Method	Precision	Recall	F1-Score	Support
TEXT CNN	0.63	0.68	0.60	33
AUDIO CNN	0.70	1.00	0.15	33
HYBRID LSTM	0.68	0.79	0.78	33
HYBRID Bi-LSTM	0.75	0.73	0.74	33

The confusion matrix can be used to predict the severity of depression. The Confusion Matrix predicts whether a patient is depressed or not by using scores between the True and Predicted Label. This matrix aims for classification. This matrix explains how the model has a tendency to predict incorrect classes. Two classes are created for depression detection: one is depressed and the other is not. The numbers 0 and 1 designate these classes. This indicates that the Confusion Matrix correctly predicts the Bi-LSTM model as shown in Table 4.

Table 4. Parameters comparison with base paper

Method	Precision	Recall	F1-Score	Support
TEXT CNN	0.56	0.61	0.58	33
AUDIO CNN	0.47	0.3	0.13	33
HYBRID LSTM	0.48	0.65	0.55	33
Bi-LSTM	0.62	0.32	0.18	33

The confusion matrix is displayed as in Table 5. In comparison to other models, Bi-LSTM predicts a higher patients with depression, as demonstrated by the confusion matrix.

Table 5. Confusion matrix labels

TRUE POSITIVE	TRUE NEGATIVE
FALSE POSITIVE	FALSE NEGATIVE

For each model, as illustrated in Figure 6, 7, 8, and 9, a graph representing accuracy, loss, val_accuracy, and val_loss is plotted to compare the performance of the four models. Figures 6(a), 7(a), 8(a), and 9(a) show a graph that plots loss against the number of epochs.

Plotting is done for the training and validation losses. Training loss decreases as the number of epochs rises. Figures 6(b), 7(b), and 8(b), as well as Figure 9(b), show a graph that plots precision in relation to the number of epochs. A plot is created using the training and validation accuracy. There are a total of 10 epochs in both scenarios. Training accuracy rises in tandem with epochs. Plotted graphs demonstrate that the textual CNN model learns more slowly than the audio CNN model, suggesting a greater learning rate for the audio CNN model. Comparing both textual and audio models the loss of audio model is small. Correctness of audio Due to its high learning feature parameters, the CNN model saturates easily after reaching its peak value quickly.

According to the results, the audio CNN model picks up features more quickly than the text CNN model. The accuracy of the Bi-LSTM model is higher than the LSTM model. Graphs clearly demonstrate that the Audio model can predict depression with a minimum loss of 1% and a maximum accuracy of 98%. This indicates that the Audio CNN model can accurately identify audio features and predict depression.

Figure 6. (a) Graphs of Textual CNN model represents training loss and Validation loss against no. of epochs; (b) Graphs of Textual CNN model REPRESENTS training accuracy and validation accuracy against no. of epochs

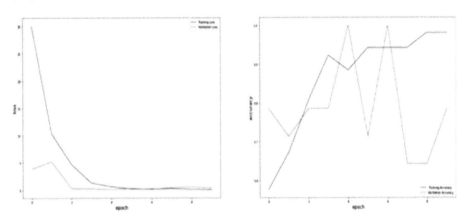

Figure 7. (a) Graphs of Audio CNN model represents training loss and validation loss against no. of epochs; (b) Graphs of Audio CNN model represents training accuracy and validation accuracy against no. of epochs

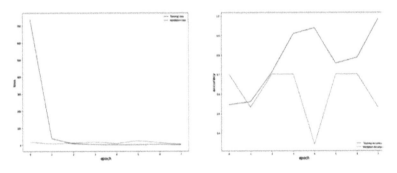

Figure 8. (a) Graphs of Hybrid LSTM model represents training loss and validation loss against no. of epochs; (b) Graphs of hybrid LSTM model represents training accuracy and validation accuracy against no. of epochs

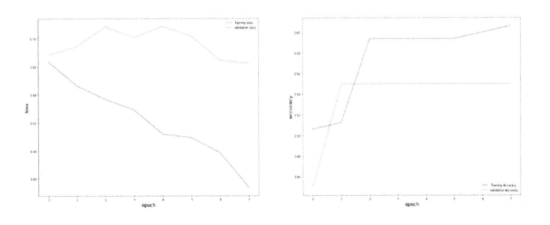

Figure 9. (a) Graphs of Hybrid Bi-LSTM model represents training loss and validation loss against no. of epochs; (b) Graphs of Hybrid Bi-LSTM model represents Training Accuracy and Validation Accuracy against no. of epochs

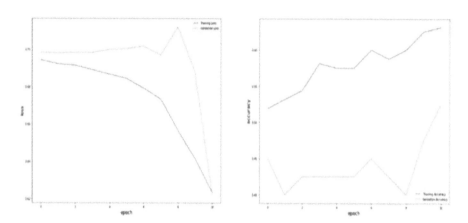

In addition, the Bi-LSTM model learns more quickly than other models. While the Bi-LSTM model requires a greater amount of pre- processing time than other models, accuracy increases and the loss decreases as the number of epochs increases. As a result, experimental findings demonstrate that Bi-LSTM has a faster learning rate and more accurate audio CNN prediction. According to the specific algorithms that each model uses, they are both good.

7. CONCLUSION

This work proposes a deep learning-based automatic depression detection system solution. The proposed work designs three models: a textual CNN model, an audio CNN model, and a hybrid LSTM and Bi-LSTM model. As per experiment results, the audio CNN model outperforms the text CNN model in deep learning depression detection. It can accurately predict the early symptoms of depression detection with 98% of accuracy and a 0.1% of loss, while the text CNN model achieves a 92% of accuracy and a 0.2% of loss as shown in Table 6.

Table 6. Confusion matrix of text CNN model

Predicted Label/True Label	Depressed	Not-Depressed
Depressed	20	13
Not-Depressed	11	3

The Text CNN model predicts 20 out of the 47 individuals in the Confusion Matrix as depressed and 3 as not-depressed, whereas the Audio CNN predicts 22 depressed and 5 not-depressed as shown in Table 7.

Table 7. Confusion matrix of audio CNN model

Predicted Label/True Label	Depressed	Not-Depressed
Depressed	22	13
Not-Depressed	7	5

Similar to this, the Bi-LSTM model's confusion matriX reveals that 30 patients are depressed and only 5 are not, whereas the LSTM model's confusion matriX demonstrates that 26 patients are depressed and 6 are not. This means that more accurate results will be obtained. As a result, it has been demonstrated that the Bi-LSTM model learns more quickly than the LSTM model, making it capable of remembering both text and audio features as shown in Table 8.

Table 8. Confusion matrix of hybrid LSTM model

Predicted Label/True Label	Depressed	Not-Depressed
Depressed	26	7
Not-Depressed	8	6

The Bi-LSTM's Confusion MatriX demonstrates that deep learning can be used to detect depression in patients. The Bi-LSTM model requires more training time than the LSTM model, which is faster than the Bi-LSTM model but less effective at long-term memory retention of text and audio features. As new data is added to the LSTM model, the previous data is lost. All models have minimal loss, which contributes to their high accuracy as shown in Table 9.

Table 9. Confusion matrix of hybrid Bi-LSTM model

Predicted Label/True Label	Depressed	Not-Depressed
Depressed	30	5
Not-Depressed	7	5

In conclusion, training and validation graphs as well as confusion matrix are used to predict depression. A few other metrics, including support, F1-score, recall, and precision, are also assessed. Bi-LSTM has the highest precision value, and more precision makes the model intelligent enough to remember past information and make predictions about the future (Khang & Medicine, 2023).

REFERENCES

Alghamdi, N. S., Hosni Mahmoud, H. A., Abraham, A., Alanazi, S. A., & Garcia-Hernandez, L. (2020). L. GarcíaHern´ andez, Predicting depression symptoms in an Arabic psychological forum. *IEEE Access: Practical Innovations, Open Solutions, 8,* 57317–57334. https://ieeexplore.ieee.org/abstract/document/9040556/. doi:10.1109/ACCESS.2020.2981834

Alhanai, T., Ghassemi, M., & Glass, J. (2018). Detecting depression with audio/text sequence modeling of interviews. *Proc. Annu. Conf. Int. Speech Commun. Assoc. INTERSPEECH (September)* (pp. 1716–1720). IEEE.

Gong, Y., & Poellabauer, C. (2017). "Topic modeling based multi-modaldepression detection. Proceedings of the 7th Annual Workshopon Audio/Visual Emotion Challenge. ACM.

Khang, A. (2023). *AI and IoT-Based Technologies for Precision Medicine* (1st ed.). IGI Global Press. doi:10.4018/979-8-3693-0876-9

Khang, A. (2024). *Medical Robotics and AI-Assisted Diagnostics for a High-Tech Healthcare Industry* (1st ed.). IGI Global Press. doi:10.4018/979-8-3693-2105-8

Khang, A., & Abdullayev, V. A. (2023). *AI-Aided Data Analytics Tools and Applications for the Healthcare Sector, "AI and IoT-Based Technologies for Precision Medicine* (1st ed.). IGI Global Press. doi:10.4018/979-8-3693-0876-9.ch018

Khang, A., & Hajimahmud, V. A. (2024). Cloud Platform and Data Storage Systems in Healthcare Ecosystem. Medical Robotics and AI-Assisted Diagnostics for a High-Tech Healthcare Industry (1st ed.). IGI Global Press. doi:10.4018/979-8-3693-2105-8.ch022

Khang, A., Rath, K. C., Anh, P. T. N., Rath, S. K., & Bhattacharya, S. (2024). Quantum-Based Robotics in High-Tech Healthcare Industry: Innovations and Applications. Medical Robotics and AI-Assisted Diagnostics for a High-Tech Healthcare Industry (1st ed.). IGI Global Press. doi:10.4018/979-8-3693-2105-8.ch001

Le, H.-N., & Boyd, R. C. (2022). Prevention of Major Depression. *Early Detection and Early Intervention in the General Population, 2006,* 23.

Lin, L., Chen, X., Shen, Y. L., & Zhang, L. (2020). Zhang, towards automatic depression detection: A bilstm/1d cnn-based model. *Applied Sciences (Basel, Switzerland), 10*(23), 1–20. doi:10.3390/app10238701

Ma, X., Yang, H., Chen, Q., Huang, D., & Wang, Y. (2016). Depaudionet:An efficient deep model for audio based depression classifica-tion, *Proceedings of the 6th International Workshop on Au-dio/Visual Emotion Challenge.* ACM.

Ma, X., Yang, H., Chen, Q., Huang, D., & Wang, Y. (2016). DepAudioNet: an efficient deep model for audio based depression classification. AVEC 2016 - Proc. 6th Int. Work. Audio/Visual Emot. Challenge, Co-located with ACM Multimed. ACM. doi:10.1145/2988257.2988267

Meng, H., Huang, D., Wang, H., Yang, H., Ai Shuraifi, M., & Wang, Y. (2013). Depression recognition based on dynamic facial and vocal expression features using partial least square regression. *Proceedings of the 3rd ACM international workshop on Audio/visual emotion challenge.* ACM. 10.1145/2512530.2512532

Narendra Kumar Rao, B. (2023). Factors influencing Mental Health due to Climate Change & Role of Artificial Intelligence. *Factors influencing Mental Health due to Climate Change & Role of Artificial Intelligence, CRC Press Taylor & Francis (T&F).* doi:10.4018/978-1-0034-2960-9

Narendra Kumar Rao, B., Partheeban, P., Naseeba, B., & Raju, H. P. (2022). ML Approaches to Detect Email Spam Anamoly. *2022 International Conference on Data Science, Agents & Artificial Intelligenc (ICDSAAI)*, Chennai, India. 10.1109/ICDSAAI55433.2022.10028911

Narendra Kumar Rao, B., Ranjana, R., Panini Challa, N., & Sreenivasa Chakravarthi, S. (2023). *Convolutional Neural Network Model for Traffic Sign Recognition.* 2023 3rd International Conference on Advance Computing and Innovative Technologies in Engineering (ICACITE), Greater Noida, India. 10.1109/ICACITE57410.2023.10182966

Sun, B., Zhang, Y., He, J., Yu, L., Xu, Q., Li, D., & Wang, Z. (2017). Arandom forest regression method with selected text feature for de-pression assessment. Proceedings of the 7th Annual Workshopon Audio/ Visual Emotion Challenge. ACM.

Wang, Z., Chen, L., Wang, L., & Diao, G. (2020). Recognition of audio depression based on convolutional neural network and generative antagonism network model. *IEEE Access : Practical Innovations, Open Solutions*, 8, 101181–101191. https://ieeexplore.ieee.org/abstract/document/9103527/. doi:10.1109/ACCESS.2020.2998532

WHO. (2023). *Depression.* World Health Organization (WHO). https://www.thelancet.com/journals/lancet/article/PIIS0140-6736(07)61415-9/fulltext?pubType=related

Yu, Z., Scherer, S., Devault, D., Gratch, J., Stratou, G., Morency, L.-P., & Cassell, J. (2013). Multimodal prediction of psychologicaldisorders: Learning verbal and nonverbal commonalities in adjacency pairs. *Semdial 2013 DialDam: Proceedings of the 17thWorkshop on the Semantics and Pragmatics of Dialogue.* ACM.

Chapter 7
Fuzzy Thresholding–Based Brain Image Segmentation Using Multi–Threshold Level Set Model

Daizy Deb
Department of Computer Sciences and Engineering, Brainware University, India

Alex Khang
https://orcid.org/0000-0001-8379-4659
Global Research Institute of Technology and Engineering, USA

Avijit Kumar Chaudhuri
https://orcid.org/0000-0002-5310-3180
Brainware University, India

ABSTRACT

Region of interest with reference to medical image is a challenging task. Clustering or grouping data objects can be used to isolate certain area of interest called image segmentation from human brain MRI scans is considered here. Together with the combination of Multilevel Otsu's thresholding and Level set approach, the most widely used fuzzy-based clustering like fuzzy C means (FCM) thresholding are taken into consideration. Here, the proper thresholding is determined using FCM thresholding. This threshold value can also be used to modify the Multilevel Otsu' method's threshold. The level set technique is then used to this segmented output image, yielding a more precise boundary level estimation. To improve brain MRI image segmentation, the proposed FTMLS system integrates the three aforementioned methods.

1. INTRODUCTION

In the modern world, early tumor detection is crucial for the best course of therapy. We have introduced a novel medical image segmentation technique with this propose algorithm, which could be helpful for accurately orienting the size and form of brain tumors from MRI brain images.

DOI: 10.4018/979-8-3693-3679-3.ch007

With the aid of the K-means and FCM algorithms already in use, the initial segmentation result was obtained. It has been recognized that the FCM approach is better suited for medical picture analysis. Next, as demonstrated in Figure2, we employed fuzzy c means thresholding to enhance the multilevel thresholding method. This suggested FCMMT technique produces superior results with better segmentation.

1.1 Fuzzy C- Means Thresholding

This research paper introduces 3-class FCM based thresholding to be used for initializing the multilevel thresholding and LS evolution and regulating the controlling parameters. C classes are created by dividing N objects using FCM clustering. N in our approach is the number of pixels in the image, therefore for 3-class FCM clustering, C=3 and N=Nx x Ny. An objective function based on a weighted similarity measure between each of the c-cluster centers and the image's pixels is iteratively optimized by the FCM algorithm. The FCM algorithm uses iterative optimization of an objective function based on a weighted similarity measure between the pixels in the image and each of the C-cluster centers. A local extremism of the objective function indicates an optimal clustering of the input data. The objective function that is minimized is given by formula (1)

$$Q = \sum_{i=1}^{C} \sum_{j=1}^{N} (u_{ij})^m \parallel z_j - v_i \parallel^2 \tag{1}$$

where $z_j \in Z$; $v = \{v_1, v_2, ..., v_c\}$ and $z = \{z_1, z_2, z, ..., z_N\}$ & $v_i \in V$ and where$\parallel * \parallel$ is a norm expressing the similarity between any measured data value and the cluster centre; m is $[1, \infty]$ is a weighting exponent and can be any real number greater than 1.

Calculations suggest that best choice of m is in the interval [1.5, 2.5], so m=2 is used here as it is widely accepted as a good choice of fuzzification parameter.

The fuzzy c-partition of given data set is the fuzzy partition matrix U= with i=1, 2....C and j=1, 2, 3...N, u_{ij} indicate the degree of membership of jth pixel to i^{th} cluster.

The membership functions are subject to satisfy the following conditions.

$$\sum_{i=1}^{C} u_{ij} = 1 \text{ for j=1,2,3,...N;}$$

$$0 < \sum_{j=1}^{N} u_{ij} < N \text{ for i=1,2,...,C; } 0 \le u_{ij} \le 1$$

The aim of FCM algorithm is to find an optimal fuzzy c-partition by evolving the fuzzy partition matrix U= $[u_{ij}]$ iteratively and computing the cluster centers. In order to achieve this, the algorithm tries to minimize the objective function Q by iteratively updating the cluster centres and the membership functions using the following equations. FCM clustering is used to partition N objects into C classes. In this method, N is equal to the number of pixels as formula 2

$$vi = \left(\sum_{j=1}^{N} (u_{ij})^m \right) / \left(z_j \sum_{j=1}^{N} (u_{ij})^m \right)$$

$$u_{ij} = 1 / \left(\sum_{k=1}^{C} \left(\frac{\| v_i - u_j \|}{\| v_i - u_k \|} \right)^{\frac{2}{m-1}} \right) \tag{2}$$

Each pixel is ultimately assigned to the cluster for which its membership value is maximum after completing FCM clustering. The threshold value is determined by taking the mean of the maximum of cluster 1 and the minimum of cluster 2, or the maximum of cluster 2 and the minimum of cluster 3, based on the intensity distribution produced from the picture histogram. The image's intensity distribution is taken into consideration while using this threshold selection technique. This method of threshold selection takes into account the intensity distribution in the image. This choice helps in obtaining optimum threshold values for different images obtained under different conditions (Masood, 2013).

1.2 Otsu's Multilevel Thresholding

The Otsu's thresholding method is used for image segmentation. This segmentation is done here with the help of image thresholding, or the reduction of a gray level image to a binary image. Thresholding can perform the task image segmentation when object and background pixels can be differentiated by their gray level values (from bi-model histogram). We have to find the threshold value and that can be calculated from total mean and variance of within-class and between-class respectively (Khang, 2023).

1.3 Level Set

Active contour is a popular approach used to estimate boundaries in medical images. Two types of algorithms lie under this category: 1) parametric active contours (Isard, 1998) which adapt a deformable curve until it fits the object boundary. 2) Geometric active contours based on level set theory. Some of the active contour models need user intervention for initialization. Thus automatic approaches like gradient vector flow algorithm based on anisotropic diffusion and robust algorithms like adaptive snakes and shape probability association model are taking important place in literature.

Level set (LS) methods, as one of the automatic process approach have shown effective results for medical image segmentation. However, intensive computational requirements and regulation of controlling parameters make it a complex and time consuming method. Fuzzy clustering has been utilized to reduce these drawbacks and enable automatic segmentation of computed tomography, magnetic resonance imaging, and ultrasound using LS segmentation. Fuzzy C mean (FCM) based thresholding and LS algorithm are different computational models that have been applied for this work is done on using clustering for initial segmentation followed by further edge preserving and refining steps for border tracing brain tumor.

2. PROPOSED METHODOLOGY OF FTMLS ALGORITHM

Medical image processing system is mainly consisting of three steps: image pre-processing, processing and post processing. The processing stage further may be subdivided into pre-processing, segmentation and analyzing. The following steps are involved in this proposed method as shown in the Figure 1.

Figure 1. Diagrammatically representation of stages involved in the FTMLS process

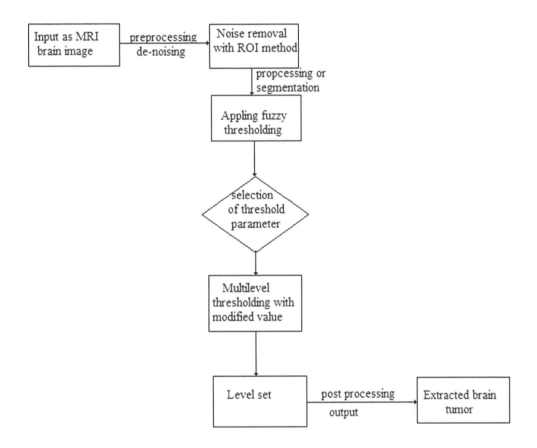

2.1 DICOM Image

DICOM, which is the most widely used medical imaging format, enables the sharing of medical information and the integration of different medical devices from different vendors through the Picture Archiving and Communication System (PACS). Here we are using MRI scan images of a brain for experimental purpose, some of them are collected from DICOM images from real time database, which usually have the patient's details and also contains some lab information. So this unwanted information which can be termed as noise here and it should be removed in preprocessing stage before processing the image further. In image processing different types of filters are used for noise removal purpose, some common filters are Gaussian Filter or Gaussian smoothing; Mean Filter and Median Filter etc. (Khang & Abdullayev, 2023).

Sometimes it is essential to process a particular area of an image, leaving other regions unaffected. This is called region-of-interest (ROI) and it is more appropriate to use here because we are removing here the artifact of four corners from MRI brain images. It should not affect the other portion of the brain because each part is equally important to detect the tumor. After noise removal we can apply the segmentation algorithm to segment the brain tumor. Here noise removal and segmentation techniques are considered and simulated using MATLAB. The results of existing algorithm and proposed algorithm are compared and presented in section. Analytical view of the result is also considered here for explanation (Khang, 2024a).

2.2 Segmentation

We used fuzzy C- means (FCM) thresholding (Masood, 2013) algorithm for segmentation purposes. Here the main aim is to detect brain tumor using image segmentation method and detecting brain tumor implies the detection of that region of interest. So clustering method is the best way to carry out the detection of affected region in an image.

In this process after noise removal the output is processed for FCM thresholding algorithm is shown in Figure 2 and values are displayed in Table 3. From this table, the most efficient threshold values are obtained out of which the best one is further used in multilevel thresholding. From the experimental value observation Fuzzy c-means thresholding gives the better output. Fuzzy thresholding algorithm is the most accepted method used in medical image segmentation because it has robust characteristics for ambiguity and can retain much more information compared to the other segmentation method. The experimental values of two level fuzzy thresholding are displayed in figure 4.3 these value can be further used in the next multilevel stage (Aslam et al., 2013; Khang et al., 2024).

These two level thresholding value of fuzzy thresholding which is called β (desire thresholding value) value is named here, we used these value to modify the multi-level thresholding as FCMMT method. This FCMMT algorithm along with Level set is used for final output of image segmentation.

Otsu's multilevel thresholding (Javeed Hussain et al., 2012) and Level set method for proper feature extraction and for the betterment of the result. Otsu's multilevel thresholding can perform the task of image segmentation when object and background pixels can be differentiated, we have to take the threshold value and that can be calculated from threshold value parameter β from the above stage of Fuzzy c-means thresholding method. Those values are taken from Table 4.3 and used for further calculation of thresholding for optimization in multi-level thresholding. From this experimental results it can be observed that the new Fuzzy c-means clustering technique works efficiently with all the sample images (Javeed Hussain et al., 2012; Khang, 2024c).

The outputs of proposed algorithm of FCM thresholding for FCMMT part are more accurate and precise. Further applied the level set method to FTMLS algorithm to enhance the image boundary region. Steps of proposed FTMLS algorithm for image segmentation

1. Read the input of MRI brain image.
2. Call or fill function for noise removal.
3. Fill the affected corner of image with different functional value.
4. Choose number of cluster
5. Initialized the Custer center
6. Calculate the membership

7. Compute the new cluster centers
8. Assign each pixel to the cluster with highest membership value
9. Calculate threshold level and perform threshold operation
10. For FCMMT method image can store into separate variable
11. Find the maximum and minimum value of gray image
12. Compute level 1, 2 and 3, and Level one can be calculated as: Level1 = threshold value * (maximum-minimum)+ minimum;
13. Also Level2= 2*level1 Level3= 3*level2
14. Than compute the automatic formation of contour using Level Set.
15. Calculate the tumor area
16. Display image

3. RESULTS AND DISCUSSION

For these experiments purpose ten different types of MRI brain images have been considered with different size and shape of the brain tumor. We have applied different filtering techniques but with ROI method gives satisfactory result. Initially we compare the output of two image segmentation result of K-means and FCM thresholding. The mathematical values of these two experimental results are shown in the Table 1 and Table 2.

Table 1. Experimental values using the K-means method

Segmentation result of K-means with morphological operator			
Input image	**Cluster No.**	**Iteration No.**	**Time**
Img1	3	23	2.73s
Img2	3	20	0.67s
Img3	3	14	0.52s
Img4	3	16	0.16s

The experimental results of K-means and FCM method are shown in the Figure 2 (a, b, c, d) and Figure 3 (a, b, c, d, e, f, g, h). In K-means algorithm, image segmentation can be done with proper clustering number and the time requirement is also less.

From FCM thresholding method we are getting the exact thresholding level value as shown in the Table 2, and that can be used for next level of the multilevel thresholding which improves the image segmentation means tumor area detection. Then Level set algorithm is used to enhance the boundary region more perfectly. This result of proposed method is also compared with the existing multilevel thresholding method as shown in the Table 3.

In Table 3 shows the different experimental values of image segmented with tumor area. Table 3 displays the three different values of existing multilevel thresholding, multilevel thresholding, FCMMT method and values of proposed method FTMLS. From these result we can observe that the image seg-

Table 2. Experimental values with the technique fuzzy c means thresholding method

I/P	Iteration No.	Fuzzy thresholding value
Img1	85	Level 0 = 0.05 Level 1 = 0.2
Img2	45	Level 0 = 0.1 Level 1 = 0.2
Img3	100	Level 0 = 0.1 Level 1 = 0.3
Img4	101	Level 0 = 0.16 Level 1 = 0.03
Img5	54	Level 0 = 0.16 Level 1 = 0.03
Img6	58	Level 0 = 0.22 Level 1 = 0.34
Img7	45	Level 0 = 0.17 Level 1 = 0.24
Img8	57	Level 0 = 0.08 Level 1 = 0.24
Img9	19	Level 0 = 0.07 Level 1 = 0.24
Img10	45	Level 0 = 0.15 Level 1 = 0.36

Figure 2. (a, b, c, d): Experimental result of K-means image segmentation with four different types of images

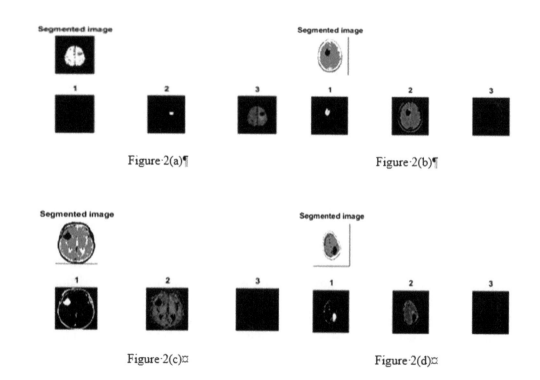

Figure·2(a)¶   Figure·2(b)¶

Figure·2(c)¤   Figure·2(d)¤

Figure 3. (a, b, c, d, e, f, g, h): Input and output image of fuzzy c-means thresholding method

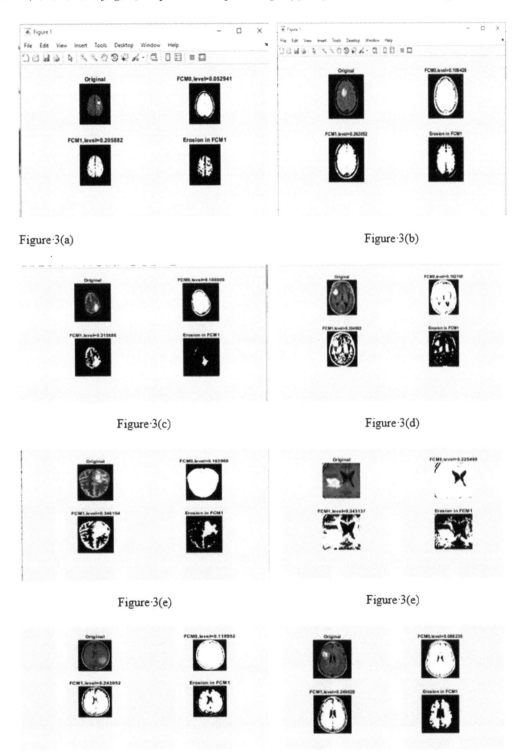

Table 3. Experimental result of multilevel thresholding, FCMMT and FTMLS method of ten distinct MRI image

Input image	Multilevel thresholding	FCMMT	Proposed FTMLS method
Img1	1722	969	922
Img2	1157	1088	924
Img3	490	478	259
Img4	271	226	226
Img5	268	282	260
Img6	2226	2226	1270
Img7	210	190	180
Img8	135	289	289
Img9	175	1113	330
Img10	1806	1002	998

mentation is definitely improved by minimizing the area of tumor more accurately with this proposed method. The output images are shown in the Figure 4 (a, b, c, d).

Alt-text: Figure 4. (a, b, c, d) display the Segmentation results of ten MRI brain image as input, along with the output of multilevel thresholding, FCMMT and proposed method (FTMLS) respectively.

Figure 4. (a, b, c, d): Segmentation results, (a [1-10]) Input image (MRI), (b [1-10]) multilevel thresholding, (c [1-10]) FCMMT, and (d [1-10]) FTMLS

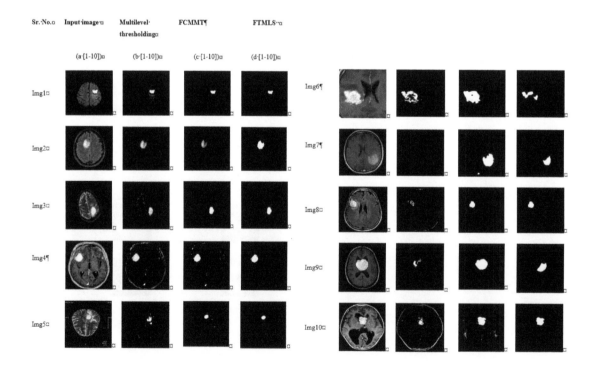

4. CONCLUSION

In today's world, for proper treatment it is very essential to detect the tumor in its early stage. With this proposed algorithm we have presented a new algorithm for medical image segmentation that would be useful for proper orientation of shape and size of brain tumor from MRI brain image. Initial result of image segmentation was obtain with the help of existing algorithm of K-means and FCM algorithm, and it has been observed that FCM algorithm is more suitable for medical image analysis (Khang, 2024b). Then we have used Fuzzy c means thresholding to improve the multilevel thresholding algorithm as a proposed FCMMT algorithm that gives better result compared with existing multilevel thresholding as shown in the Figure 5.

Figure 5. Graphical representation for three methods: MLT, FCMMT, and FTMLS

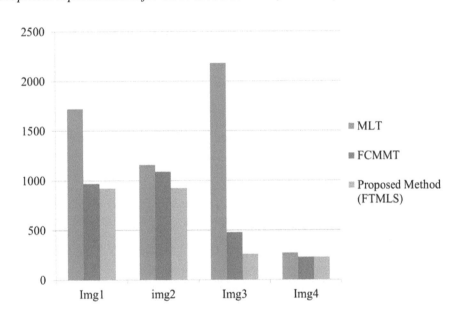

The graphical representations of the segmented values with different methods are also shown in the Figure 5.

Finally the reconstructing with proposed FTMLS method that gives quite satisfactory result that can be understood from the area of segmented results analysis from the Table 4. In this experiment, this proposed method performs better result. This FTMLS algorithm is presented for MRI brain tumor segmentation. It combines the advantages of clustering, multilevel thresholding and level set method, for getting more accurate segmentation results (Khang & Hajimahmud, 2024).

REFERENCES

Aslam, H., Ramashri, T., & Mohammed, I. (2013). A New Approach to Image Segmentation. *International Journal of Advanced Research in Computer and Communication Engineering, 2*(3), 1429-1436.

Bandyopadhyay, S. (2011). Detection of Brain Tumor – A Proposed Method. *Journal of Global Research in Computer Science, 2*(1), 55-63.

BrainTumorInfo. (n.d.). *Info.* Brain Tumor Community.

Dhanalakshmi, P., & Kanimozhi, T. (2013). Automatic Segmentation of Brain Tumor using K-Means Clustering and its Area Calculation. *International Journal of Advanced Electrical and Electronics Engineering*, 130-134.

Isard, A. B. A. M. (1998). *Active Contours.* Springer Verlag.

Islam, M., Hossain, M., & Haque, I. (2021). Mathematical Comparison of Defuzzification of Fuzzy Logic Controller for Intelligence Air Conditioning System. *Int. J. Sci. Res. Math. Stat. Sci., 8*, 29–37.

Javeed Hussain, S., Satya Savitr, T., & Sree Devi, P. (2012). Segmentation of Tissues in Brain MRI Images using Dynamic Neuro – Fuzzy Technique. *International Journal of Soft Computing and Engineering.*

Khang, A. (2023). *AI and IoT-Based Technologies for Precision Medicine* (1st ed.). IGI Global Press. doi:10.4018/979-8-3693-0876-9

Khang, A. (Ed.). (2024a). *AI and IoT Technology and Applications for Smart Healthcare Systems* (1st ed.). Auerbach Publications. doi:10.1201/9781032686745

Khang, A. (2024b). The Era of Digital Healthcare System and Its Impact on Human Psychology. In *AI and IoT Technology and Applications for Smart Healthcare Systems.* Taylor and Francis. doi:10.1201/9781032686745-1

Khang, A. (2024c). *Medical Robotics and AI-Assisted Diagnostics for a High-Tech Healthcare Industry* (1st ed.). IGI Global Press. doi:10.4018/979-8-3693-2105-8

Khang, A., & Abdullayev, V. A. (2023). AI-Aided Data Analytics Tools and Applications for the Healthcare Sector. In AI and IoT-Based Technologies for Precision Medicine (1st ed.). IGI Global Press. doi:10.4018/979-8-3693-0876-9.ch018

Khang, A., & Hajimahmud, V. A. (2024). Cloud Platform and Data Storage Systems in Healthcare Ecosystem. In Medical Robotics and AI-Assisted Diagnostics for a High-Tech Healthcare Industry (1st ed.). IGI Global Press. doi:10.4018/979-8-3693-2105-8.ch022

Khang, A., Rath, K. C., Anh, P. T. N., Rath, S. K., & Bhattacharya, S. (2024). Quantum-Based Robotics in High-Tech Healthcare Industry: Innovations and Applications. In Medical Robotics and AI-Assisted Diagnostics for a High-Tech Healthcare Industry (1st ed.). IGI Global Press. doi:10.4018/979-8-3693-2105-8.ch001

Li, X., Chen, Q., Hao, J.-H., Chen, X., & He, K.-L. (2019). Heat current method for analysis and optimization of a refrigeration system for aircraft environmental control system. *International Journal of Refrigeration, 106*, 163–180. doi:10.1016/j.ijrefrig.2019.06.004

Logswari, T., & Karnan, M. (2010). An improved implementation of brain tumor detection using segmentation based on soft computing. *Journal of Cancer Research and Experimental Oncology, 2*(1), 6-14.

Masood, A. (2013). Fuzzy C Mean Thresholding based Level Set for Automated Segmentation of Skin Lesions. *Journal of Signal and Information Processing, 4*, 66-71. https://www.scirp.org/journal/jsip doi:10.4236/jsip.2013.43B012

Nagalkar, V.J. & Asole, S.S. (2012). Brain tumor detection using digital image processing based on soft computing. *Journal of Signal and Image Processing, 3*(3).

Natarajan, P., Krishnan, N., Kenkre, N. S., Nancy, S., & Singh, B. P. (2012). Tumor detection using threshold operation in MRI brain images. *Computational Intelligence & Computing Research (ICCIC).* IEEE. 10.1109/ICCIC.2012.6510299

Priyanka, B. (2013). A Review on Brain Tumor Detection using segmentation. *International Journal of Computer Science and Mobile Computing, 2*(7).

Rash, B. (2010). The Brain MR Image Segmentation Techniques And Use Of Diagnostic Packages. *Proceedings Of The Academic Radiology, 17*(May).

Rohit, S. (2013). Segmentation of Brain Tumor and Its Area Calculation in Brain MR Images using K – Mean Clustering and Fuzzy C – Mean Algorithm. *International Journal of Computer Science & Engineering Technology, 4*(5).

Singh, P., & Bhadauria, H. S. (2014). Automatic brain MRI image segmentation using FCM and LSM", Reliability, Infocom Technologies and Optimization. *2014 3rd International Conference on.* IEEE.

Suchita, G. (2013). Brain Tumor Detection using Unsupervised Learning based Neural Network. In *International conference on communication system and networking technologies.* IEEE.

Szilagyi, L. (2003). *MR brain image segmentation using an enhanced fuzzy c-means algorithm.* Engineering in Medicine and Biology Society. doi:10.1109/IEMBS.2003.1279866

Withey, D. J., & Koles, Z. J. (2008). A review of medical image segmentation: method and available software. International Journal of Bioelectromagnetism, 10(3).

Zulpe, N. S. (2012). Level set and Thresholding for Brain Tumor Segmentation. *International Journal of Computer and Electrical Engineering, 4*(1).

Chapter 8
Healthcare Performance in Predicting Type 2 Diabetes Using Machine Learning Algorithms

Khushwant Singh

Maharshi Dayanand University, Rohtak, India

Dheerdhwaj Barak

Vaish College of Engineering, Rohtak, India

ABSTRACT

The body's imbalanced glucose consumption caused type 2 diabetes, which in turn caused problems with the immunological, neurological, and circulatory systems. Numerous studies have been conducted to predict this illness using a variety of clinical and pathological criteria. As technology has advanced, several machine learning approaches have also been used for improved prediction accuracy. This study examines the concept of data preparation and examines how it affects machine learning algorithms. Two datasets were built up for the experiment: LS, a locally developed and verified dataset, and PIMA, a dataset from Kaggle. In all, the research evaluates five machine learning algorithms and eight distinct scaling strategies. It has been noted that the accuracy of the PIMA data set ranges from 46.99 to 69.88% when no pre-processing is used, and it may reach 77.92% when scalers are used. Because the LS data set is tiny and regulated, accuracy for the dataset without scalers may be as low as 78.67%. With two labels, accuracy increases to 100%.

1. INTRODUCTION

Diabetic mellitus (DM) is one of the most common non-communicable diseases globally. It is observed that, 46% of people with diabetes are not diagnosed at early stage. By the year of 2040, it is expected that the count may rise to 642 million all over the globe (Diabetes.co, n.d.). India contributes about 49% of world's burden. In Southeast Asia region, out of 88 million people with diabetes, India contributes 77 million people which is expected to increase to 134.2 in 2045 (WHO, n.d.).

DOI: 10.4018/979-8-3693-3679-3.ch008

The number of people with diabetes in India increased from 26·0 million (95% UI 23·4–28·6) in 1990 to 65·0 million (58·7–71·1) in 2016 (Harris et al., 2017). In Maharashtra, overall reported prevalence of diabetes in urban and rural area is 10.9% and 6.5% respectively (WHO, n.d.).

Enormous data and increased complexities have led to rising interest in the use of machine learning (ML) in healthcare. It develops on existing statistical methods and finds patterns in the data. Ml uses different models for prediction of Type 2 diabetes. The accuracy of these models are of prime importance as analysis is directly impacting patient's life (Khang, Rath, Anh et al, 2024). The aim of this research is to design a predictive model for estimation of diabetes in healthy people with diverse age groups based on different life style related factors i.e. stress, food habit, smoking, profession and exercise. The impact of data pre-processing with different scalers on ML model performance is studied methodically to improve decision support systems for physician (Khang, 2024a).

Some of the important pre-processing steps include data cleaning, pruning, feature selection, and scaling. Many researchers considered diverse ML algorithms along with feature selection (Kaur & Kumari, 2018; Lai et al., 2019) few considered the effect of the data scaling process on overall model performance (Srinivas et al., 2010). Thus, the primary purpose of this study is to evaluate the effect of different data scaling methods on different ML algorithms and develop a prediction model for healthy patients with early diabetes symptoms.

In the present study, five machine learning algorithms like - Logistic regression, K Neighbours (KNN), Gaussian Naïve Bias (GNB), Decision Tree (DT) and Random Forest (RF) and 7 data scaling methods like MinMaxScaler, Sandard scalar, RobustScaler, QuantileTransformer (QT), PowerTransformer (PT) and Normalizer are used together to find the best match for type 2 diabetes prediction. The effect of different data scaling techniques is observed using the UCI PIMA India dataset (Pima Indians Diabetes dataset, n.d.) and LS data set (Patil & Shah, 2019) where data is collected through survey in Indian environment.

2. LITERATURE SURVEY

2.1 Survey on Machine Learning Algorithm for Type-2 Diabetes

Contreas et al. (2018) study focuses on all AI techniques for diabetic prediction and management. Study shows an AI is powerful tool applicable for prediction and prevention of complications due to diabetes. AI techniques are being progressively utilized in area of medicine containing complex sets of diagnostic and clinical information. This tool helps in improving quality of patient's life through predictive approach which helps for improving health outcomes (Anh, 2024).

Sneha and Tarun (2019) proposed method for selecting the attributes which will be used in early detection of Diabetes and showed Random forest model and decision tree model has specificity of 98.00% and 98.20%

In Sisodia et al. (2018) designed a system which can prognosticate the likelihood of diabetes in patients by achieving with higher accuracy. Dataset used in this study is PIDD from UCI repository. Experimentation done using weka tool by applying NB, DT and SVM classifier for early detection of diabetes. Model performance measured using accuracy, precision, and recall and F-score. As reported in the paper, NB achieved the best performance results, with a maximum accuracy of 76.3% and highest ROC value of 81.9.

In Mahabub et al. (2019) designed a system which can prognosticate the diabetes by improving an accuracy. Used 11 classifiers as, NB, KNN, SVM, DT, RF, ANN, LR, GB, AdaBoosting etc. on PIMA dataset. Evaluations of all models are examined on various measures like accuracy, precision, F-measure and recall. Ensemble voting classifier developed using 3 best classifiers as SVM, MLP and KNN by applying hyper parameter tuning and cross validation. The proposed ensemble framework gives an accuracy of almost 86%.

Ahmed et al. (2021) designed a system for predicting DM using ML algorithms, namely, DT, KNN, NB, RF, GB, LR, and SVM. Label–encoding and data normalization, are used for improving an accuracy. Two different datasets are used, PIMA and Tigga and Garg. PIMA dataset provides the highest accuracy for SVM and RF with 80.26% and for another dataset, the highest accuracy achieved by DT and RF with 96.81%. Developed a web app. Model is compared with other studies, and the findings reveal that, the suggested model can offer greater accuracy of 2.71% to 13.13%.

2.2 Survey for Application of Different Scalers for Data Pre-Processing for ML Models

There are many data scaling techniques available for ML algorithms and they have different impact on efficacy of the ML model (Ambarwari et al., 2020; Shahriyari, 2019). Study conducted by Ambarwari et al. (2020) showed that data scaling techniques such as minimax normalization and standardization have also significant effects on data analysis (Ambarwari et al., 2020). The study was carried out using ML algorithms such as KNN, Naïve Bayesian, ANN, and SVM with RB. The result discovered that MinMax scaling with SVM performed better than other algorithms (Khang & Hajimahmud, 2024b).

Another study conducted by Balabaeva et al. (2019) addressed the effect of different scaling methods on heart failure patient datasets. Their study uses more robust ML algorithms such as XGB, LR, DT, and RF with scaling methods such as Standard Scaler, MinMax Scaler, Max Abs Scaler, Robust scaler, and Quantile Transformer. In their study, RF showed higher performance with Standard and Robust Scaler (Khang & Abdullayev, 2023).

3. METHODOLOGY

To maintain integrity of research accurate data collection is necessary. To investigate efficacy of machine learning algorithms at the earlier stages of predicting risk of diabetes following datasets were used in this study

- UCI repository diabetes dataset - PIMA Indian diabetes dataset, Self-collected questionnaire based dataset – LS_ diabetes dataset (Pima Indians Diabetes dataset, n.d.).
- Standard Dataset: P dataset is a UCI Repository dataset, consist of 768 records with female centric data. It contains both 268 diabetic instances and 500 non-diabetic instances. Dataset comprises of numeric-valued 8 attributes. Data contain both medical examination data as well as personal health data. Age (age), Body mass index (bmi), Diastolic blood pressure (pres),Number of times pregnant (preg), 2-h serum insulin (insu),Plasma glucose concentration at 2 h in an oral glucose tolerance test (plas), Skin fold thickness (skin), Pedigree function (pedi), Class variable (class)

- LS dataset- Self-collected Questionnaire-based Dataset for the Study (Patil & Shah, 2019). The dataset was developed by web-based questionnaires. LS_diabetes dataset comprising of 374 people with of 35 features the questions were related to demographic information, dietary pattern, life style, pathological and stress related factors as shown in Figure 1.

Figure 1. Features collected through online survey in indian environment for LS dataset

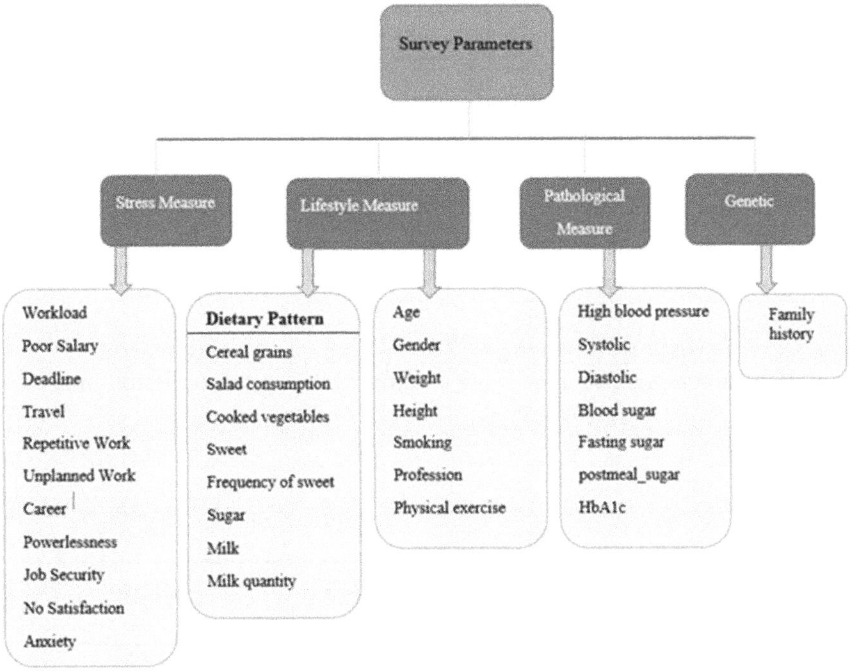

Alt-text: Figure 1 displays the features Collected through Online Survey in Indian Environment for LS Dataset.

4. IMPLEMENTATION

The experiment was carried out by splitting the dataset into 80% and 20% for the training and testing set, respectively. The performance of the model was evaluated using 10-fold cross- validations, and the performance of the model is presented by averaging the outcomes of all 10 folds (Khang, 2023). The results took place using the Anaconda modules with Python 3.7 and were run on an office- grade laptop with common specifications (Windows 11, AMD RYZEN 7 6800H, and 64 GB of RAM). Instead of developing different preprocessing steps, this study uses built-in preprocessing libraries provided by Scikit-learn tools: Normalization, Standardization, MinMax Scale, MaxAbs scale, Robust Scaler, Quantile Transformer (Khang, 2024b).

Following is a process flow where different scalers like Minimax Scaler, Standard Scaler, MaxAbs Scaler Robust Scaler, Quantile Transformer Scaler, Power Transformer Scaler and Normalizer Scale rare applied for data cleaning on both datasets with five diverse ML model like Logistic Regression, KNN, NB, DT and RF for predicting the type 2 diabetes.

Alt-text: Figure 2 shown the process of Comparing Performance of ML Model with the Influence of Scalers as a Part of Preprocessing Stage

Figure 2. Shows the process flow of the experiment

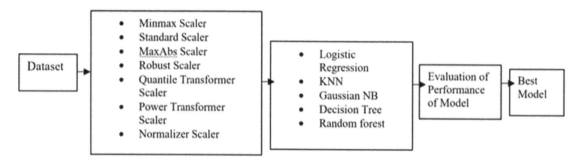

The Performance parameters of the model are calculated based on confusion matrix (Visa, 2011) as shown in Figure 3.

Figure 3. Confusion matrix

		Predicted·Class¤	
	Total·Population¤	Positive·Prediction¤	Negative·Prediction¤
ActualClass¤	Diabetes¤	True·Positive·(TP)¤	False·Negative·(FN)¤
	Non-diabetes¤	False·Positive·(FP)¤	True·Negative·(TN)¤

The performance was evaluated based on accuracy, precision, recall, and F1 score. The matrix outcomes are as follows:

- True positive (Tp) – TP denote the number of patients having diabetes and are predicted as diabetes individuals.
- False positive (Fp) –FP denote the number of patients having diabetes and are predicted as healthy individuals.
- True negative (Tn) –TN denote the number of patients not having diabetes and are predicted as healthy individuals.

- False negative (Fn) –FN denote the number of patients not having diabetes and are predicted as diabetes individuals.
- The Accuracy, Precision and recall are defined as follows

$Accuracy = Tp + Tn$

$Tn + Tp + Fp + Fn$

$Precision = Tp$

$Tp + Fp$

$Recall/Sensitivity = Tp$

$Tp + Fn$

Characteristics of Different Scalers used for Preprocessing are

- MinMax Scaler: It just scales all the data between 0 and 1.

x_scaled = (x – x_min)/(x_max – x_min)

- Standard Scaler- Z score

For each feature, the Standard Scaler scales the values such that the mean is 0 and the standard deviation is 1.

x_ scaled = x – mean/std_dev

- the MaxAbs scaler takes the absolute maximum value of each column and divides each value in the column by the maximum value. Range [-1,1]
- Robust Scaler is not sensitive to outliers

It removes the median from the data and scales the data by the InterQuartile Range(IQR)

- Q1= First half of data and its median
- Q2= Actual median
- Q3= Second half of data and its median IQR = Q3 – Q1

x_scaled = (x – Q1)/(Q3 – Q1)

- Quantile Transformer Scaler is best to use this for non-linear data.

- The Power Transformer actually automates this decision making by introducing a parameter called lambda. It decides on a generalized power transform by finding the best value of lambda
- Normalizer: If we are using L1 norm, the values in each column are converted so that the sum of their absolute values along the row = 1

5. RESULTS AND DISCUSSION

The experiments were carried out on both datasets PIMA and LS with 80% training and 20% testing data. Following Table 1 to 5 shows the performance of PIMA dataset.

It is observed that data cleaning and pre-processing with different scalers have remarkable impact on the accuracy of the ML models in PIMA dataset. In Logistic Regression model efficiency improved by 39.69% with standard and robust scaler. In KNN Minmax scaler performed better than all other scalers and improve efficiency by 9.1%. In GNB the accuracy is improved by 35.5% and QT scaler performs better than other scalers. In DT the MaxAbs scaler performs better with improvement in efficiency by 18.89% and in RF the efficacy improvement is 39.49% with Robust scaler performing better. The performance in different ML model is based on data base characteristics and spread of data in features. Table 6 to 10 shows the performance of LS data set with respect to various scalers and different ML models.

Table 1. Logistic regression model is applied with various scalers in data preprocessing stage PIMA data set

Sr No.	Scaler Name	F1 Score	Precision	Recall	Accuracy (%)
1	No Scaler	0.45	0.47	0.43	46.99
2	Minmaxscaler	0.83	0.77	0.90	76.19
3	Sandard Scalar	0.84	0.80	0.88	77.92
4	Maxabsscaler	0.83	0.77	0.90	76.19
5	Robustscaler	0.84	0.80	0.88	77.92
6	Quantiletransformer	0.83	0.80	0.87	77.76
7	Powertransformer	0.82	0.79	0.85	75.76

Table 2. KNN Model is applied with various scalers in data preprocessing stage PIMA data **Set**

Sr No.	Scaler Name	F1 Score	Precision	Recall	Accuracy (%)
1	No scaler	0.68	0.73	0.63	69.88
2	MinMaxScaler	0.82	0.8	0.85	76.19
3	Sandard scalar	0.8	0.75	0.86	72.29
4	MaxAbsScaler	0.81	0.76	0.87	74.09
5	RobustScaler	0.8	0.76	0.85	72.73
6	QuantileTransformer	0.8	0.77	0.85	73.16
7	PowerTransformer	0.85	0.75	0.88	73.59

Table 3. GNB model is applied with various scalers in data pre-processing stage PIMA data Set

Sr No.	Scaler Name	F1 Score	Precision	Recall	Accuracy (%)
1.	No scaler	0.49	0.49	0.48	49.4
2.	MinMaxScaler	0.82	0.79	0.85	75.76
3.	Sandard scalar	0.82	0.79	0.85	75.76
4.	MaxAbsScaler	0.82	0.79	0.85	75.76
5.	RobustScaler	0.82	0.79	0.85	75.76
6.	QuantileTransformer	0.82	0.81	0.83	76.62
7.	PowerTransformer	0.82	0.81	0.83	76.62

Table 4. DT model is applied with various scalers in data preprocessing stage PIMA data Set

Sr No.	Scaler Name	F1 Score	Precision	Recall	Accuracy (%)
1.	No scaler	0.55	0.58	0.53	57.23
2.	MinMaxScaler	0.76	0.75	0.76	68.04
3.	Sandard scalar	0.76	0.75	0.77	68.83
4.	MaxAbsScaler	0.78	0.76	0.81	70.56
5.	RobustScaler	0.76	0.74	0.77	67.97
6.	QuantileTransformer	0.76	0.75	0.77	68.04
7.	PowerTransformer	0.78	0.76	0.76	70.56

Table 5. RF Model is applied with various scalers in data preprocessing stage PIMA data set

Sr No.	Scaler name	F1 score	Precision	Recall	Accuracy (%)
1.	No scaler	0.45	0.47	0.43	46.99
2.	MinMaxScaler	0.61	0.78	0.85	74.8
3.	Sandard scalar	0.62	0.79	0.84	74.89
4.	MaxAbsScaler	0.82	0.77	0.87	74.89
5.	RobustScaler	0.83	0.81	0.85	77.66
6.	QuantileTransformer	0.82	0.79	0.86	75.76
7.	PowerTransformer	0.81	0.78	0.84	74.46

It is observed that data cleaning and preprocessing with different scalers have remarkable impact on the accuracy of the ML models in LS dataset. In Logistic Regression model efficiency improved by 14.67%, in KNN accuracy improves by 21.33%, In GNB efficiency improves by 16%, in DT accuracy improves by 8% and RF accuracy improves by 6.66%. The variations in accuracy through different scalers is less in LS dataset as its controlled dataset collected by researchers so missing values are very less compared to PIMA dataset.

Table 6. Logistic regression model is applied with various scalers in data preprocessing stage LS data set

Sr No.	Scaler name	F1 score	Precision	Recall	Accuracy (%)
1.	No scaler	0.59	0.8	0.47	85.33
2.	MinMaxScaler	1	1	1	99.87
3.	Sandard scalar	1	1	1	100
4.	MaxAbsScaler	1	1	1	100
5.	RobustScaler	1	1	1	100
6.	QuantileTransformer	1	1	1	98.92
7.	PowerTransformer	1	1	1	100

Table 7. KNN model is applied with various scalers in data preprocessing stage LS data Set

Sr No.	Scaler name	F1 score	Precisionn	Recall	Accuracy (%)
1.	No scaler	0.43	0.55	0.35	78.67
2.	MinMaxScaler	1	1	1	100
3.	Sandard scalar	1	1	1	100
4.	MaxAbsScaler	1	1	1	100
	RobustScaler	1	1	1	100
5.	QuantileTransformer	1	1	1	100
6.	PowerTransformer	1	1	1	100

Table 8. GNB model is applied with various scalers in data preprocessing stage LS data Set

Sl. No.	Scaler Name	F1 Score	Precision	Recall	Accuracy (%)
1.	No Scaler	0.71	0.60	0.88	84.0
2.	Minmaxscaler	1	1	1	100
3.	Sandard Scalar	1	1	1	100
4.	Maxabsscaler	1	1	1	98.99
5.	Robustscaler	1	1	1	100
6.	Quantiletransformer	1	1	1	99.98
7.	Powertransformer	1	1	1	100

6. CONCLUSION

As the stress and lifestyle parameters of individual are changing very rapidly towards negative curve the occurrences of diabetes at early age are expected in India and across the globe. For predicting the disease accurately at early stage, the experiment is done with Two datasets PIMA standard dataset and LS locally generated dataset. It is observed that data cleaning methods have high level of impact on accuracy of prediction in all models. Without scalar the accuracy of PIMA data set is from 46.99 to 69.88%, which

Table 9. DT Model is applied with various scalers in data preprocessing stage LS data Set

Sl. No.	Scaler name	F1 score	Precision	Recall	Accuracy (%)
1.	No scaler	0.81	0.87	0.76	92.0
2.	MinMaxScaler	1	1	1	99.8
3.	Sandard scalar	1	1	1	100
4.	MaxAbsScaler	1	1	1	100
5.	RobustScaler	1	1	1	100
6.	QuantileTransformer	1	1	1	100
7.	PowerTransformer	1	1	1	99.46

Table 10. RF Model is applied with various scalers in data preprocessing stage LS data Set

Sl. No.	Scaler name	F1 score	Precision	Recall	Accuracy (%)
1.	No scaler	0.83	1	0.71	93.33
2.	MinMaxScaler	1	1	1	100
3.	Sandard scalar	1	1	1	100
4.	MaxAbsScaler	1	1	1	100
5.	RobustScaler	1	1	1	100
6.	QuantileTransformer	1	1	1	100
7.	PowerTransformer	1	1	1	100

improves with scalers up to 77.92%. For LS dataset without scalers accuracy is as low as 78.67 which improves to 100% with two labels as the LS data set is small and controlled.

It is concluded that scaler have observable impact on the ML model prediction efficiency and as per the data spread if appropriate scaler is selected the accuracy of predication can be surely improving. Future work: The data scaling methods can be applied to other datasets in health care domain to improve the accuracy of prediction of decease to help mankind (Khang, 2024c).

REFERENCES

Ahmeda, N., Ahammeda, R., Islama, M., & Uddina, A. (2021). Machine learning based diabetes prediction and development of smart web application. *International Journal of Cognitive Computing in Engineering*, 2, 229–241. doi:10.1016/j.ijcce.2021.12.001

Ambarwari, A., Adrian, Q.J., & Herdiyeni, Y. (2020). Analysis of the Effect of Data Scaling on the Performance of the Machine Learning Algorithm for Plant Identification. *J. Resti (Rekayasa Sist. Dan Teknol. Inf.), 4*, 117–122.

Anh, P. T. N. (2024). *AI Models for Disease Diagnosis and Prediction of Heart Disease with Artificial Neural Networks. In Computer Vision and AI-integrated IoT Technologies in Medical Ecosystem* (1st ed.). CRC Press. doi:10.1201/9781003429609-9

Balabaeva, K., & Kovalchuk, S. (2019). Comparison of Temporal and Non-Temporal Features Effect on Machine Learning Models Quality and Interpretability for Chronic Heart Failure Patients. *Procedia Computer Science, 156,* 87–96. doi:10.1016/j.procs.2019.08.183

Contreas, I., & Vehi, J. (2018). Artificial intelligence for diabetes management and decision support: Literature review. *Journal of Medical Internet Research, 20*(5), e10775. doi:10.2196/10775 PMID:29848472

Diabetes.co. (n.d.). *Welcome!* Diabetes.co.uk. https://www.diabetes.co.uk/

Harris, M.L., Oldmeadow, C., Hure, A., Luu, J., Loxton, D., & Attia, J. (2017). Stress increases the risk of type 2 diabetes onset in women: A 12-year longitudinal study using causal modelling. *PLoS One, 12*(2), e0172126. doi:.pone.0172126 doi:10.1371/journal

Kaur, H., & Kumari, V. (2018). Predictive Modelling and analytics for diabetes using a machine learning approach. *Applied Computing and Informatics, 12*(1/2), 90–100. doi:10.1016/j.aci.2018.12.004

Khang, A. (2023). *AI and IoT-Based Technologies for Precision Medicine* (1st ed.). IGI Global Press. doi:10.4018/979-8-3693-0876-9

Khang, A. (2024a). *Medical Robotics and AI-Assisted Diagnostics for a High-Tech Healthcare Industry* (1st ed.). IGI Global Press. doi:10.4018/979-8-3693-2105-8

Khang, A. (2024b). Using Big Data to Solve Problems in the Field of Medicine. In Computer Vision and AI-integrated IoT Technologies in Medical Ecosystem (1st ed.). CRC Press. doi:10.1201/9781003429609-21

Khang, A. (2024c). Medical and BioMedical Signal Processing and Prediction. In Computer Vision and AI-integrated IoT Technologies in Medical Ecosystem (1st ed.). CRC Press. doi:10.1201/9781003429609-7

Khang, A., Abdullayev, V., Hrybiuk, O., & Shukla, A. K. (2024). *Computer Vision and AI-Integrated IoT Technologies in the Medical Ecosystem* (1st ed.). CRC Press. doi:10.1201/9781003429609

Khang, A., & Abdullayev, V. A. (2023). AI-Aided Data Analytics Tools and Applications for the Healthcare Sector. In AI and IoT-Based Technologies for Precision Medicine (1st ed.). IGI Global Press. doi:10.4018/979-8-3693-0876-9.ch018

Khang, A., & Hajimahmud, V. A. (2024a). Cloud Platform and Data Storage Systems in Healthcare Ecosystem. Medical Robotics and AI-Assisted Diagnostics for a High-Tech Healthcare Industry (1st ed.). IGI Global Press. doi:10.4018/979-8-3693-2105-8.ch022

Khang, A., & Hajimahmud, V. A. (2024b). *Application of Computer Vision in the Healthcare Ecosystem. Computer Vision and AI-integrated IoT Technologies in Medical Ecosystem* (1st ed.). CRC Press. doi:10.1201/9781003429609-1

Khang, A., Rath, K. C., Anh, P. T. N., Rath, S. K., & Bhattacharya, S. (2024). Quantum-Based Robotics in High-Tech Healthcare Industry: Innovations and Applications. Medical Robotics and AI-Assisted Diagnostics for a High-Tech Healthcare Industry (1st ed.). IGI Global Press. doi:10.4018/979-8-3693-2105-8.ch001

Lai, H., Huang, H., Keshavjee, K., Guergachi, A., & Gao, X. (2019). Predictive models for diabetes mellitus using machine learning techniques. *BMC Endocrine Disorders*, *19*(1), 1–9. doi:10.1186/s12902-019-0436-6 PMID:31615566

Mahabub, A. (2019). A robust voting approach for diabetes prediction using traditional machine learning techniques. *SN Applied Sciences*, *1*(12), 1667. doi:10.1007/s42452-019-1759-7

Patil, P., & Shah, L. (2019). Assessment of risk of type 2 diabetes mellitus with stress as a risk factor using classification algorithms. *International Journal of Recent Technology and Engineering*, *8*(4), 11273–11277. doi:10.35940/ijrte.D9509.118419

Shahriyari, L. (2019). Effect of normalization methods on the performance of supervised learning algorithms applied to HTSeq-FPKM-UQ data sets: 7SK RNA expression as a predictor of survival in patients with colon adenocarcinoma. *Briefings in Bioinformatics*, *20*(3), 985–994. doi:10.1093/bib/bbx153 PMID:29112707

Sisodia, D., & Sisodia, D. (2018). Prediction of diabetes using classification algorithms. *Procedia Computer Science*, *132*, 1578–1585. doi:10.1016/j.procs.2018.05.122

Sneha, N., & Gangil, T. (2019). Analysis of diabetes mellitus for early prediction using optimal features selection. *Journal of Big Data*, *6*(1), 13. doi:10.1186/s40537-019-0175-6

Srinivas, K., Rani, B. K., & Govrdhan, A. (2010). Applications of data mining techniques in healthcare and prediction of heart attacks. *International Journal on Computer Science and Engineering*, *2*, 250–255.

Pima Indians Diabetes dataset. (n.d.). UC Irving. http://archive.ics.uci.edu/ml/machine learning-databases/pima-indiansdiabetes/pima-indians-diabetes

Visa, S. (2011). *Confusion Matrix-based Feature Selection*. Conference: Proceedings of the 22nd Midwest Artificial Intelligence and Cognitive Science Conference 2011, Cincinnati, OH, USA.

WHO. (n.d.). *Diabetes Fact Sheet*. WHO. https://www.who.int/en/news-room/fact-sheets/detail/diabetes

Chapter 9
Leveraging Deep Learning for Early Diagnosis of Alzheimer's Using Comparative Analysis of Convolutional Neural Network Techniques

Namria Ishaaq

(iD) https://orcid.org/0009-0009-9239-4986

Jamia Hamdard, India

Md Tabrez Nafis

(iD) https://orcid.org/0000-0002-3395-8448

Jamia Hamdard, India

Anam Reyaz

Jamia Hamdard, India

ABSTRACT

Alzheimer's disease, a debilitating neurodegenerative condition, poses a formidable challenge in healthcare, necessitating early and precise detection for effective intervention. This study delves into the realm of Alzheimer's detection, leveraging the prowess of deep learning. A novel convolutional neural network (CNN) model is proposed for AD detection. This model achieves a remarkable accuracy of 99.99% on the test dataset, outperforming established pre-trained models like ResNet50, DenseNet201, and VGG16. The outcomes distinctly highlight the CNN model's superior precision in AD identification, marking a watershed moment in neurodegenerative disease detection. The findings of this research have important implications for the development of a more accurate and sensitive diagnostic tool, which could lead to significant advancements in the early diagnosis and treatment of Alzheimer's disease. This research not only presents a novel diagnostic approach for AD but also demonstrates its resilience and potential for accurate classification of early Alzheimer's disease diagnosis.

DOI: 10.4018/979-8-3693-3679-3.ch009

1. INTRODUCTION

Alzheimer's disease is a progressive neurodegenerative disorder that causes progressive cognitive decline, memory loss, and reduced everyday functioning. It is currently more dreaded than cancer and is the fourth leading cause of mortality worldwide (Raees & Thomas, 2021; Zhang et al., 2019). Alzheimer's disease represents a profound and pressing challenge within the healthcare landscape. This relentless neurodegenerative disorder robs individuals of their cognitive abilities, disrupts the lives of their families, and exerts a substantial socioeconomic burden on society. People with AD may have trouble speaking, solving problems, and short-term memory as the condition worsens. They may also become withdrawn and irritable. AD can eventually lead to a complete loss of independence and death (Zeng et al., 2017).

Early detection and precise prediction of Alzheimer's have emerged as critical objectives in the quest to mitigate its devastating impact. In this context, the convergence of advanced data analytics and healthcare offers a beacon of hope, and this research paper seeks to illuminate the transformative role of machine learning in Alzheimer's prediction and its broader implications for the healthcare domain (Al-Shoukry, Rassem, & Makbol, 2020; Al-Shoukry, Rassem, & Makbol, 2020).

The urgency of effective Alzheimer's prediction is underscored by the soaring prevalence of the disease, which affects millions globally, and the projected exponential growth as population's age. Machine learning, a subfield of artificial intelligence, has emerged as a powerful instrument capable of gleaning invaluable insights from vast and complex healthcare datasets. Its ability to identify subtle patterns, draw meaningful correlations, and generate predictive models has propelled it to the forefront of Alzheimer's research (Altinkaya et al., 2020).

In this era of rapid technological advancement, the fusion of healthcare and artificial intelligence has provided unprecedented opportunities for the development of innovative diagnostic tools (Puente-Castro et al., 2020). A branch of artificial intelligence called machine learning has shown to be a potent ally in the fight to identify Alzheimer's early on. By harnessing the potential of diverse data sources, including neuroimaging, genetic markers, and clinical data, machine learning algorithms have demonstrated the ability to discern subtle patterns and associations that elude human perception (Feng et al., 2019; Ghazal, 2022). These advances hold the promise of more accurate, non-invasive, and cost-effective diagnostic methods (Khang, Abdullayev, Hrybiuk et al, 2024).

In order to forecast Alzheimer's disease, this study conducts a thorough investigation of machine learning, shedding light on the technology's promise as well as its limitations with regard to influencing healthcare in the future. The study focuses on Alzheimer's disease diagnosis using recent machine learning methods such as Convolutional Neural Networks (CNNs) and transfer learning techniques (Khang & Hajimahmud, 2024).

A pivotal revelation in this study is the proposition of a CNN model, demonstrating accuracy on par with, if not surpassing, established models like DenseNet201, VGG16 and ResNet50. This finding signifies the CNN model's competence in accurate Alzheimer's disease prediction, potentially offering a more robust alternative for diagnosis. Concurrently, the study addresses prevalent challenges, including the ethical imperative of generalizability across diverse populations, charting a course for future research and clinical application. This paper's insights not only emphasize the significance of the CNN model in healthcare but also define the trajectory for enhanced diagnostic precision in Alzheimer's disease detection.

2. LITERATURE REVIEW

In recent years, deep learning techniques have been widely used for the diagnosis of and they have shown high accuracy rates in disease diagnosis from Brain MRI images. A thorough analysis of the application of deep learning methods for the identification of Alzheimer's and dementia disorders using MRI images was conducted by Helaly et al. It highlights the importance of early detection and appropriate treatment for these diseases. It provides insights into the advancements in biomedical imaging for patient care and the study of biological structure and function (Helaly et al., 2022).

3D-CNN and FSBi-LSTM are two methods that the Deep Learning Framework can utilize to diagnose Alzheimer's disease. The framework utilizes a combination of 3D-CNN and FSBi-LSTM to extract deep feature representation from MRI and PET data, improving the performance of AD diagnosis this study was proposed by Feng et al. (2019) which highlights the successful application of the deep learning framework in accurately diagnosing AD and its prodromal states using MRI and PET data.

Deep learning has grown in popularity for detecting Alzheimer's disease since 2013, with a boom in published articles in this subject since 2017. In terms of accuracy, deep learning models have been demonstrated to surpass classic machine learning methods. Ebrahimighahnavieh et al. (2020) conducted a review of the useful biomarkers and features utilized for Alzheimer's disease identification, such as personal information, genetic data, and brain scans. It also covers the essential pre-processing stages as well as the various ways for dealing with neuroimaging data from single-modality and multi-modality investigations (Khang, Rath, Anh et al, 2024).

The CNN model architecture provided by Ebrahim et al produced promising results in terms of train loss, validation loss, train accuracy, and validation accuracy at each training session. The study also evaluates the accuracy of several CNN models, such as GoogLeNet and ResNet, in classifying Alzheimer's disease using MRI images. The highest accuracy achieved was 98.88% by GoogLeNet, while ResNet-18 and ResNet-152 achieved accuracies of 98.01% and 98.14% respectively (Ebrahim et al., 2020).

The use of structural MRIs, which are more accessible and cost-effective compared to PET imaging techniques, makes the proposed approach more feasible for widespread clinical use. Bi et al. (2020) created a deep learning model that achieved an area-under-the-curve (AUC) of 85.12 when differentiating between cognitive normal people and subjects with mild cognitive impairment (MCI) or mild Alzheimer's disease.

Jo et colleagues examined 16 research that employed deep learning techniques and neuroimaging data to diagnose and predict the progression from moderate cognitive impairment (MCI) to Alzheimer's disease (AD). Accuracy of up to 98.8% for AD classification and 83.7% for MCI to AD conversion prediction was achieved using a combination of standard machine learning and stacked auto-encoder (SAE). Deep learning techniques, such as convolutional neural network (CNN) or recurrent neural network (RNN), demonstrated accuracies of up to 96.0% for AD classification and 84.2% for MCI conversion prediction without pre-processing (Jo et al., 2019).

A unique approach to data interpretation is presented by Venugopalan et al. (2021); it uses perturbation analysis and clustering to identify the best-performing features that the deep models have learned. Imaging models based on 3D convolutional neural networks (CNNs) perform better than shallow models and obtain the highest mean F1 scores and precision when applied to MRI images. An example of how deep learning works well for processing imaging data is the analysis of Alzheimer's illness that comes from using a 3D convolutional neural network architecture to MRI image data.

Feng et al. (2020) suggested a method that uses Transfer Learning (TL) approaches to automatically identify Alzheimer's disease (AD) in sagittal magnetic resonance imaging (MRI). According to the results obtained with DL models employing sagittal MRIs, sagittal-plane MRIs can be just as useful as other planes in diagnosing AD in its early stages as horizontal-plane MRIs.

A deep learning method based on retinal photos was proposed by Cheung et al. (2022) and demonstrated good accuracy in identifying Alzheimer's disease, with an area under the receiver operating characteristic curve (AUROC) of 0.93 and an internal validation accuracy of 83.6%. With accuracy ranging from 79.6% to 92.1% and AUROCs ranging from 0.73 to 0.91, it also fared well in testing datasets.

Laura Mccrakin did a study that introduces a 3D multichannel CNN for predicting symptomatic Alzheimer's using dMRI data. The model was extended to incorporate longitudinal scans, enhancing accuracy and prognosis. Despite a small dataset, data augmentation methods enhance robustness. The approach marks a promising step towards early Alzheimer's prediction through advanced computational methods (Bagheri et al., 2018).

A study by Trambaiolli et al. used quantitative EEG (qEEG) processing and Support Vector Machine (SVM) to distinguish AD patients from controls. The analysis of EEG epochs yielded a sensitivity of 83.2% and an accuracy of 79.9%. The analysis considering the diagnosis of each individual patient reached an accuracy of 87.0% and sensitivity of 91.7% (Trambaiolli et al., 2011).

A study by Petersen et al. with 819 participants included people with moderate cognitive impairment (MCI), people with Alzheimer's disease (AD), and cognitively normal people. The researchers found that the memory impairment levels of the MCI subjects were in between those of the normal and AD groups. The 12-month progression rate to dementia for MCI was 16.5% per year, consistent with predictions. Baseline cerebrospinal fluid (CSF) measures effectively distinguished the three groups and accurately predicted 12-month cognitive changes. The Alzheimer's Disease Neuroimaging Initiative successfully recruited and characterized these cohorts, providing valuable insights into cognitive decline and progression (Petersen et al., 2010).

3. DATA PRE-PROCESSING

In preparing our model to detect Alzheimer's disease, we took a crucial step in organizing our dataset. We divided our dataset into three essential parts: training, testing, and validation. This separation allows our model to learn from one portion, test its skills on another, and validate its understanding on a third. The data split occurred with an 80-10-10 ratio, meaning 80% for training, 10% for testing, and 10% for validation. This division ensures our model gets a good mix of examples to learn from and then challenges it with new, unseen cases (Khang & Abdullayev, 2023).

Our dataset includes 6400 MRI images separated into four classes indicating distinct phases of dementia: Mild Demented, Moderate Demented, Non-Demented, and Very Mild Demented. After this split, we loaded the data into our model using TensorFlow, a powerful tool for handling such information. The TensorFlow tool helped us organize the images into batches, making it easier for our model to process them.

Additionally, we made sure all the images were of the same size, 224x224 pixels, allowing our model to 'see' each image in a consistent way. This standardization helps the model focus on the important details without getting distracted by differences in image sizes. We used a technique called one-hot encoding for the labels, which essentially provides a clear way for our model to understand the different classes

Figure 1. Flowchart representation for the proposed framework

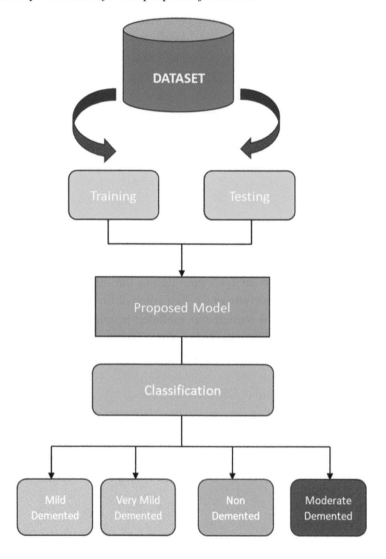

of dementia. The training set contained 5119 images, the test set had 642 images, and the validation set held 639 images, each file representing a real-world example our model learns from.

To ensure consistency in our work, we used specific seed values (123 and 1345). These seeds act like a fingerprint, ensuring that every time we run our code, the data is split in the same way. This consistency is essential for research as it allows us to compare results accurately and make sure our model is learning and improving. This process not only organized our dataset but also set the stage for our model's training, testing, and evaluation, laying a strong foundation for our journey in Alzheimer's disease detection.

Several other steps were also performed in this stage of model development like data augmentation techniques are applied such as the images are rescaled, calculated class weights to address imbalanced datasets, rotated, zoomed, flipped horizontally and vertically, and split. This dataset was divided into four categories: mild demented, very mild demented, non-demented, and moderate demented. After applying these pre-processing steps, the dataset was available for further processing (Khang, 2024).

4. DATASET

The training process consisted of 50 epochs, which signifies 50 complete iterations through the entire dataset. This number was chosen to allow the model to converge and learn patterns in the data and a batch size of 64 was used meaning the training dataset was divided into batches of 64 images, and the model's weights were updated after processing each batch. The dataset had 6,400 photos that were divided into four categories: Mild Demented, Very Mild Demented, Non-Demented, and Moderate Demented. These classes indicate various stages of Alzheimer's disease. The number of photos for each class is 896,64, 3200, and 2240 for Mild Demented, Very Mild Demented, Non-Demented, and Moderate Demented, respectively.

Figure 2. Number of images for each class

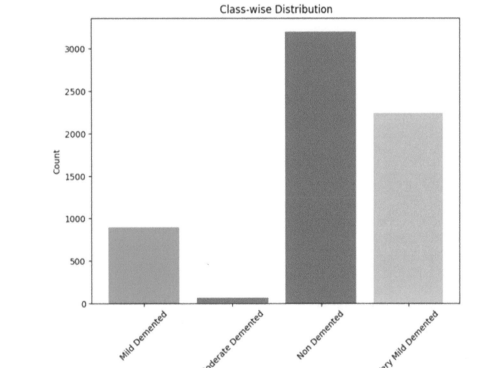

5. PROPOSED CNN MODEL

Our proposed model employs a sequential structure of layers, optimized for discerning intricate patterns within medical images related to different stages of Alzheimer's disease. The architectural specifics include:

- Image Pre-processing: The initial layer of our model encompasses a Rescaling function, standardizing pixel values within the images to a normalized range (1/255). This step optimizes computational efficiency and ensures uniformity in input data.

- Convolutional Layers: Subsequent to rescaling, a series of convolutional layers, each with 16, 32, and 64 filters respectively, operate on image data resized to 224x224 pixels. These layers are equipped with the ReLU activation function and he normal weight initialization. Their role is to identify and extract intricate features crucial for discerning different stages of Alzheimer's.

- ReLU activation function: $ReLU(x)=\max(0,x)$. This function sets all negative values to zero and leaves positive values unchanged. The derivative of ReLU is 0 for all negative values and 1 for all positive values.

- Pooling Layers: Following each convolutional stage, MaxPooling2D layers with a pool size of (2, 2) effectively condense the information, summarizing the identified features and retaining vital image details, contributing to computational efficiency.

- Dropout Layers: Strategically positioned, Dropout layers (rate 0.25) help prevent overfitting by intermittently deactivating a fraction of neurons during training, ensuring the model's adaptability and preventing dependence on specific image attributes.

- Fully Connected Layers: Transitioning to the densely connected layers, a Flatten layer prepares the feature-extracted data for subsequent analysis. The Dense layers with 128 and 32 neurons and ReLU activation provide a more intricate analysis of the abstracted features, enabling the model to comprehend complex patterns within the images.

- Output Layer: The final layer, utilizing a softmax activation function, yields a probability distribution across the four distinct classes, enabling precise classification of different Alzheimer's stages based on the standardized 224x224 pixel images. Softmax activation function:

$$Softmax\left(x_i\right)=\frac{e^{x_i}}{\sum_{j=1}^{N}e^{x_j}}$$

Here, for a vector of N elements, it exponentiates each element and normalizes it by the sum of all exponentiated values, providing a probability distribution over the N classes.

6. PERFORMANCE EVALUATION

When evaluating Alzheimer's disease (AD) classification, the confusion matrix is pivotal. It helps us understand how well the model is performing in identifying AD and non-AD cases. (Table.2).It comprises four components: true positives (properly recognized positive cases), true negatives (correctly identified negative cases), false positives (incorrectly identified as positive), and false negatives (incorrectly identified as negative).Four more classifiers were employed in our model evaluation.

Accuracy measures the overall correctness of the model's predictions. It signifies the ratio of correctly identified cases (both AD and non-AD) to the total instances.

$$Accuracy=\frac{TP+TN}{TP+FP+FN+TN}\times100\%$$

Table 1. CNN model architecture used for AD diagnosis

Layer (type)	Output Shape	Param #
rescaling (Rescaling)	(None, 224, 224, 3)	0
conv2d (Conv2D)	(None, 224, 224, 16)	448
max_pooling2d (MaxPooling2D)	(None, 112, 112, 16)	0
conv2d_1 (Conv2D)	(None, 112, 112, 32)	4640
max_pooling2d_1 (MaxPooling2D)	(None, 56, 56, 32)	0
dropout (Dropout)	(None, 56, 56, 32)	0
conv2d_2 (Conv2D)	(None, 56, 56, 64)	18496
max_pooling2d_2 (MaxPooling2D)	(None, 28, 28, 64)	0
dropout_1 (Dropout)	(None, 28, 28, 64)	0
flatten (Flatten)	(None, 50176)	0
dense (Dense)	(None, 128)	6422656
dense_1 (Dense)	(None, 32)	4128
dense_2 (Dense)	(None, 4)	132

Total params: 6450500 (24.61 MB)
Trainable params: 6450500 (24.61 MB)
Non-trainable params: 0 (0.00 Byte)

Precision in AD detection refers to the accuracy of the model's positive predictions, specifically its ability to correctly identify AD cases among all predicted AD cases. High precision signifies fewer false positives, which is crucial in AD detection as misdiagnosing a non-AD case as AD can have significant consequences for the patient.

$$Precision = \frac{TP}{TP + FP} \times 100\%$$

Recall quantifies the proportion of accurately recognized AD cases to the total number of real AD cases. High recall implies that the model effectively captures a higher proportion of AD cases, reducing the chances of missing an actual AD diagnosis.

$$Recall = \frac{TP}{TP + FN} \times 100\%$$

The F1 score, which is derived from the harmonic mean of precision and recall, offers a fair evaluation of the model's effectiveness in AD detection. It's particularly valuable when there's an imbalance between AD and non-AD cases. A high F1 score indicates a balance between precision and recall, ensuring both accurate identification of AD cases and a reduced likelihood of missing actual AD cases.

$$F1\ score = 2 \times \frac{Precision \times Recall}{Precision + Recall} \times 100\%$$

7. RESULTS AND DISCUSSION

A comparison study was conducted as part of the research to highlight how well the suggested CNN model classified MRI brain images associated with Alzheimer's disease. Table 2 provides a comprehensive comparison, clearly indicating that our model outperforms previous classification methods, achieving the highest accuracy rate. The classification task involves categorizing MRI brain images into subtypes such as Mild Demented, Moderate Demented, Non-Demented, and Very Mild Demented (Figure 6).

Figure 3. Training and validation loss against the number of epochs for (a) proposed model (b) DenseNet121 (c) Resnet50 (d) VGG 16 prediction models

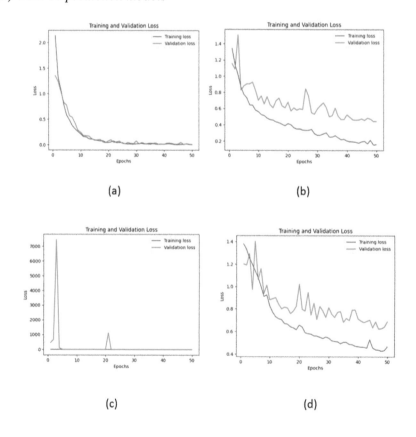

Figure 4. Training and validation accuracy against the number of epochs for (a) proposed model (b) DenseNet121 (c) Resnet50 (d) VGG 16 prediction models

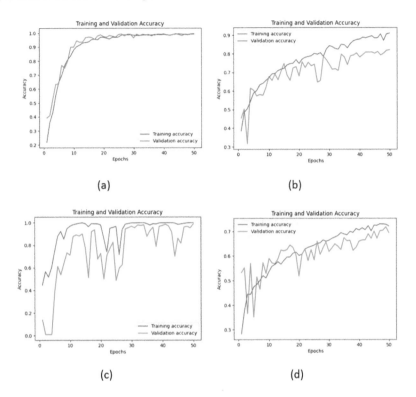

Moreover, the study juxtaposed our model with other CNNs utilizing transfer learning models, specifically VGG16, ResNet50, and DenseNet201 architectures. These networks, pretrained on the ImageNet dataset, were used as baselines for comparison. This comparison investigation highlights the higher performance and efficacy of our proposed CNN model over existing models that use transfer learning in correctly categorizing MRI brain images associated with Alzheimer's disease.

The figure presents a visual comparison between the original MRI brain images and their respective predicted counterparts generated by our CNN model. The comparison offers a compelling visualization of the CNN model's effectiveness in Alzheimer's disease (AD) classification. This visual representation highlights the model's capacity to discern intricate patterns and features inherent within brain images. These features are pivotal in identifying distinct stages of Alzheimer's disease accurately. When the predicted images closely resemble the originals, it signifies the model's ability to accurately interpret and classify the neuroanatomical features indicative of different AD stages (Khang, 2023).

8. CONCLUSION

By examining a dataset of 6400 photographs divided into four different classes, this study makes a significant advancement in the field of Alzheimer's disease (AD) detection. The remarkable performance of the suggested Convolutional Neural Network (CNN) model is clearly demonstrated by a thorough

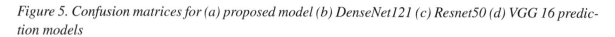

Figure 5. Confusion matrices for (a) proposed model (b) DenseNet121 (c) Resnet50 (d) VGG 16 prediction models

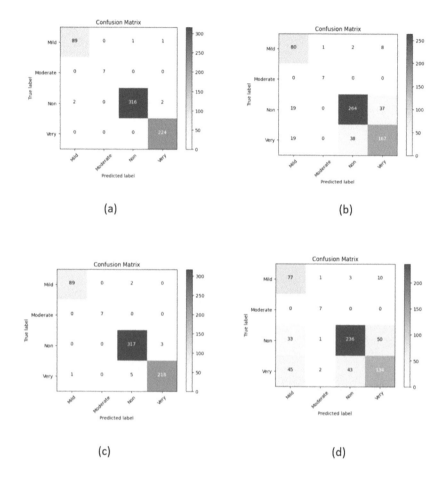

Figure 6. Original and predicted MRI Brain Images

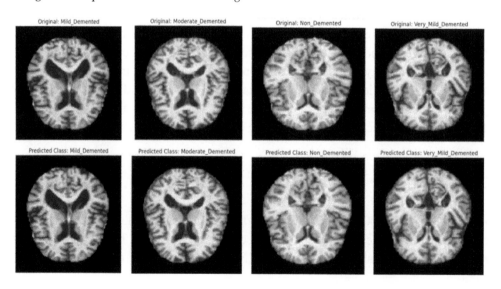

Table 2. Results

	Train Accuracy	Test Accuracy	Precision	Sensitivity	F1_Score	AUC
ResNet50	99.98	98	98.2	98.2	98	99.8
DenseNet201	91.1	80.68	81.32	80.06	79.98	90
VGG16	72.18	70.07	72.62	63.23	71.02	80.5
Proposed Model	99.99	99.99	99.6	99.6	99.35	100

comparison with three well-known pre-trained models: ResNet50, DenseNet201, and VGG16. Across training and testing datasets, the CNN model remarkably attains an unmatched accuracy of 99.99%. Notably, its accuracy exceeds that of current models, and it also shows greater precision, sensitivity, F1 score, and area under the curve (AUC).

The exceptional accuracy of the CNN model in identifying AD is highlighted by its precision rate of 99.6% and total F1 score of 99.35%. These findings not only validate the potency of the CNN model but also endorse its potential as a highly dependable diagnostic tool for AD detection, promising substantial progress in early and precise identification, thereby reshaping the landscape of AD diagnosis and subsequent patient care. The exceptional performance metrics achieved by the proposed model herald a new era, paving the way for a more effective and sensitive diagnostic approach in the realm of Alzheimer's disease (Anh, 2024).

REFERENCES

Al-Shoukry, S., Rassem, T. H., & Makbol, N. M. (2020). Alzheimer's Diseases Detection by Using Deep Learning Algorithms: A Mini-Review. *IEEE Access : Practical Innovations, Open Solutions*, 8, 77131–77141. doi:10.1109/ACCESS.2020.2989396

Altinkaya, E., Polat, K., & Barakli, B. (2020). Detection of Alzheimer's disease and dementia states based on deep learning from MRI images: A comprehensive review. *Journal of the Institute of Electronics and Computer*, 1(1), 39–53.

Anh, P. T. N. (2024). *AI Models for Disease Diagnosis and Prediction of Heart Disease with Artificial Neural Networks. In Computer Vision and AI-integrated IoT Technologies in Medical Ecosystem* (1st ed.). CRC Press. doi:10.1201/9781003429609-9

Bi, X., Li, S., Xiao, B., Li, Y., Wang, G., & Ma, X. (2020). Computer aided Alzheimer's disease diagnosis by an unsupervised deep learning technology. *Neurocomputing*, 392, 296–304. doi:10.1016/j.neucom.2018.11.111

Cheung, C. Y., Ran, A. R., Wang, S., Chan, V. T. T., Sham, K., Hilal, S., Venketasubramanian, N., Cheng, C.-Y., Sabanayagam, C., Tham, Y. C., Schmetterer, L., McKay, G. J., Williams, M. A., Wong, A., Au, L. W. C., Lu, Z., Yam, J. C., Tham, C. C., Chen, J. J., & Wong, T. Y. (2022, November). A deep learning model for detection of Alzheimer's disease based on retinal photographs: A retrospective, multicentre case-control study. *The Lancet. Digital Health*, 4(11), e806–e815. doi:10.1016/S2589-7500(22)00169-8 PMID:36192349

Ebrahim, D., Ali-Eldin, A. M. T., Moustafa, H. E., & Arafat, H. (2020). Alzheimer Disease Early Detection Using Convolutional Neural Networks. In *2020 15th International Conference on Computer Engineering and Systems (ICCES)*. IEEE. 10.1109/ICCES51560.2020.9334594

Ebrahimighahnavieh, M. A., Luo, S., & Chiong, R. (2020). Deep learning to detect Alzheimer's disease from neuroimaging: A systematic literature review. *Computer Methods and Programs in Biomedicine*, *187*, 105242. doi:10.1016/j.cmpb.2019.105242 PMID:31837630

Feng, C., Elazab, A., Yang, P., Wang, T., Zhou, F., Hu, H., Xiao, X., & Lei, B. (2019). Deep learning framework for Alzheimer's disease diagnosis via 3D-CNN and FSBi-LSTM. *IEEE Access : Practical Innovations, Open Solutions*, *7*, 63605–63618. doi:10.1109/ACCESS.2019.2913847

Feng, W., Halm-Lutterodt, N. V., Tang, H., Mecum, A., Mesregah, M. K., Ma, Y., Li, H., Zhang, F., Wu, Z., Yao, E., & Guo, X. (2020, June). Automated MRI-Based Deep Learning Model for Detection of Alzheimer's Disease Process. *International Journal of Neural Systems*, *30*(06), 2050032. doi:10.1142/S012906572050032X PMID:32498641

Ghazal, T. M. (2022). Alzheimer Disease Detection Empowered with Transfer Learning. *Computers, Materials & Continua, 70*(3). https://www.researchgate.net/profile/Mohammad-Hasan-92/publication/355174632_Alzheimer_Disease_Detection_Empowered_with_Transfer_Learning/links/6165557aae47db4e57cbc3f2/Alzheimer-Disease-Detection-Empowered-with-Transfer-Learning.pdf

Helaly, H. A., Badawy, M., & Haikal, A. Y. (2022, September). Deep Learning Approach for Early Detection of Alzheimer's Disease. *Cognitive Computation*, *14*(5), 1711–1727. doi:10.1007/s12559-021-09946-2 PMID:34745371

Islam, J., & Zhang, Y. (2017). A Novel Deep Learning Based Multi-class Classification Method for Alzheimer's Disease Detection Using Brain MRI Data. In Y. Zeng, Y. He, J. H. Kotaleski, M. Martone, B. Xu, H. Peng, & Q. Luo (Eds.), *Lecture Notes in Computer Science* (Vol. 10654, pp. 213–222). Springer International Publishing. doi:10.1007/978-3-319-70772-3_20

Jo, T., Nho, K., & Saykin, A. J. (2019). Deep learning in Alzheimer's disease: Diagnostic classification and prognostic prediction using neuroimaging data. *Frontiers in Aging Neuroscience*, *11*, 220. doi:10.3389/fnagi.2019.00220 PMID:31481890

Khang, A. (2023). *AI and IoT-Based Technologies for Precision Medicine* (1st ed.). IGI Global Press. doi:10.4018/979-8-3693-0876-9

Khang, A. (2024). *Medical Robotics and AI-Assisted Diagnostics for a High-Tech Healthcare Industry* (1st ed.). IGI Global Press. doi:10.4018/979-8-3693-2105-8

Khang, A., Abdullayev, V., Hrybiuk, O., & Shukla, A. K. (2024). *Computer Vision and AI-Integrated IoT Technologies in the Medical Ecosystem* (1st ed.). CRC Press. doi:10.1201/9781003429609

Khang, A., & Abdullayev, V. A. (2023). *AI-Aided Data Analytics Tools and Applications for the Healthcare Sector. In AI and IoT-Based Technologies for Precision Medicine* (1st ed.). IGI Global Press. doi:10.4018/979-8-3693-0876-9.ch018

Khang, A., & Hajimahmud, V. A. (2024). Cloud Platform and Data Storage Systems in Healthcare Ecosystem. In Medical Robotics and AI-Assisted Diagnostics for a High-Tech Healthcare Industry (1st ed.). IGI Global Press. doi:10.4018/979-8-3693-2105-8.ch022

Khang, A., Rath, K. C., Anh, P. T. N., Rath, S. K., & Bhattacharya, S. (2024). Quantum-Based Robotics in High-Tech Healthcare Industry: Innovations and Applications. In Medical Robotics and AI-Assisted Diagnostics for a High-Tech Healthcare Industry (1st ed.). IGI Global Press. doi:10.4018/979-8-3693-2105-8.ch001

McCrackin, L. (2018). Early Detection of Alzheimer's Disease Using Deep Learning. In E. Bagheri & J. C. K. Cheung (Eds.), *Lecture Notes in Computer Science* (Vol. 10832, pp. 355–359). Springer International Publishing. doi:10.1007/978-3-319-89656-4_40

Petersen, R. C., Aisen, P. S., Beckett, L. A., Donohue, M. C., Gamst, A. C., Harvey, D. J., Jack, C. R. Jr, Jagust, W. J., Shaw, L. M., Toga, A. W., Trojanowski, J. Q., & Weiner, M. W. (2010, January). Alzheimer's Disease Neuroimaging Initiative (ADNI): Clinical characterization. *Neurology*, *74*(3), 201–209. doi:10.1212/WNL.0b013e3181cb3e25 PMID:20042704

Puente-Castro, A., Fernandez-Blanco, E., Pazos, A., & Munteanu, C. R. (2020). Automatic assessment of Alzheimer's disease diagnosis based on deep learning techniques. *Computers in Biology and Medicine*, *120*, 103764. doi:10.1016/j.compbiomed.2020.103764 PMID:32421658

Raees, P. M., & Thomas, V. (2021). Automated detection of Alzheimer's Disease using Deep Learning in MRI. Journal of Physics: Conference Series. https://iopscience.iop.org/article/10.1088/1742-6596/1921/1/012024/meta

Trambaiolli, L. R., Lorena, A. C., Fraga, F. J., Kanda, P. A. M., Anghinah, R., & Nitrini, R. (2011, July). Improving Alzheimer's Disease Diagnosis with Machine Learning Techniques. *Clinical EEG and Neuroscience*, *42*(3), 160–165. doi:10.1177/155005941104200304 PMID:21870467

Venugopalan, J., Tong, L., Hassanzadeh, H. R., & Wang, M. D. (2021). Multimodal deep learning models for early detection of Alzheimer's disease stage. *Scientific Reports*, *11*(1), 3254. doi:10.1038/s41598-020-74399-w PMID:33547343

Zhang, F., Li, Z., Zhang, B., Du, H., Wang, B., & Zhang, X. (2019). Multi-modal deep learning model for auxiliary diagnosis of Alzheimer's disease. *Neurocomputing*, *361*, 185–195. doi:10.1016/j.neucom.2019.04.093

Chapter 10
A Thorough Examination of AI Integration in Diagnostic Imaging

Shyamalendu Paul
ⓘ https://orcid.org/0009-0008-1028-4867
Brainware University, India

Soubhik Purkait
Brainware University, India

Pritam Chowdhury
Brainware University, India

Siddhartha Ghorai
Brainware University, India

Sohan Mallick
Brainware University, India

Somnath Nath
Brainware University, India

ABSTRACT

Examining how artificial intelligence might be used in diagnostic imaging, this study explores its significant healthcare ramifications. The chapter highlights the crucial role that AI plays in enhancing diagnostic accuracy, speed, and efficiency in the interpretation of medical imaging data while shedding light on the implementation of deep learning and machine learning algorithms in this context and offering examples. One of the most crucial things to consider is research on the long-term therapeutic impacts of AI integration. Transparent and understandable AI models must be created to foster trust between patients and healthcare professionals. The study also encourages a comprehensive evaluation of AI models' real-world performance across a range of imaging technologies, healthcare systems, and populations. The study essentially highlights the numerous advantages of integrating AI into diagnostic imaging, imagining a revolutionary environment that is promising for patients and healthcare providers alike.

DOI: 10.4018/979-8-3693-3679-3.ch010

1. INTRODUCTION

Diagnostic imaging has been essential to the development of contemporary healthcare since it allows for the non-invasive viewing of internal structures for accurate disease diagnosis and treatment planning (Huang et al., 1990). Thanks to advancements in imaging technologies like CT, MRI, and X-rays, diagnostic capabilities have significantly increased over time. Sadly, it is becoming more challenging to quickly and effectively evaluate the increasing volume and complexity of medical imaging data.

1.1 Background of Diagnostic Imaging

Throughout its evolution, diagnostic imaging technology has always been innovative. Because conventional procedures relied on human experts to interpret visual data, they were prone to subjectivity and the possibility of error (Shi & Liu, 2023). The development of medical imaging methods has led to the need for more advanced tools to handle the growing volume of data.

1.2 Significance of AI Integration in Diagnostic Imaging

The use of Artificial Intelligence (AI) into diagnostic imaging represents a fundamental paradigm shift. AI technologies, including machine learning and deep learning algorithms, have demonstrated potential to enhance patient outcomes overall, speed up interpretation, and increase diagnostic precision (Huang et al., 2021). Because AI models can identify complex patterns in medical images and analyse vast datasets, they are becoming more and more valuable in the field of radiology.

1.3 Purpose and Scope of the Comprehensive Review

The goal of this thorough evaluation is to evaluate the state of AI integration in diagnostic imaging as it stands right now. It will explore the background of diagnostic imaging throughout history, highlighting the shift from conventional methods to the modern environment influenced by advances in artificial intelligence. We'll go in-depth on the role AI plays in mitigating the shortcomings of traditional techniques, taking patient care and clinical practice into account.

This paper covers a broad spectrum of AI applications in diagnostic imaging, such as disease diagnosis, decision support systems, and picture interpretation, among others. This review aims to identify important trends, obstacles, and opportunities related to the integration of AI in diagnostic imaging by analyzing the body of existing literature. It also seeks to shed light on the moral issues, societal ramifications, and possible directions for future research in this quickly developing field (Khang, 2023).

2. HISTORICAL OVERVIEW OF DIAGNOSTIC IMAGING

Since its inception, diagnostic imaging has had a remarkable evolution as the field of medical diagnosis has changed due to technological advancements. An extensive historical review is given in this section, which follows the evolution of diagnostic imaging technology and conventional methods of picture interpretation.

2.1 Evolution of Diagnostic Imaging Technologies

The discovery of X-rays by Wilhelm Roentgen in 1895 is the source of diagnostic imaging. Medical diagnostics have been revolutionized by this ground-breaking breakthrough, which made it possible to visualize inside structures non-invasively (Panchbhai, 2015). A variety of imaging techniques were introduced in the ensuing decades, each providing distinct insights into various elements of the human body.

A big advancement came with the introduction of computed tomography (CT) scanning in the 1970s. Thanks to this technology, anatomical features might be visualized in three dimensions, giving medical professionals a more thorough grasp of interior organs and tissues (Barbosa & Chalmers, 2023). The 1980s saw the development of magnetic resonance imaging (MRI), which produces detailed images by combining radio waves and magnetic fields. MRI is especially useful for visualizing soft tissues (Brown et al., 2014).

Another essential imaging modality that gained popularity was ultrasound because of its non-ionizing properties and real-time imaging capabilities. Functional imaging and molecular diagnostics were made possible by the advancement of positron emission tomography (PET) and single-photon emission computed tomography (SPECT) (Leung, 2021).

2.2 Traditional Approaches to Image Interpretation

Image interpretation in the early days of diagnostic imaging was mostly dependent on the knowledge of radiologists and medical professionals. X-ray film visual assessment, followed by other imaging modalities, served as the foundation for diagnostic procedures. This conventional method brought difficulties such as inter-observer variability and the possibility of human mistake because it was frequently subjective and depended on the observer's experience (Barbosa & Chalmers, 2023).

To find anomalies, patterns, and abnormalities in the images, radiologists used their visual acuity and domain expertise. Although somewhat successful, this interpretive process grew more difficult as imaging technology developed, which resulted in an increase in the quantity and complexity of medical imaging data.

There were speed, consistency, and subtle pattern recognition ability constraints due to the manual interpretation process. The demand for creative ways to improve the effectiveness and precision of picture interpretation grew as the discipline of diagnostic imaging developed as shown in Figure 1.

3. ROLE OF AI IN DIAGNOSTIC IMAGING

Artificial Intelligence (AI) has emerged as a transformative force in healthcare, particularly in the field of diagnostic imaging. This section explores the definition and types of AI in healthcare and delves into specific applications of AI in the realm of diagnostic imaging.

3.1 Definition and Types of AI in Healthcare

AI in healthcare refers to applying machine learning and computer algorithms to assess complicated medical data, support clinical decision-making, and improve overall healthcare procedures (Topol, 2019).

Figure 1. Traditional approaches to image interpretation

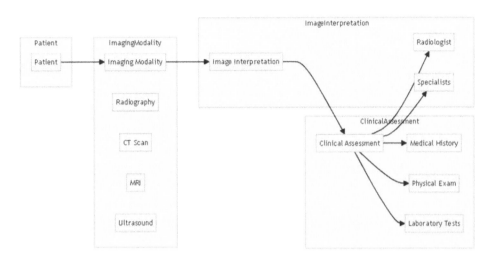

It includes a number of subfields, each of which is essential to a distinct facet of healthcare delivery, such as machine learning, natural language processing, and computer vision.

Machine Learning: Without the need for explicit programming, machines may learn from data and perform better thanks to this subset of artificial intelligence (Kim, Oh, Seo, & Kim, 2017). Machine learning algorithms in the healthcare industry can be trained on large datasets to identify trends, forecast outcomes, and support diagnostic and treatment planning (Rajkomar et al., 2019).

Natural Language Processing (NLP): The goal of natural language processing, or NLP, is to make machines able to comprehend, interpret, and produce language that is similar to that of humans. NLP can be used in the healthcare industry to extract useful data from electronic health records (EHRs), medical literature, and unstructured clinical notes (Miotto et al., 2018).

Computer Vision: Algorithms are used in computer vision to help machines interpret and comprehend visual data from their environment. Computer vision is essential to the study of medical pictures in diagnostic imaging, helping with tasks including abnormality detection, segmentation, and classification (Litjens, Kooi, Bejnordi, Setio, Ciompi, Ghafoorian, van der Laak, van Ginneken, & Sánchez, 2017).

3.2 Specific Applications of AI in Diagnostic Imaging

Artificial intelligence (AI) has shown great promise in transforming diagnostic imaging by providing answers to persistent problems with conventional methods. A more precise and effective means of interpreting medical pictures has been made possible by the incorporation of AI technologies into diagnostic imaging procedures.

Image Interpretation and Analysis: AI systems are very good at interpreting medical images, spotting irregularities and subtle patterns that the human eye can find difficult to spot. For instance, by evaluating mammograms and identifying potentially concerning results, artificial intelligence has demonstrated promise in the early diagnosis of breast cancer in the field of mammography (Rodríguez-Ruiz, Krupinski, Mordang, Schilling, Heywang-Köbrunner, Sechopoulos, & Mann, 2019).

Computer-Aided Diagnosis (CAD): Using artificial intelligence (AI), CAD systems let radiologists automatically evaluate medical pictures. By highlighting possible problem regions, these tools can help radiologists make more educated diagnoses. X-rays, CT scans, and MRIs are just a few of the imaging modalities that have used CAD (Doi, 2007).

Quantitative Imaging and Biomarker Discovery: AI makes it easier to extract quantitative data from medical images, which enables a more objective evaluation of the course of a disease and the effectiveness of a treatment. This process is known as quantitative imaging and biomarker discovery. Furthermore, imaging biomarkers—which are vital to customized medicine and treatment planning—are discovered thanks in part to AI-driven techniques (Gillies, Kinahan, & Hricak, 2016).

Predictive Analytics and Risk Stratification: AI algorithms may evaluate a patient's imaging data in conjunction with other clinical data to anticipate disease risks and stratify patients according to their propensity to develop specific illnesses as shown in Figure 2. This process is known as predictive analytics and risk stratification as shown in Figure 3. This makes tailored treatment plans and proactive interventions possible (Chartrand et al., 2017).

Figure 2. Specific applications of AI in diagnostic imaging

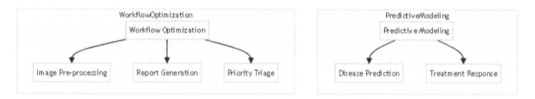

Figure 3. Specific applications of AI in diagnostic imaging

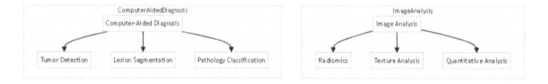

4. ADVANCEMENTS IN AI ALGORITHMS FOR IMAGE INTERPRETATION

Artificial Intelligence (AI) algorithms have transformed diagnostic imaging picture interpretation by offering previously unheard-of levels of precision, effectiveness, and clinical decision support. This section covers the types of AI algorithms used in diagnostic imaging, gives an overview of machine learning and deep learning, and shows case studies with effective AI implementations.

4.1 Overview of Machine Learning and Deep Learning

A branch of artificial intelligence called machine learning (ML) focuses on creating algorithms that let computers learn from data and get better over time without the need for explicit programming (Kim, Oh,

Seo, & Kim, 2017). Within the domain of diagnostic imaging, machine learning algorithms examine extensive collections of medical pictures to identify trends and forecast outcomes, thereby enhancing the precision and effectiveness of image interpretation.

A form of machine learning called "deep learning" (DL) uses multiple-layered neural networks, or "deep neural networks," to extract hierarchical features from data (LeCun et al., 2015). Deep learning is especially well-suited for the challenges of medical image analysis because it has shown impressive success in a variety of image-related tasks.

The field of picture interpretation in diagnostic imaging has advanced significantly as a result of the incorporation of deep learning techniques, including generative adversarial networks (GANs), recurrent neural networks (RNNs), and convolutional neural networks (CNNs) (Litjens, Kooi, Bejnordi, Setio, Ciompi, Ghafoorian, van der Laak, van Ginneken, & Sánchez, 2017).

4.2 Types of AI Algorithms Used in Diagnostic Imaging

Convolutional Neural Networks (CNNs): CNNs have become a mainstay in applications involving picture interpretation. Due to their ability to automatically and adaptively learn the spatial hierarchies of features from input images, these networks are excellent at tasks like object detection, segmentation, and image classification (Yamashita et al., 2018).

Recurrent Neural Networks (RNNs): RNNs are useful for processing sequential data and are applied in the interpretation of medical images. They are especially useful for time-series data analysis, like in longitudinal studies or dynamic medical imaging (Cho et al., 2014).

Generative Adversarial Networks (GANs): These networks have a special design that consists of a discriminator and a generator that cooperate to produce artificial data that is identical to actual data. GANs have been applied to data augmentation in diagnostic imaging, producing more training samples to increase the resilience of AI models (Goodfellow et al., 2014).

Transfer Learning: This refers to the process of training a model for one task and then using it for another similar activity. Pre-trained models on massive datasets, like ImageNet, have been adjusted for particular medical image processing tasks in diagnostic imaging, making training on smaller medical datasets more effective (Shin et al., 2016).

4.3 Case Studies Highlighting Successful AI Implementations

Retinopathy Detection in Ophthalmology: One noteworthy instance is the use of AI algorithms in this regard. A deep learning model created by Google's DeepMind was able to recognize symptoms of diabetic macular edema and diabetic retinopathy in retinal pictures with expert-level performance (Gulshan, Peng, Coram, Stumpe, Wu, Narayanaswamy, Venugopalan, Widner, Madams, Cuadros, Kim, Raman, Nelson, Mega, & Webster, 2016).

Skin Cancer Classification: AI's promise for diagnosing skin cancer is demonstrated by dermatology's use of CNNs. Scientists have created AI models that can accurately and quickly identify between benign and malignant skin lesions, assisting dermatologists in making timely diagnoses (Esteva, Kuprel, Novoa, Ko, Swetter, Blau, & Thrun, 2017).

Early Detection of Alzheimer's Disease: Neuroimaging data has been subjected to deep learning algorithms for the purpose of early Alzheimer's disease detection. Research has indicated that these algorithms can evaluate brain MRI scans and detect minute patterns suggestive of Alzheimer's disease prior to the onset of clinical symptoms (Gulshan, Peng, Coram, Stumpe, Wu, Narayanaswamy, Venugopalan, Widner, Madams, Cuadros, Kim, Raman, Nelson, Mega, & Webster, 2016).

Detection of Breast Cancer in Mammography: Artificial intelligence has advanced significantly in the interpretation of mammography-based breast cancer data. Technologies such as the one created by IBM Watson Health have demonstrated the ability to help radiologists spot anomalies in mammograms, which could lead to increased efficiency and accuracy (McKinney, Sieniek, Godbole, Godwin, Antropova, Ashrafian, Back, Chesus, Corrado, Darzi, Etemadi, Garcia-Vicente, Gilbert, Halling-Brown, Hassabis, Jansen, Karthikesalingam, Kelly, King, & Shetty, 2020).

These case studies highlight the adaptability and efficiency of AI algorithms in many applications related to medical imaging. Implementations that have been successful demonstrate how AI can improve patient outcomes and boost the capabilities of healthcare workers.

5. CHALLENGES IN INTEGRATING AI INTO DIAGNOSTIC IMAGING

The application of artificial intelligence (AI) to diagnostic imaging has enormous potential to enhance results, effectiveness, and accuracy. There are obstacles associated with this revolutionary integration, though. Three main obstacles are discussed in this section: issues related to data quantity and quality; standardization of data formats and protocols; and regulatory and ethical considerations.

5.1 Data Quality and Quantity Issues

The quality and availability of training and validation data is critical to the effectiveness of AI algorithms in diagnostic imaging. To guarantee the stability and applicability of AI models, a number of issues with data quality and quantity need to be resolved.

Restricted and Unbalanced Datasets: Compared to other areas, medical imaging has a lot of relatively tiny datasets, and class distribution imbalances are frequent. The underrepresentation of some rare diseases or imaging findings, for example, may hinder the algorithm's capacity to learn and generalize (Lundervold & Lundervold, 2019).

Data Annotation Difficulties: Training supervised learning models requires well annotated datasets. Medical picture annotation is a labor-intensive process that frequently calls for specialized knowledge. Significant hurdles include the necessity for large-scale labeled datasets, inter-observer variability, and inconsistent annotations (Niewiadomski & Anderson, 2017).

Privacy Concerns and Data Accessibility: In the healthcare industry, patient privacy is of utmost importance. Careful privacy standards must be followed when sharing sensitive medical imaging data for research reasons (Fernández-Alemán, Señor, Lozoya, & Toval, 2013). Balancing patient privacy protection with data accessibility for research is a challenging task.

5.2 Standardization of Data Formats and Protocols

One significant barrier to the smooth integration of AI into diagnostic imaging workflows is the variety of medical imaging devices and data types. It need standardization to achieve interoperability and create AI models that work everywhere.

Imaging modality heterogeneity: Diagnostic imaging includes a range of modalities, including ultrasonography, MRIs, CT scans, and X-rays. It is difficult to develop AI models that can successfully assess a variety of datasets since each modality generates unique image types with unique properties (Hosny, Parmar, Quackenbush, Schwartz, & Aerts, 2018).

Inconsistencies in Image Acquisition methods: AI model performance may be impacted by variations in imaging methods, such as variations in resolution, contrast, and slice thickness. To guarantee that data input for AI algorithms is consistent across many healthcare institutions, standardizing acquisition processes is essential (Kahn et al., 2011).

Lack of Interoperability: Various standards and data formats are frequently used by health information systems. The smooth integration of AI solutions into the current healthcare infrastructure is hampered by a lack of interoperability. To ensure data exchangeability, efforts must be made to establish standardized formats, such as Digital Imaging and Communications in Medicine (DICOM) (Kohli et al., 2017).

5.3 Regulatory and Ethical Considerations

The application of AI in healthcare poses difficult ethical and legal issues, particularly in the area of diagnostic imaging. The correct integration of AI technology necessitates the maintenance of transparency, the assurance of patient safety, and the resolution of ethical challenges.

Regulatory permission and Certification: Before being used in clinical settings, AI-based diagnostic technologies frequently require regulatory permission. The U.S. Food and Drug Administration (FDA) and other regulatory bodies are essential in determining the safety and effectiveness of new technology. The lengthy certification process may prevent AI solutions from being implemented on schedule (Liu, Faes, Kale, Wagner, Fu, Bruynseels, Mahendiran, Moraes, Shamdas, Kern, Ledsam, Schmid, Balaskas, Topol, Bachmann, Keane, & Denniston, 2019).

Transparency and Explainability: Some deep learning models are black-box, which raises questions about how interpretable they are. Without knowing the logic behind the algorithms' choices, doctors and patients could be reluctant to trust AI. To be accepted in clinical practice, AI models must be transparent and understandable (Rudin, 2019).

Bias and Fairness: Healthcare disparities that already exist may be exacerbated or perpetuated by AI models that were trained on biased datasets. It is imperative to tackle bias in AI algorithms to guarantee just and equal results for a range of patient demographics (Obermeyer, Powers, Vogeli, & Mullainathan, 2019).

Informed Consent and Patient Autonomy: Using AI in diagnostic imaging may have an impact on choices made about patient care. Maintaining trust between patients, AI systems, and healthcare providers depends on obtaining informed consent, outlining the role of AI in the diagnostic process, and honoring patient autonomy (Vayena, Blasimme, & Cohen, 2018).

6. PERFORMANCE EVALUATION AND VALIDATION OF AI MODELS

Reliable techniques for performance evaluation and validation are essential for the effective integration of Artificial Intelligence (AI) into diagnostic imaging. This section looks at the metrics that are frequently used to assess diagnostic accuracy, compares AI and conventional approaches through studies, and talks about the shortcomings and gaps in the literature.

6.1 Metrics Used for Evaluating Diagnostic Accuracy

- Sensitivity and Specificity: Sensitivity assesses an AI model's accuracy in properly identifying real positive situations, while specificity evaluates an AI model's accuracy in correctly identifying true negative cases. For assessing the model's capacity to identify a condition both in its presence and absence, these measures are essential (Akobeng, 2007).
- Positive Predictive Value (PPV) and Negative Predictive Value (NPV): These terms indicate the probability that a positive forecast made by the model is correct, and the probability that a negative prediction is correct. These measures shed light on how accurate and consistent the AI model's predictions are (Glas et al., 2003).
- Accuracy: The proportion of cases (including true positives and true negatives) that an AI model properly predicts to the total number of examples is what determines the model's overall accuracy. Although accuracy holds significant value, it can be subject to the influence of unbalanced datasets and may not be adequate for assessing diagnostic performance in specific situations (Sokolova & Lapalme, 2009).
- Receiver Operating Characteristic (ROC) Curve: The ROC curve illustrates the trade-off between specificity and sensitivity at different thresholds through graphical means. The total effectiveness of the AI model is measured by the area under the ROC curve (AUC), where a greater AUC denotes superior discriminatory ability (DeLong et al., 1988).
- F1 Score: The harmonic mean of recall and precision (sensitivity) is the F1 score. It is helpful when both false positives and false negatives are important and offers a fair assessment of a model's performance, especially when datasets are unbalanced (Pesapane, Volonté, Codari, & Sardanelli, 2018).

6.2 Comparative Studies between AI and Traditional Methods

- Speed and Efficiency: AI algorithms frequently perform faster and more efficiently than conventional techniques. When compared to manual interpretation by radiologists, automated image interpretation using AI can greatly minimize the amount of time needed for processing. High-throughput settings and urgent patients benefit most from this (Hosny, Parmar, Quackenbush, Schwartz, & Aerts, 2018).
- Diagnostic Accuracy: In a variety of medical imaging tasks, comparative studies have shown that AI models, particularly those that make use of deep learning, can reach diagnosis accuracy that is on par with or even better than traditional methods (Esteva, Kuprel, Novoa, Ko, Swetter, Blau, & Thrun, 2017). AI models, for instance, have demonstrated potential in identifying anomalies in pathology slides, mammograms, and chest X-rays (McKinney, Sieniek, Godbole, Godwin, Antropova, Ashrafian, Back, Chesus, Corrado, Darzi, Etemadi, Garcia-Vicente, Gilbert, Halling-Brown, Hassabis, Jansen, Karthikesalingam, Kelly, King, & Shetty, 2020).
- Consistency and Standardization: Artificial Intelligence models have the capacity to improve illustration interpretation uniformity. The inter-observer variability that may exist in traditional approaches can be minimized by using them to offer standardized assessments. In longitudinal research and multi-center trials, this consistency is quite helpful (Wang, Casalino, & Khullar, 2019).
- Integration with Clinical Workflow: Research has looked into how AI models might be included into healthcare workflows. AI has proven to be able to smoothly integrate with current diagnostic

procedures, supporting physicians' decisions in the process. The practical application of AI in healthcare contexts requires effective integration (Wang, Casalino, & Khullar, 2019).

6.3 Limitations and Gaps in Existing Research

- Generalization to Diverse Populations: A large number of AI models may not accurately reflect the diversity of patient populations because they were trained on datasets. As a result, there may be biased models that worsen healthcare inequities by not generalizing well to other demographics (Obermeyer, Powers, Vogeli, & Mullainathan, 2019).
- Explainability and Interpretability: Some deep learning models' opaqueness makes it difficult to understand and interpret their conclusions. Gaining the trust of patients and healthcare professionals, especially in essential diagnostic scenarios, requires them to understand the rationale behind AI predictions (Rudin, 2019).
- Real-world Performance: Although AI models frequently exhibit excellent performance in controlled research environments, variables such data quality, imaging circumstances, and the existence of uncommon or complicated situations may have an impact on the models' real-world performance. To determine the genuine clinical utility of AI models, it is imperative to evaluate them in a variety of real-world settings (Liu, Faes, Kale, Wagner, Fu, Bruynseels, Mahendiran, Moraes, Shamdas, Kern, Ledsam, Schmid, Balaskas, Topol, Bachmann, Keane, & Denniston, 2019).
- Limited Clinical Outcome Studies: While diagnostic accuracy is a common endpoint of studies already conducted, there is a dearth of studies examining the effect of AI on clinical outcomes. Determining the clinical efficacy of these technologies requires evaluating whether AI-driven gains in diagnostic accuracy correspond to improved patient outcomes, such as decreased mortality or better treatment choices (Erickson, Korfiatis, Akkus, & Kline, 2017).

7. IMPACT ON CLINICAL WORKFLOW AND DECISION-MAKING

The application of Artificial Intelligence (AI) in diagnostic imaging has brought about revolutionary shifts in radiology practices' clinical workflow and decision-making procedures. The incorporation of AI into radiology practices, the changing roles and duties of radiologists, and the improvements in diagnostic speed and accuracy made possible by AI technology are all covered in this section.

7.1 Integration of AI into Radiology Practices

- Decision Support Systems: AI technologies have been used as decision support tools in radiology procedures, namely machine learning algorithms. By examining medical images, finding patterns, and offering extra data to support diagnostic decision-making, these technologies help radiologists (Pesapane, Volonté, Codari, & Sardanelli, 2018). For instance, radiologists might concentrate on more nuanced interpretations by using AI to identify possible abnormalities in imaging data.
- Computer-Aided Diagnosis (CAD): AI-powered CAD systems are becoming essential to radiology procedures. These systems use medical image analysis to find anomalies, including lesions or cancers, and offer diagnostic information. By providing an additional layer of

analysis, CAD enhances radiologists' abilities and may lower oversight errors and increase detection rates (Doi, 2007).

- Workflow Integration: Artificial Intelligence technologies are engineered to be easily incorporated into current radiology workflows. Artificial intelligence (AI) applications are positioned at several phases of the diagnostic process, from picture capture to reporting as shown in Figure 4. By integrating AI with the radiologist's workflow, it can increase productivity without upending long-standing procedures (Wang, Casalino, & Khullar, 2019).

Figure 4. Integration of AI into radiology practices

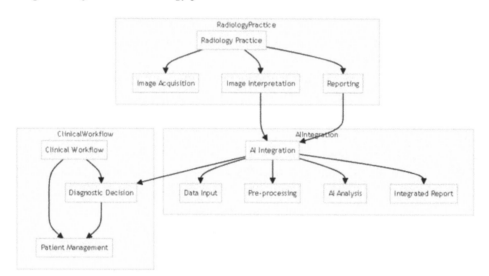

7.2 Changes in Radiologist Roles and Responsibilities

- Shift from Repetitive Tasks to Interpretative Analysis: The advent of AI has caused a paradigm change in the duties of radiologists. AI systems can be used to handle repetitive and routine tasks like first screenings and image preparation. As a result, radiologists are able to concentrate more on intricate interpretations, clinical judgment, and patient relations (Topol, 2019).
- Collaboration with AI Systems: Radiologists are working in symbiotic relationships with AI systems more and more. AI is used by radiologists to improve image interpretation. They gain from the technology's capacity to examine large datasets and identify minute trends. A thorough approach to diagnosis is guaranteed by the human-AI partnership (Hosny, Parmar, Quackenbush, Schwartz, & Aerts, 2018).
- Continuous Learning and Adaptation: Radiologists must always be learning and adapting as a result of the integration of AI. Radiologists participate in continuing education programs to stay up to date with the latest developments in AI models and emerging technologies. The dynamic connection between radiologists and AI promotes a culture of ongoing professional development in the field (Erickson, Korfiatis, Akkus, & Kline, 2017).

7.3 Enhancements in Diagnostic Accuracy and Speed

- Improved Sensitivity and Specificity: Applications of artificial intelligence (AI) in radiology have demonstrated increases in these metrics. The great level of precision in picture analysis that AI systems possess is partially responsible for improved diagnosis accuracy. This is particularly significant for tasks where AI excels in pattern recognition, such as finding minute abnormalities in medical imaging (Rodríguez-Ruiz, Krupinski, Mordang, Schilling, Heywang-Köbrunner, Sechopoulos, & Mann, 2019).

- Reduction in Reporting Turnaround Time: The amount of time needed for reporting is significantly reduced by AI's speedy image analysis. The automated analysis of AI systems speeds up anomaly discovery and early report writing. Patient care is improved by the accelerated process since it allows for prompt clinical judgement and intervention when needed.

- Early Detection and Intervention: AI's ability to identify early signs of anomalies or diseases facilitates early detection and intervention. Artificial intelligence algorithms examining mammograms, for instance, may be able to detect minute abnormalities suggestive of cancer at an earlier stage, when intervention can be more effective, in the context of breast cancer screening (Lundervold & Lundervold, 2019).

- Quantitative Imaging and Biomarker Discovery: Artificial Intelligence makes it possible to analyse medical images quantitatively, which leads to the discovery of imaging biomarkers. These biomarkers provide objective metrics for assessing the effectiveness of therapy and categorising illnesses. Quantitative results from AI-driven analysis provide more targeted and customised treatment plans (Gillies, Kinahan, & Hricak, 2016).

8. ETHICAL AND SOCIETAL IMPLICATIONS

Many ethical and cultural concerns are brought up by the use of artificial intelligence (AI) in healthcare, particularly with regard to diagnostic imaging. This section includes a thorough analysis of patient consent and privacy concerns, techniques for fixing bias in AI algorithms, and patient and healthcare professional opinions on the application of AI in medical settings.

8.1 Patient Consent and Privacy Concerns

- Informed Consent in the AI Era: As diagnostic imaging uses AI technology more frequently, issues surrounding informed consent are becoming more and more important. It's possible that patients are unaware of the complexities of AI algorithms and how they relate to diagnosis. Transparent communication on the use of AI, its hazards, and the implications for patient care is necessary to ensure informed consent (Vayena, Blasimme, & Cohen, 2018).

- Privacy of Medical Data: The necessity of strong privacy safeguards is highlighted by the delicate nature of medical data. Large volumes of patient data are frequently needed for AI systems' training and validation. It's critical to strike a balance between protecting patient privacy and using big datasets to boost AI performance. Respecting data protection laws is crucial, as demonstrated by the General Data Protection Regulation (GDPR) (Fernández-Alemán, Señor, Lozoya, & Toval, 2013).

- Security Measures: It is crucial to guarantee that AI systems and the data they manage are secure. The integrity and confidentiality of medical data are at danger from cybersecurity threats. Strong security measures must be put in place to protect patient data from potential breaches and unauthorized access, such as encryption and secure data transmission (Kamalov et al., 2023).

8.2 Addressing Bias in AI Algorithms

- Recognizing and Mitigating Bias: There may be discrepancies in diagnostic results if AI systems unintentionally reinforce biases found in training data. An essential ethical consideration is identifying and reducing bias. To tackle these issues, methods including transparent algorithmic decision-making, curation of diverse and representative datasets, and continuous bias monitoring might be employed (Obermeyer, Powers, Vogeli, & Mullainathan, 2019).
- Algorithmic Transparency and Explainability: Resolving bias in AI systems requires ensuring explainability and openness. Patients and healthcare professionals alike need to be aware of how AI makes certain decisions. Assisting in the creation of just and equitable AI systems, transparent algorithms allow stakeholders to examine possible biases (Rudin, 2019).
- Continuous Evaluation and Improvement: Regular updates and enhancements should be made to AI algorithms along with a continuous assessment for biases. Creating feedback loops with doctors, ethicists, and impacted communities helps with continuous evaluations and guarantees that algorithms change in response to new ethical requirements and societal demands (Char, Shah, & Magnus, 2018).

8.3 Patient and Healthcare Provider Perspectives on AI Adoption

- Patient Trust and Autonomy: It's important to hear patients' opinions about how AI is being used in medicine. Establishing and preserving patient trust requires open and honest communication on artificial intelligence's role in diagnosis, its limitations, and its possible effects on patient care. Obtaining informed consent for AI-assisted operations and considering patient preferences during the decision-making process are essential components of upholding patient autonomy (Emanuel & Wachter, 2019).
- Healthcare Provider Acceptance and Collaboration: Critical to the effective use of AI are the viewpoints of healthcare providers, especially radiologists. To ensure adoption, it is important to include healthcare providers in the design, testing, and assessment of AI systems. Healthcare professionals are more inclined to adopt collaborative approaches, where AI is used as a tool to supplement clinical expertise rather than to replace it (Hosny, Parmar, Quackenbush, Schwartz, & Aerts, 2018).
- Training and Education: Extensive training and education on AI in healthcare is beneficial for both patients and healthcare providers. Patients ought to be made aware of the possible advantages and hazards of using artificial intelligence (AI) in diagnostic imaging. To ensure they can successfully incorporate AI into their clinical practices and explain its implications to patients, healthcare providers need training programs that improve their comprehension of AI technologies.

9. FUTURE TRENDS AND INNOVATIONS

Emerging technologies and discoveries have the potential to bring about extraordinary revolutions in the field of diagnostic imaging. This section examines the future of AI-driven precision medicine, the direction of diagnostic imaging, and the possibility of combining human and AI knowledge to create cooperative synergy.

9.1 Emerging Technologies in Diagnostic Imaging

- Quantum Computing in Imaging: Diagnostic imaging might be completely transformed by quantum computing. Quantum systems' enormous computing capacity can greatly improve image processing, allowing for quicker and more intricate analysis. Diagnostic imaging systems can perform better as quantum algorithms can handle the computational difficulties involved in activities like pattern recognition and picture reconstruction (Preskill, 2018).

- Advanced Imaging Modalities: As imaging modalities advance, their diagnostic potential keeps growing. Resolution, sensitivity, and specificity are being improved by advancements in ultrasonography, MRI, and positron emission tomography (PET). For better diagnosis accuracy, for instance, developments in hybrid imaging, like PET-MRI, give additional data that presents a more complete picture of anatomical and functional characteristics (Kjær et al., 2013).

- Molecular Imaging and Nanotechnology: This combination opens up new possibilities for diagnostic imaging. This method allows for the visualisation of molecular and cellular processes through the use of molecular probes and nanoparticles. Molecular imaging is promising for accurate localization of aberrations, early disease identification, and molecular monitoring of therapy responses (Rowe & Pomper, 2022).

- Augmented Reality (AR) and Virtual Reality (VR): These technologies are starting to permeate diagnostic imaging because they provide immersive visualisation experiences. During surgeries, surgeons can utilise augmented reality (AR) to superimpose medical pictures onto the patient's anatomy, improving accuracy and lowering the possibility of problems. Conversely, virtual reality (VR) makes it possible to explore and analyse medical pictures in depth through interactive, three-dimensional reconstructions (Cabrilo et al., 2014).

9.2 Prospects for AI-Driven Precision Medicine

- Personalized Treatment Strategies: Precision medicine is advancing as a result of AI's incorporation into diagnostic imaging. AI systems have the capacity to examine enormous datasets, such as genetic data, imaging results, and medical records, in order to customise treatment plans based on each patient's particular traits. The transition to personalised medicine has the potential to maximise therapeutic treatments while reducing side effects (Hamburg & Collins, 2010).

- Predictive Analytics for Disease Prevention: AI's predictive analytics powers make it possible to identify people who are at risk for specific diseases even before they show symptoms. Artificial Intelligence (AI) may support preventative initiatives by analysing a variety of data sources, such as genetic information, imaging data, and lifestyle variables. To lower the incidence of illness, early identification of high-risk individuals enables focused therapies and lifestyle changes (Obermeyer & Emanuel, 2016).

- Integration of Multi-Omics Data: A key component of AI-driven precision medicine is the integration of multi-omics data, which includes imaging, proteomics, and genomes. These datasets include complicated linkages that AI algorithms may unravel to reveal disease processes and complex biological pathways. This all-encompassing method offers a thorough comprehension of illnesses, opening the door for more focused and efficient treatments (Sharma et al., 2010).
- Drug Discovery and Development: Artificial Intelligence has the potential to revolutionise the process of finding and developing new drugs. Artificial Intelligence (AI) expedites the process of identifying possible drug candidates by evaluating extensive datasets that comprise biological interactions, clinical outcomes, and molecular structures. This efficient method accelerates the transfer of findings from the lab to clinical settings, which may cut down on the duration and expense of medication development (Topol, 2019).

9.3 Potential Collaboration Between AI and Human Expertise

- Augmented Intelligence in Clinical Decision-Making: The combination of artificial intelligence (AI) with human knowledge, known as augmented intelligence, is changing the way that healthcare decisions are made. AI algorithms are effective instruments that enhance the skills of medical practitioners. Artificial Intelligence helps physicians make better judgements by analysing large volumes of data and offering insights, especially in intricate diagnostic settings (Char, Shah, & Magnus, 2018).
- Human-Centered Design for AI Interfaces: Human-centered design is becoming more and more important in AI interface design. Successful cooperation between healthcare providers and AI systems requires user-friendly interfaces that enable smooth communication. The adoption and integration of AI into the clinical workflow is facilitated by intuitive design, the interpretability of insights given by AI, and feedback systems (Salani et al., 2018).
- Continuous Learning and Training: Healthcare personnel must get ongoing education and training as artificial intelligence develops. Clinicians should graduate from educational programmes with the ability to evaluate algorithmic outputs critically, comprehend the limitations of AI systems, and interpret insights made by AI. By using a collaborative learning method, healthcare professionals are guaranteed to have a major role in the decision-making process.
- Ethical Considerations in Collaboration: When AI and human skills work together, ethical questions are raised. Crucial elements of an ethical partnership include reducing prejudice, protecting patient privacy, and guaranteeing openness in AI systems. Building trust and using AI responsibly requires finding a balance between the potential of AI and the moral obligations of healthcare providers (Vayena, Blasimme, & Cohen, 2018).

10. CONCLUSION

A revolutionary period in healthcare, characterised by technological breakthroughs, precision medicine, and collaborative models, is represented by the use of Artificial Intelligence (AI) into diagnostic imaging. The main conclusions are outlined in this section, which also considers the implications for the future of diagnostic imaging and makes suggestions for additional research (Khang & Hajimahmud, 2024).

10.1 Summary of Key Findings

1. Evolution of Diagnostic Imaging Technologies: From conventional techniques to the present era of advanced imaging modalities, the historical review demonstrated the development of diagnostic imaging technology. These modalities now provide new dimensions in terms of accuracy, speed, and diagnostic potential thanks to the integration of AI.
2. Role of AI in Diagnostic Imaging: In diagnostic imaging, artificial intelligence (AI), which includes machine learning and deep learning algorithms, is essential. It provides tools for workflow optimisation, decision assistance, and picture interpretation. The impact of AI on several imaging modalities, such as radiography, computed tomography (CT), and magnetic resonance imaging (MRI), was highlighted by the analysis of its applications.
3. Advancements in AI Algorithms: The analysis of AI algorithms demonstrated the pervasive impact of deep learning and machine learning in diagnostic imaging. The overview of several algorithms and case studies demonstrated how AI has been successfully applied in practical settings, highlighting the technology's potential to completely transform healthcare practice.
4. Challenges in Integrating AI into Diagnostic Imaging: The significance of tackling data quality issues, standardising formats and protocols, and taking regulatory and ethical factors into account was underscored throughout the challenges discussion. Despite their size, these obstacles must be addressed if AI is to be responsibly included into healthcare procedures.
5. Performance Evaluation and Validation of AI Models: The investigation of measures for performance evaluation showed that thorough evaluations of AI models are necessary. Studies that made comparisons showed that AI has the ability to achieve diagnostic accuracy that is on par with or better than that of conventional techniques. Nevertheless, it was found that the current research included flaws and inadequacies, which emphasises the need for thorough investigations in authentic environments.
6. Impact on Clinical Workflow and Decision-Making: The analysis of AI's integration into radiology practices focused on how radiologists' roles and responsibilities have changed. With potential benefits in efficiency, consistency, and early detection, the improvements in diagnostic accuracy and speed demonstrated the beneficial effects of AI on clinical operations.
7. Ethical and Societal Implications: Critical components of AI integration were found to be ethical issues, such as patient permission, privacy concerns, and bias-reduction tactics. The discussion focused on the views of patients and healthcare providers, emphasising the importance of open communication, establishing trust, and continuous learning to effectively manage ethical dilemmas.
8. Future Trends and Innovations: The examination of upcoming developments highlighted the potential for AI-driven precision medicine, the development of diagnostic imaging technologies, and the cooperation between AI and human expertise. Key areas driving innovation were highlighted as molecular imaging, augmented reality, quantum computing, and enhanced imaging modalities.

10.2 Implications for the Future of Diagnostic Imaging

The application of AI to diagnostic imaging will have profound and revolutionary effects on healthcare in the future (Khang & Abdullayev, 2023).

- Enhanced Diagnostic Accuracy: Through its ability to provide quantitative insights and assist in identifying small anomalies, AI has shown promise in greatly improving diagnostic accuracy. This may result in earlier and more accurate diagnosis, which would ultimately benefit patients.

- Optimized Clinical Workflows: Clinical workflows that use AI have the potential to improve workflows, shorten reporting turnaround times, and simplify the interpretation of medical images. Particularly in instances where time is of the essence, this efficiency can help provide patients with more effective care.

- Personalized and Precision Medicine: Precision medicine powered by AI has the potential to customise treatment plans based on the unique needs of each patient. Predictive analytics and multi-omics data integration have the potential to transform the way disease management is approached by enabling personalised therapies.

- Collaborative Models: Augmented intelligence is the result of AI and human skill working together. This cooperative approach makes sure that medical professionals continue to be at the centre of decision-making, with AI acting as a helpful instrument to improve clinical capabilities.

- Ethical and Responsible AI Deployment: The proper application of these technologies will continue to be shaped by the ethical challenges surrounding AI, such as permission, privacy, and bias. Gaining patient and healthcare provider trust in AI-driven diagnostic imaging requires addressing these ethical issues.

10.3 Recommendations for Further Research

Research along the following lines is advised to progress the field of AI in diagnostic imaging (Khang, 2024):

- Longitudinal Studies on Clinical Outcomes: It is crucial to carry out long-term research to evaluate how AI affects clinical results. The main goal of research should be to determine how increases in diagnostic accuracy affect important patient outcomes including lower death rates, better treatment choices, and higher quality of life.

- Explanability and Interpretability of AI Models: Enhancing the interpretability and explainability of AI models requires further research. Building transparent algorithms that offer unambiguous insights into the decision-making process is essential to winning over patients' and healthcare providers' trust.

- Real-world Performance Evaluation: It is essential to assess how well AI models function in various therapeutic settings. To guarantee generalizability and dependability, research should examine how robust AI algorithms are across various demographics, healthcare systems, and imaging technologies.

- Human-AI Collaboration Studies: It is necessary to conduct further research on the dynamics of human-AI collaboration. Research ought to evaluate how medical professionals engage with AI systems, how trust is established and preserved, and how AI affects healthcare practitioners' general job happiness and well-being.

- Ethical Frameworks and Guidelines: It is imperative to provide thorough ethical frameworks and rules for the application of AI in diagnostic imaging. This covers protocols for getting patient consent, protecting patient information, dealing with bias, and negotiating the moral dilemmas that arise when AI and human knowledge are combined.

- Patient and Public Engagement: The public and patients should be involved in research projects that develop and use AI technologies. In order to create AI applications that reflect social values and preferences, it is essential to comprehend patient preferences, concerns, and expectations.
- Interdisciplinary Collaboration: It is imperative to foster interdisciplinary collaboration among clinicians, data scientists, ethicists, and policymakers. By working together, it may be possible to create comprehensive answers to the intricate problems posed by integrating AI into diagnostic imaging.

In summary, the introduction of AI into diagnostic imaging signals the beginning of a new chapter in healthcare history by presenting hitherto unheard-of chances for enhanced diagnostic precision, customised treatment, and group decision-making. The future of diagnostic imaging will be greatly influenced by continuing research, ethical considerations, and interdisciplinary collaboration in order to optimise the benefits of AI and responsibly navigate its obstacles. AI will prove to be a priceless ally in the fight for improved patient outcomes and healthcare delivery if research and ethical standards are upheld as technology advances (Khang et al., 2024).

REFERENCES

Akobeng, A. K. (2007, May). Understanding diagnostic tests 3: Receiver operating characteristic curves. *Acta Paediatrica (Oslo, Norway)*, *96*(5), 644–647. doi:10.1111/j.1651-2227.2006.00178.x PMID:17376185

Barbosa, M., & Chalmers, J. D. (2023). Bronchiectasis. *La Presse Medicale*, *52*(3), 104174. doi:10.1016/j.lpm.2023.104174 PMID:37778637

Brown, R., Cheng, Y., Haacke, M., Thompson, M., & Venkatesan, R. (2014). *Magnetic Resonance Imaging: Physical Principles and Sequence Design*. Wiley. doi:10.1002/9781118633953

Cabrilo, I., Bijlenga, P., & Schaller, K. (2014, September). Augmented reality in the surgery of cerebral arteriovenous malformations: Technique assessment and considerations. *Acta Neurochirurgica*, *156*(9), 1769–1774. doi:10.1007/s00701-014-2183-9 PMID:25037466

Char, D. S., Shah, N. H., & Magnus, D. (2018, March 15). Implementing Machine Learning in Health Care - Addressing Ethical Challenges. *The New England Journal of Medicine*, *378*(11), 981–983. doi:10.1056/NEJMp1714229 PMID:29539284

Chartrand, G., Cheng, P. M., Vorontsov, E., Drozdzal, M., Turcotte, S., Pal, C. J., Kadoury, S., & Tang, A. (2017, November-December). Deep Learning: A Primer for Radiologists. *Radiographics*, *37*(7), 2113–2131. doi:10.1148/rg.2017170077 PMID:29131760

Cho, K., Van Merriënboer, B., Gülçehre, Ç., Bahdanau, D., Bougares, F., Schwenk, H., & Bengio, Y. (2014). Learning Phrase Representations using RNN Encoder-Decoder for Statistical Machine Translation. *arXiv (Cornell University)*. /arxiv.1406.1078 doi:10.3115/v1/D14-1179

DeLong, E. R., DeLong, D. M., & Clarke-Pearson, D. L. (1988, September). Comparing the areas under two or more correlated receiver operating characteristic curves: A nonparametric approach. *Biometrics*, *44*(3), 837–845. doi:10.2307/2531595 PMID:3203132

Doi, K. (2007, June-July). Computer-aided diagnosis in medical imaging: Historical review, current status and future potential. *Computerized Medical Imaging and Graphics*, *31*(4-5), 198–211. doi:10.1016/j.compmedimag.2007.02.002 PMID:17349778

Emanuel, E. J., & Wachter, R. M. (2019, June 18). Artificial Intelligence in Health Care: Will the Value Match the Hype? *Journal of the American Medical Association*, *321*(23), 2281–2282. doi:10.1001/jama.2019.4914 PMID:31107500

Erickson, B. J., Korfiatis, P., Akkus, Z., & Kline, T. L. (2017, March-April). Machine Learning for Medical Imaging. *Radiographics*, *37*(2), 505–515. doi:10.1148/rg.2017160130 PMID:28212054

Esteva, A., Kuprel, B., Novoa, R. A., Ko, J., Swetter, S. M., Blau, H. M., & Thrun, S. (2017, February 2). Dermatologist-level classification of skin cancer with deep neural networks. *Nature*, *542*(7639), 115–118. doi:10.1038/nature21056 PMID:28117445

Fernández-Alemán, J. L., Señor, I. C., Lozoya, P. Á., & Toval, A. (2013, June). Security and privacy in electronic health records: A systematic literature review. *Journal of Biomedical Informatics*, *46*(3), 541–562. doi:10.1016/j.jbi.2012.12.003 PMID:23305810

Gillies, R. J., Kinahan, P. E., & Hricak, H. (2016, February). Radiomics: Images Are More than Pictures, They Are Data. *Radiology*, *278*(2), 563–577. doi:10.1148/radiol.2015151169 PMID:26579733

Glas, A. S., Lijmer, J. G., Prins, M. H., Bonsel, G. J., & Bossuyt, P. M. (2003, November). The diagnostic odds ratio: A single indicator of test performance. *Journal of Clinical Epidemiology*, *56*(11), 1129–1135. doi:10.1016/S0895-4356(03)00177-X PMID:14615004

Goodfellow, I. J., Pouget-Abadie, J., Mirza, M., Xu, B., Warde-Farley, D., Ozair, S., Courville, A., & Bengio, Y. (2014). Generative adversarial networks. *arXiv (Cornell University)*. https://doi.org//arxiv.1406.2661 doi:10.48550

Gulshan, V., Peng, L., Coram, M., Stumpe, M. C., Wu, D., Narayanaswamy, A., Venugopalan, S., Widner, K., Madams, T., Cuadros, J., Kim, R., Raman, R., Nelson, P. C., Mega, J. L., & Webster, D. R. (2016, December 13). Development and Validation of a Deep Learning Algorithm for Detection of Diabetic Retinopathy in Retinal Fundus Photographs. *Journal of the American Medical Association*, *316*(22), 2402–2410. doi:10.1001/jama.2016.17216 PMID:27898976

Hamburg, M. A., & Collins, F. S. (2010, July 22). The path to personalized medicine. *The New England Journal of Medicine*, *363*(4), 301–304. doi:10.1056/NEJMp1006304 PMID:20551152

Hosny, A., Parmar, C., Quackenbush, J., Schwartz, L. H., & Aerts, H. J. W. L. (2018, August). Artificial intelligence in radiology. *Nature Reviews. Cancer*, *18*(8), 500–510. doi:10.1038/s41568-018-0016-5 PMID:29777175

Huang, H. K., Aberle, D. R., Lufkin, R., Grant, E. G., Hanafee, W. N., & Kangarloo, H. (1990, February 1). Advances in medical imaging. *Annals of Internal Medicine*, *112*(3), 203–220. doi:10.7326/0003-4819-112-3-203 PMID:2404446

Huang, J., Saleh, S., & Liu, Y. (2021). A review on Artificial intelligence in education. *Academic Journal of Interdisciplinary Studies*, *10*(3), 206. doi:10.36941/ajis-2021-0077

Kahn, C. E. Jr, Langlotz, C. P., Channin, D. S., & Rubin, D. L. (2011, January-February). Informatics in radiology: An information model of the DICOM standard. *Radiographics*, *31*(1), 295–304. doi:10.1148/rg.311105085 PMID:20980665

Kamalov, F., Pourghebleh, B., Gheisari, M., Liu, Y., & Moussa, S. (2023). Internet of Medical Things Privacy and Security: Challenges, Solutions, and Future Trends from a New Perspective. *Sustainability (Basel)*, *15*(4), 3317. doi:10.3390/su15043317

Khang, A. (2023). *AI and IoT-Based Technologies for Precision Medicine* (1st ed.). IGI Global Press. doi:10.4018/979-8-3693-0876-9

Khang, A. (2024). *Medical Robotics and AI-Assisted Diagnostics for a High-Tech Healthcare Industry* (1st ed.). IGI Global Press. doi:10.4018/979-8-3693-2105-8

Khang, A., & Abdullayev, V. A. (2023). *AI-Aided Data Analytics Tools and Applications for the Healthcare Sector. In AI and IoT-Based Technologies for Precision Medicine* (1st ed.). IGI Global Press. doi:10.4018/979-8-3693-0876-9.ch018

Khang, A., & Hajimahmud, V. A. (2024). *Cloud Platform and Data Storage Systems in Healthcare Ecosystem. In Medical Robotics and AI-Assisted Diagnostics for a High-Tech Healthcare Industry* (1st ed.). IGI Global Press. doi:10.4018/979-8-3693-2105-8.ch022

Khang, A., Rath, K. C., Anh, P. T. N., Rath, S. K., & Bhattacharya, S. (2024). *Quantum-Based Robotics in High-Tech Healthcare Industry: Innovations and Applications. In Medical Robotics and AI-Assisted Diagnostics for a High-Tech Healthcare Industry* (1st ed.). IGI Global Press. doi:10.4018/979-8-3693-2105-8.ch001

Kim, D., Oh, G., Seo, Y., & Kim, Y. (2017). Reinforcement Learning-Based optimal flat spin recovery for unmanned aerial vehicle. *Journal of Guidance, Control, and Dynamics*, *40*(4), 1076–1084. doi:10.2514/1.G001739

Kjær, A., Loft, A., Law, I., Berthelsen, A. K., Borgwardt, L., Löfgren, J., Johnbeck, C. B., Hansen, A. E., Keller, S., Holm, S., & Højgaard, L. (2013, February). PET/MRI in cancer patients: First experiences and vision from Copenhagen. *Magma (New York, N.Y.)*, *26*(1), 37–47. doi:10.1007/s10334-012-0357-0 PMID:23266511

Kohli, M., Prevedello, L. M., Filice, R. W., & Geis, J. R. (2017, April). Implementing Machine Learning in Radiology Practice and Research. *AJR. American Journal of Roentgenology*, *208*(4), 754–760. doi:10.2214/AJR.16.17224 PMID:28125274

LeCun, Y., Bengio, Y., & Hinton, G. (2015, May 28). Deep learning. *Nature*, *521*(7553), 436–444. doi:10.1038/nature14539 PMID:26017442

Leung, K. Y. (2021, July 6). Applications of Advanced Ultrasound Technology in Obstetrics. *Diagnostics (Basel)*, *11*(7), 1217. doi:10.3390/diagnostics11071217 PMID:34359300

Litjens, G., Kooi, T., Bejnordi, B. E., Setio, A. A. A., Ciompi, F., Ghafoorian, M., van der Laak, J. A. W. M., van Ginneken, B., & Sánchez, C. I. (2017, December). A survey on deep learning in medical image analysis. *Medical Image Analysis*, *42*, 60–88. doi:10.1016/j.media.2017.07.005 PMID:28778026

Liu, X., Faes, L., Kale, A. U., Wagner, S. K., Fu, D. J., Bruynseels, A., Mahendiran, T., Moraes, G., Shamdas, M., Kern, C., Ledsam, J. R., Schmid, M. K., Balaskas, K., Topol, E. J., Bachmann, L. M., Keane, P. A., & Denniston, A. K. (2019, October). A comparison of deep learning performance against healthcare professionals in detecting diseases from medical imaging: A systematic review and meta-analysis. *The Lancet. Digital Health*, *1*(6), e271–e297. doi:10.1016/S2589-7500(19)30123-2 PMID:33323251

Lundervold, A. S., & Lundervold, A. (2019, May). An overview of deep learning in medical imaging focusing on MRI. *Zeitschrift für Medizinische Physik*, *29*(2), 102–127. doi:10.1016/j.zemedi.2018.11.002 PMID:30553609

McKinney, S. M., Sieniek, M., Godbole, V., Godwin, J., Antropova, N., Ashrafian, H., Back, T., Chesus, M., Corrado, G. S., Darzi, A., Etemadi, M., Garcia-Vicente, F., Gilbert, F. J., Halling-Brown, M., Hassabis, D., Jansen, S., Karthikesalingam, A., Kelly, C. J., King, D., & Shetty, S. (2020, January). International evaluation of an AI system for breast cancer screening. *Nature*, *577*(7788), 89–94. doi:10.1038/s41586-019-1799-6 PMID:31894144

Miotto, R., Wang, F., Wang, S., Jiang, X., & Dudley, J. T. (2018, November 27). Deep learning for healthcare: Review, opportunities and challenges. *Briefings in Bioinformatics*, *19*(6), 1236–1246. doi:10.1093/bib/bbx044 PMID:28481991

Niewiadomski, R., & Anderson, D. (2017). The rise of artificial intelligence. In Advances in computational intelligence and robotics book series (pp. 29–49). IGI Global. doi:10.4018/978-1-5225-1656-9.ch003

Obermeyer, Z., & Emanuel, E. J. (2016, September 29). Predicting the Future - Big Data, Machine Learning, and Clinical Medicine. *The New England Journal of Medicine*, *375*(13), 1216–1219. doi:10.1056/NEJMp1606181 PMID:27682033

Obermeyer, Z., Powers, B., Vogeli, C., & Mullainathan, S. (2019, October 25). Dissecting racial bias in an algorithm used to manage the health of populations. *Science*, *366*(6464), 447–453. doi:10.1126/science.aax2342 PMID:31649194

Panchbhai, A. S. (2015). Wilhelm Conrad Röntgen and the discovery of X-rays: Revisited after centennial. *Journal of Indian Academy of Oral Medicine and Radiology*, *27*(1), 90-95. doi:10.4103/0972-1363.167119

Pesapane, F., Volonté, C., Codari, M., & Sardanelli, F. (2018, October). Artificial intelligence as a medical device in radiology: Ethical and regulatory issues in Europe and the United States. *Insights Into Imaging*, *9*(5), 745–753. doi:10.1007/s13244-018-0645-y PMID:30112675

Preskill, J. (2018, August 6). Quantum Computing in the NISQ era and beyond. *Quantum : the Open Journal for Quantum Science*, *2*, 79. doi:10.22331/q-2018-08-06-79

Rajkomar, A., Dean, J., & Kohane, I. (2019, April 4). Machine Learning in Medicine. *The New England Journal of Medicine*, *380*(14), 1347–1358. doi:10.1056/NEJMra1814259 PMID:30943338

Rodríguez-Ruiz, A., Krupinski, E., Mordang, J. J., Schilling, K., Heywang-Köbrunner, S. H., Sechopoulos, I., & Mann, R. M. (2019, February). Detection of Breast Cancer with Mammography: Effect of an Artificial Intelligence Support System. *Radiology*, *290*(2), 305–314. doi:10.1148/radiol.2018181371 PMID:30457482

Rowe, S. P., & Pomper, M. G. (2022, July). Molecular imaging in oncology: Current impact and future directions. *CA: a Cancer Journal for Clinicians*, *72*(4), 333–352. doi:10.3322/caac.21713 PMID:34902160

Rudin, C. (2019). Stop explaining black box machine learning models for high stakes decisions and use interpretable models instead. *Nature Machine Intelligence*, *1*(5), 206–215. doi:10.1038/s42256-019-0048-x PMID:35603010

Salani, M., Roy, S., & Fissell, W. H. IV. (2018, November). Innovations in Wearable and Implantable Artificial Kidneys. *American Journal of Kidney Diseases*, *72*(5), 745–751. doi:10.1053/j.ajkd.2018.06.005 PMID:30146422

Sharma, S., Kelly, T. K., & Jones, P. A. (2010, January). Epigenetics in cancer. *Carcinogenesis*, *31*(1), 27–36. doi:10.1093/carcin/bgp220 PMID:19752007

Shi, Y., & Liu, Z. (2023). Evolution from Medical Imaging to Visualized Medicine. *Advances in Experimental Medicine and Biology*, *1199*, 1–13. doi:10.1007/978-981-32-9902-3_1 PMID:37460724

Shin, H., Roth, H. R., Gao, M., Lü, L., Xu, Z., Nogues, I., Yao, J., Mollura, D. J., & Summers, R. M. (2016). Deep Convolutional Neural Networks for Computer-Aided Detection: CNN architectures, dataset characteristics and transfer learning. *IEEE Transactions on Medical Imaging*, *35*(5), 1285–1298. doi:10.1109/TMI.2016.2528162 PMID:26886976

Sokolova, M., & Lapalme, G. (2009). A systematic analysis of performance measures for classification tasks. *Information Processing & Management*, *45*(4), 427–437. doi:10.1016/j.ipm.2009.03.002

Topol, E. J. (2019, January). High-performance medicine: The convergence of human and artificial intelligence. *Nature Medicine*, *25*(1), 44–56. doi:10.1038/s41591-018-0300-7 PMID:30617339

Vayena, E., Blasimme, A., & Cohen, I. G. (2018, November 6). Machine learning in medicine: Addressing ethical challenges. *PLoS Medicine*, *15*(11), e1002689. doi:10.1371/journal.pmed.1002689 PMID:30399149

Vayena, E., Blasimme, A., & Cohen, I. G. (2018, November 6). Machine learning in medicine: Addressing ethical challenges. *PLoS Medicine*, *15*(11), e1002689. doi:10.1371/journal.pmed.1002689 PMID:30399149

Wang, F., Casalino, L. P., & Khullar, D. (2019, March 1). Deep Learning in Medicine-Promise, Progress, and Challenges. *JAMA Internal Medicine*, *179*(3), 293–294. doi:10.1001/jamainternmed.2018.7117 PMID:30556825

Yamashita, R., Nishio, M., Do, R. K. G., & Togashi, K. (2018, August). Convolutional neural networks: An overview and application in radiology. *Insights Into Imaging*, *9*(4), 611–629. doi:10.1007/s13244-018-0639-9 PMID:29934920

Chapter 11
Internet of Things– Combined Deep Learning for Electroencephalography– Based E–Healthcare

Sima Das
Maulana Abul Kalam Azad University of Technology, West Bengal, India

Ahona Ghosh
🆔 https://orcid.org/0000-0003-0498-285X
Maulana Abul Kalam Azad University of Technology, West Bengal, India

Sriparna Saha
🆔 https://orcid.org/0000-0002-7312-2450
Maulana Abul Kalam Azad University of Technology, West Bengal, India

ABSTRACT

Deep Learning (DL) is the most popular subset of machine learning, with many applications in healthcare and other areas. On the other hand, electroencephalography has effectively solved different brain activity-related healthcare applications. This non-invasive data collection method can monitor and diagnose brain-based health conditions as it is painless and safe. This chapter discusses different smart healthcare applications of DL. Different DL models applied in the existing literature have been described also, from which future researchers will benefit by having a clear insight into the concerned area. Then a smart health framework has been proposed where step by step-by-step process of designing the system has been presented using the Internet of Things (IoT) combined with DL.

1. INTRODUCTION

Nowadays, Deep Learning (DL) is the prevalent technique applied in a wide variety of domains, including speech recognition, object recognition, disorder forecasting, bioinformatics, biomedicine, etc. Programs relating to fitness care and health technology are rapidly expanding. Incredible development of data sci-

DOI: 10.4018/979-8-3693-3679-3.ch011

ence, Internet of Things (IoT) related gadgets, and good-performing processors operating graphical and tensor processing units are the foremost reasons behind the introduction of DL (Bolhasani et al., 2021).

The adage "Health is Wealth" is very much appropriate in the current world. The fast-paced lifestyle, rising pollution, and the emergence of epidemic and pandemic diseases have resulted in a poor and unhealthy quality of human life. Mental health in this concern is as important as physical health. Brain activity analysis is typically regarded as a crucial area in neuroscience. Keeping mental and cognitive health in consideration, Electroencephalography (EEG) data is gathered noninvasively from people in diverse behavioral circumstances (Nahmias et al., 2020). EEG is a kind of brain signal recording device, activated during electrical activities by neuronic firing and taken by electrode channels located on the participant's scalp. The taken signal is further processed through different stages with the final intention of categorizing the disease (Das & Bhattacharya, 2021; Das et al., 2020).

One of the demanding situations in recognition tasks is understanding powerful representations with consistent performances from EEG signals (Das et al., 2022). DL carried out on EEG data to find patterns associated with different disorders are being utilized in developing diagnostic technique and predicting disease (Aghaeeaval, 2021). To keep away bias, the captured signal can be classified by a DL technique. The quantitative EEG and scientific information comprise prognostic data for patient outcomes. Human emotion should significantly contribute to human-computer interaction with promising programs in Artificial Intelligence (AI). EEG is broadly applied to analyze tense situations like epilepsy, neurodegenerative illnesses, and sleep-related issues (Aqeel et al., 2022). Establishing semantic information sharing among heterogeneous data is a crucial problem in dealing with the incredible capacity of various medical systems (Chong & Ali, 2021). The affected person's status tracking and the EEG processing consequences are shared with healthcare carriers, who can verify the affected person's condition and provide emergency assistance as per the need (Amin, Hossain, Muhammad, Alhussein, & Rahman, 2019).

The next section analyses some existing smart healthcare applications inducing DL techniques. Section 3 step by step presents the proposed work. Section 4 discusses the corresponding experimental results. Section 5 finally concludes the work.

2. SMART HEALTHCARE APPLICATIONS INDUCING DEEP LEARNING

According to recent research, almost 90% of the population is exposed to a contaminated environment (Sharma & Joshi, 2021). Furthermore, most people live in poverty due to the industrial revolution and population boom. As a result, it is vital to monitor, improve, and promote a healthy lifestyle. Along with physical health, mental health analysis is also important at every stage of life, from childhood and adolescence through adulthood. Schizophrenia (Sz) is a brain condition that significantly impacts people's thoughts, behavior, and moods worldwide. EEG is a useful biomarker in the detection of Sz, which is a non-linear time-series signal, and because of its non-linear structure, using it for research is extremely important. Sharma *et al*. (2021) used a DL framework to increase EEG-based Sz detection efficiency. Schizophrenia Hybrid Neural Network (Sz HNN), a new hybrid DL framework merging Long Short-Term Memory (LSTM) and Convolutional Neural Networks (CNN), has been proposed in their work where the CNN is used for local feature extraction and the LSTM is used in classification. The suggested model was compared against traditional machine learning (ML) and DL models tested on two distinct datasets, with the first dataset having 19 participant's data and the second dataset having 16 participants. Electrodes are applied to the scalp and cleaned with a conducting gel to assess the electrical activity of neuronal populations (scalp electrodes) to collect EEG data. Several studies were carried out with varied parametric tunings on various frequency bands and several groups of scalp electrodes. Based on the results of all the tests, the hybrid framework has a better classification accuracy of 89.9% compared to other models. With only five electrodes, the suggested model overwhelms the effect of multiple frequency bands and achieves a 91% accuracy. The model is also tested for smart healthcare and remote monitoring applications using the Internet of Medical Things framework.

DL and Transfer Learning (TL) are subsections of AI, specifically ML. Multiple layers record relevant data that increasingly extract advanced-level features from the primary data and based on similarity pattern, classifies those resulting in useful information. DL models are employed in various fields, including smart health monitoring, and telemedicine (Cai et al., 2020), while TL is used to apply the knowledge gained from past situations. However, it causes negative transfer issues in the study for researchers and engineers, which refers to the reduction of the accuracy of a DL model after re-training. The combination of IoT and DL has been widely recognized as a potential solution for easing the strain on healthcare systems and thus has an emphasis on contemporary research in these systems.

2.1 Posture Detection

Body positions and gesture detection are key DL applications in smart household setups. Desai et al. (2015) developed a Restricted Boltzmann Model for detecting body positions from wearable data. Weizmann human silhouette-based action database was used to test the model which consists of nine films representing nine different behaviors from nine participants. The body postures were recognized with 80% accuracy by the model.

2.2 Activity Detection

Sensor-based human activity detection has become more prevalent as sensor and ubiquitous computing frameworks have grown popular. Wang et al. (2016) developed a Stacked Autoencoder (SAE) model to distinguish individual actions. They tested their findings using three open-source datasets containing sensory records from three smart houses. The model was tested against the k-Nearest Neighbour (kNN), Support Vector Machine (SVM), Naive Bayes, and Hidden Markov Model (HMM) algorithms, and the SAE outperformed all the shallow models. The authors suggested adjusting hyper-parameters like the number of hidden units and layers could improve the model. Park *et al.* (2016) used the Recurrent Neural Network (RNN) to recognize human behavior in another study. The researchers tested their findings on the MSRC-12 gesture dataset, depicting human activities as temporal modifications at distinct joint angles. With a 92.55% accuracy rate, the model could detect twelve activities. The study also compared RNN's performance to the HMM and Deep Belief Network (DBN), finding that RNN surpasses HMM by 7.06% and the DBN by 2.01%.

2.3 Disease Prediction

A functional anomaly or disruption is referred to as a disorder and it is classified into two types: mental and physical. While being independent and self-sufficient is everyone's dream, persons suffering from mental disorders, like depression (Biswas et al., 2022), anxiety, and stress leading to various personality traits (Mitra et al., 2022), must be diagnosed early for quick recovery of their brain functionality.

2.4 Health Monitoring

For examining and recovering one's health, health monitoring is essential. This category of applications uses DL to provide critical advice to people with health problems and alert healthcare personnel in an emergency. Amin et al. (2019) proposed a healthcare architecture based on the IoT and the cloud for real-time patient monitoring. Using an EEG classification use case, the framework was assessed. The patient's EEG waves were sent to the cloud, where a DL module with CNNs separated the signals into two categories: abnormal and normal. Visual Geometry Group 16 (VGG16) and Alexnet, two pre-trained CNN models, were applied. The SVM classifier replaced the final classification layer in both topologies. The authors showed that their suggested Alexnet performed better than the VGG-16 and different existing approaches. The authors in Xue et al. (2018) developed an RNN-based model to predict obesity positions on step count, demographics, and blood pressure. Having a 0.5 dropout rate, the model had twenty-five hidden units. A total of 150 epochs were used to train the model. Experiments revealed that the model was effective in projecting obesity status improvement. The model can be used to predict the status of diabetes and hypertension, according to Qinghan *et al.* However, to increase forecast accuracy, the scientists may include additional characteristics such as nutrition.

In the context of missing data, Nguyen et al. (2018) used RNN to model the evolution of Alzheimer's disease. The researchers presented a 256-unit RNN with Adam as an optimizer and categorical cross-entropy as a loss function. Variational dropout and L2 regularisation were utilized to prevent model overfitting. Using 100 epochs, the model was trained. The RNN performed better than the traditional architectures in the experiments. To identify distinct stages of sleep, they built a system using Stacked SAE (Najdi et al., 2017). Three layers made up the model: a two-layered Stacked SAE and a soft-max layer. There were 20 concealed units in the first layer of the Stacked SAE. In the second layer, there were 12 when the suggested model's performance was compared to that of the kNN and SoftMax classifiers. Their model performed better than the existing models of classification.

3. PROPOSED WORK

This section describes the step-by-step proposed work. The proposed work is based on the IoT combined with DL for the electronic healthcare (e-healthcare) system (Chakraborty et al., 2020), as shown in Figure 1. In this chapter, our proposed system is based on three steps. In Step 1, input is taken from the brain using an EEG sensor, and raw data is pre-processed. In Step 2, data is analyzed with the help of an expert knowledge database. In Step 3, classification is performed using several DL-based techniques for disease detection. Finally, the classification results are forwarded to healthcare professionals who monitor the patient's status, and remedies to the health issues are prescribed accordingly when needed.

3.1 Dataset Collection

The dataset collection is the first and initial step for any healthcare diagnosis system. The raw dataset is collected from the human scalp by an EEG sensor focusing on the P300 signal. An event-related potential (ERP) (Flöck & Walla, 2020) component triggered during the decision-making process is the P300 (P300) (Zhong et al., 2019) wave. It is regarded as an endogenous potential since the cause of its existence is linked to a person's response to the stimulus rather than the stimulus's physical characteristics. The P300 is supposed to reflect unique processes involved in categorization or sensory evaluation. The oddball paradigm, which combines high-probability non-target (or "standard") items with low-probability target items, is typically used to elicit it. EEG recordings show it to manifest as a positive voltage deflection with a latency (delay between stimulus and reaction) of approximately 250 to 500 ms (Olichney et al., 2022). After raw dataset collection, the next step is to store data in a cloud database.

3.2 Data Analysis and Feature Extraction

After dataset collection and storage, the next step is the analysis of the raw data stored in the cloud. The data analysis is done by filtering, artifact removal, and feature extraction. As the EEG signals are found to be contaminated with noise, a band pass filter (BPF) is employed in the (4-16 Hz), covering the theta band (4-8 Hz), the alpha band (8-12 Hz), and the beta band (12-16 Hz) (Newson & Thiagarajan, 2019). Several prototype models of BPF, including Butterworth, Chebyshev, and the like, are available in the literature (Kawala-Sterniuk et al., 2020). First, the Chebyshev filter of order 16 is chosen for its low ripples and narrow sidebands in comparison to its competitors like Butterworth. After filtering, as an artifact removal tool, the Independent Component Analysis (ICA) (Tharwat, 2021) is applied to the filtered data to identify the location of actual signal sources as shown in Figure 1.

Figure 1. Proposed work for DL-based e-healthcare

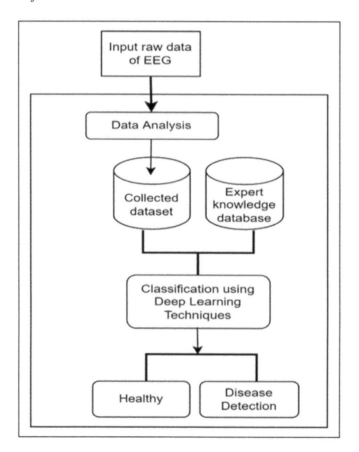

Traditional feature extraction strategies are effective and lengthy systems; however, aiming at new applications, a DL model like CNN (Ghosh & Saha, 2022) enables acquiring new powerful feature illustrations from expert knowledge databases. The CNN model in our experiment extracts features using one convolutional layer followed by one max pooling and one convolutional layer. For the RNN (Ghosh & Saha, 2021) and Back Propagation Neural Network (BPNN) (Wright et al., 2022) based frameworks, Power Spectral Density (PSD) (Muhammad et al., 2021) has been considered to extract frequency domain features from the noise-free EEG data, where the feature matrix includes the sum, the mean, the standard deviation, the kurtosis, the skewness, and the root mean square of alpha, beta, and theta frequency bands of the obtained EEG samples (Bag et al., 2023).

3.3 Classification using DL techniques

This section discusses DL-based classification techniques like CNN, RNN, and BPNN applied to diagnose the subject in our e-health framework.

3.3.1 Convolutional Neural Network

In DL, a CNN is a category of Artificial Neural Network (ANN) (Abiodun et al., 2019), most usually carried out in image processing and signal processing applications. CNNs are normalized variations of multilayer perceptron (MLP) (Almeida, 2020). MLP generally means connected networks, in which each neuron in a single layer is associated with all neurons in the subsequent layer. Filter in the CNN framework refers to the weights found by the convolutions. For instance, a 3×3 convolution is called a filter, which has ten weights including one bias. Those networks' full connectivity makes them vulnerable to overfitting facts (Arora et al., 2020; Goularas & Kamis, 2019). After successful feature extraction by the first three layers, the fully connected layer finally classifies the data in the CNN framework of our experiment. The block diagram is presented in Figure 2.

Figure 2. Block diagram of convolutional neural network

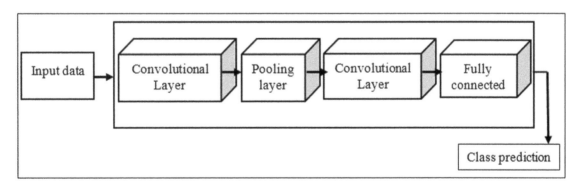

3.3.2 Recurrent Neural Network

An RNN is a category of ANN wherein connections between nodes shape a directed or undirected graph in conjunction with a temporal collection. This lets it exhibit temporal dynamic conduct. As a derivative of feedforward neural networks (Suganthan & Katuwal, 2021), RNNs can use their inside storage system to method variable period collection of inputs (Chowdhury & Kashem, 2008; Shao, 2008). The block diagram is presented in Figure 3. Since it is ideal for sequential data processing, the time series EEG data has considered the RNN architecture as the proposed classifier.

3.3.3 Backpropagation Neural Network

BPNN is the core of the neural network. It is the method of tuning a neural network's weights based on the error acquired from the earlier epoch (new release). Appropriate tuning of the weights lessens error values and makes the model dependable by increasing its simplification. Backpropagation in a neural network is short for backward propagation of errors. This approach allows calculating the gradient of a loss feature with appreciation to all the weights inside the network (Jiang & Shen, 2019; Lydia & Francis, 2019) as shown in Figure 3 and Figure 4.

Figure 3. Block diagram of recurrent neural network

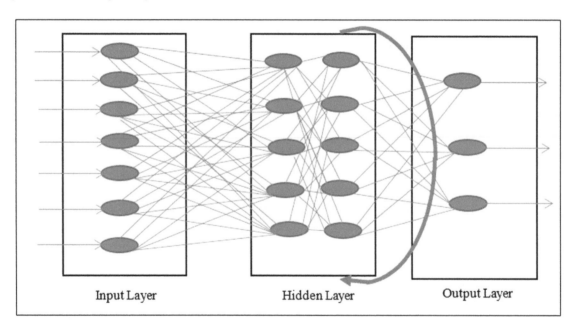

Input Layer   Hidden Layer   Output Layer

Alt-text: Figure 3 presents the block diagram of RNN architecture.
Alt-text: Figure 4 presents the block diagram of BPNN architecture.

3.4 Introduction to the Internet-of-Things

Internet-of-Things (IoT) has primarily integrated cloud computing capabil*ities and initiated the creation of ubiquitous connectivity in our framework. The Google Cloud Services has been employed with Message Queuing Telemetry Transport (MQTT) based IoT platform to avail this (Wardana et al., 2019). The

Figure 4. Block diagram of backpropagation neural network

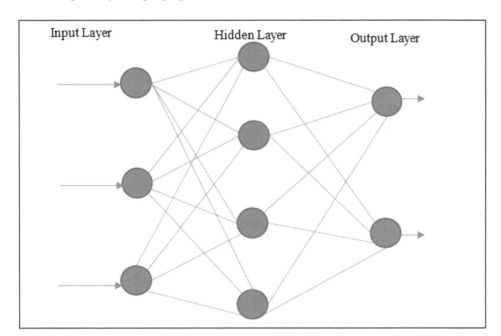

forwarded diagnosis results are used by the doctors or concerned healthcare professionals for checking and confirming them and suggesting required steps to the patient for the betterment of life.

4. DISCUSSIONS AND RESULTS

The experimental outcomes have been discussed in this section. Also, a comparative analysis has been performed between the proposed model and its competitors already discussed as shown in Figure 5.

Figure 5. User display in the experimental paradigm

A	B	C	D	E	F
G	H	I	J	K	L
M	N	O	P	Q	R
S	T	U	V	W	X
Y	Z	1	2	3	4
5	6	7	8	9	-

4.1 Dataset Description

A patient database has been downloaded from a publicly available dataset (Riccio et al., 2013) where EEG data from eight channels according to the 10/10 standard (Fz, Cz, Pz, Oz, P3, P4, PO7, and PO8) has been acquired from eight Amyotrophic Lateral Sclerosis (ALS) (Newell et al., 2022) patients to investigate the support of attentional and memory processes in controlling a P300-based Brain Computing Interface (BCI) paradigm (Gao, Wang, Chen et al, 2021).

The experimental data for the healthy subjects is acquired in the Human-Computer Interaction (HCI) (Ren & Bao, 2020; Sampath, 2023) Laboratory of MAKAUT, WB following the pattern of (Riccio et al., 2013) using the BrainTech Traveler EEG device. From the twenty-one-channel data, the most relevant eight-channel data has been selected. Here, the data has been collected from 5 healthy subjects where the subjects are asked to copy and spell seven predefined words of five characters each (runs), by controlling a P300 speller. Figure 5 illustrates the 6✕6 matrix of characters shown to the subjects where the desired character was present in two of the twelve intensifications of rows or columns (i.e., one specific row and one specific column). The reactions induced by these infrequent stimuli (i.e., the two stimuli out of twelve having the desired character) differ from those evoked by the stimuli that do not contain the desired character and are comparable to the P300 responses (Namita, 2023).

4.2 Data Analysis

Since it is not feasible to present feature extraction results from all the epochs due to space constraints, Table 1 shows feature space (mentioned in Section 3.2) generated from epoch 1, trial 1, class 1, and subject 1.

Table 1. Features extracted from the first epoch, first trial, first class, and the first subject

	Mean	Standard deviation	RMS	Skewness	Kurtosis	Sum
Frequency of Alpha wave (Hz)	10	5	7	12	11	103
Frequency of Beta wave (Hz)	15	12	13	21	23	169
Frequency of Gamma wave (Hz)	50	21	53	18	32	124

4.3 CNN-Based Classification Results

The activation function denoted by f, and used for the classification task has been considered a hyperparameter and has been varied between sigmoid, hyperbolic tangent (tanh), and Rectified Linear Unit (ReLU) (Rasamoelina et al., 2020). Among these functions, ReLU is the most common one and has outperformed the others as shown in the Receiver Operating Characteristics (ROC) curves of Figure 6. Apart from the activation function, the optimizer (o) also has varied between Stochastic Gradient Descent (SGD), Adaptive Moment (Adam) Estimation, Root Mean Square (RMS Prop), Adadelta, Adaptive Gradient Descent (AdaGrad), and Adamax (Bera & Shrivastava, 2020). Figure 6 signifies that the combination of ReLU and AdaGrad as the activation function and optimizer respectively has best suited the model and the curve has been marked bold (Namita, 2023).

4.4 RNN-Based Classification Results

The ROC curves shown in Figure 7 indicate that the tanh as the activation function and Adam as the optimizer have outperformed the other combinations, since, 0.84 as the Area Under the Curve (AUC) value is higher than the optimized CNN and BPNN and the curve has been marked bold. Thus, the choice of RNN as the time series EEG classifier has been suitable in the concerned scenario (Eswaran, 2023).

4.5 BPNN-Based Classification Results

The BPNN classifier in our e-healthcare framework also has considered two hyperparameters for possible tuning to improve its performance. Figure 6 signifies that among all the possible combinations, ReLU and Adamax as activation function and optimizer respectively have worked better and the curve has been marked bold (Khang et al., 2023).

4.6 Performance Comparison

All the DL models are applied to the validation and test data and the result is shown in Figure 8. RNN proved to be an excellent supportive method because it has the best accuracy (98.56% in validation and 96.79% in testing) values among other DL techniques (Khang, 2023b). The proposed method has the following advantages

- The chapter examines the usage of different kinds of DL methods in e-healthcare.
- EEG-based brain-computer interfaces can practically implement the proposed system.

Thus, the proposed system is suitable to be applied in real-time e-healthcare scenarios as shown in Figure 9.

5. CONCLUSION

The IoT generally upholds the smart medical care field; combined with computer vision, ML, and DL strategies; it offers quick and exact types of assistance for mechanized patient inconvenience observing or location predicting frameworks. Customary patient-checking frameworks are normally made of wearable sensors and vision-based strategies. Remote health monitoring and analysis can be acknowledged through smart healthcare (Bera & Shrivastava, 2020). First, this chapter summarizes smart healthcare-related existing DL techniques and IoT techniques, which help specialists by working on the conclusion of smart healthcare status in clinical practice. Then it uses a DL-based method to introduce an IoT-based non-invasive automatic patient uneasiness observing/ recognition framework.

The framework depends on EEG data and the features extracted from it are transmitted to a cloud server using the Internet. The server stores the feature space and transfers it to the DL-based classification model for further processing (Khang, 2023a). It has been proved that for the current EEG-based electronic healthcare framework, RNN is the most suitable technique for classifying the mental status of a patient into two classes, uneasiness, and normal. By employing cloud facilities, it is effective in larger e-heathcare scenario also, when remote monitoring is needed (Khang & Muthmainnah, 2023).

Figure 6. ROC curves generated from tuned hyperparameters of CNN

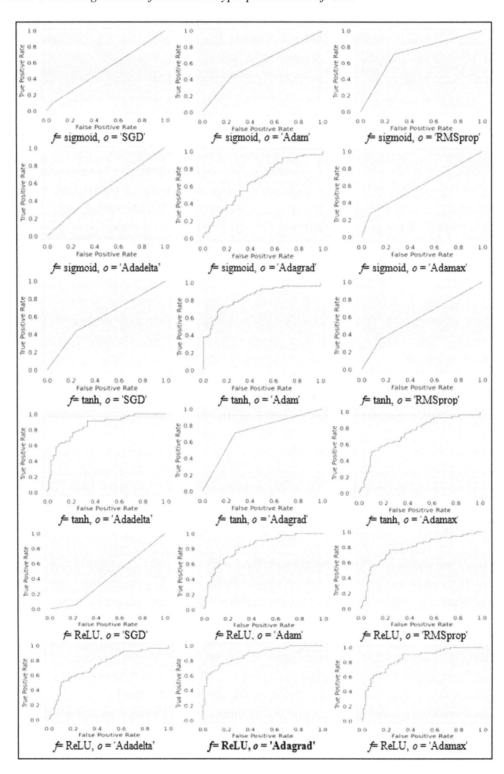

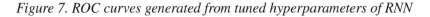

Figure 7. ROC curves generated from tuned hyperparameters of RNN

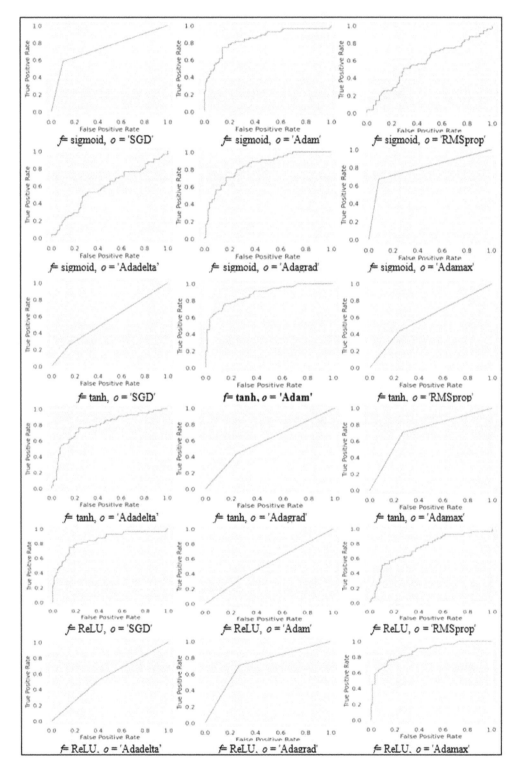

Figure 8. ROC curves generated from tuned hyperparameters of BPNN

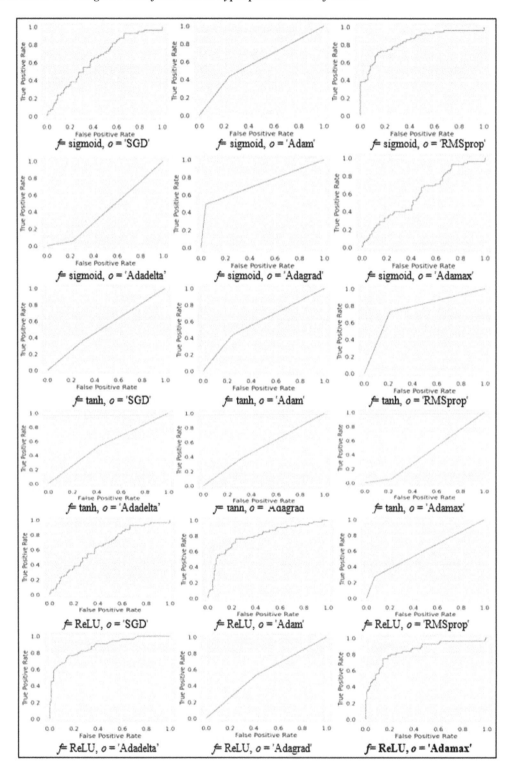

Figure 9. Disease prediction results using DL models

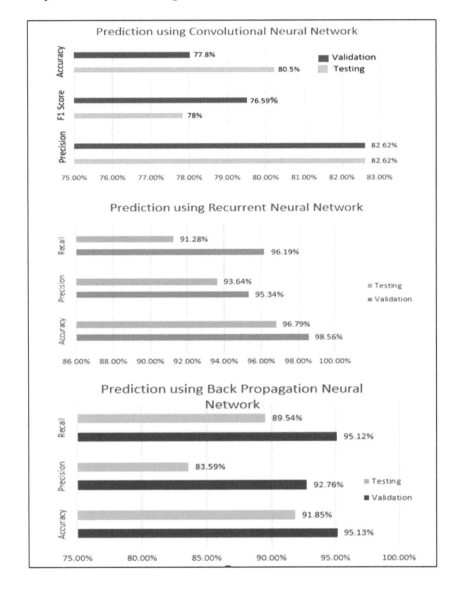

The generalizability of our findings to larger datasets and the effectiveness of different ML algorithms for finding the EEG patterns require more study (Khang & Abdullayev, 2023).

6. ACKNOWLEDGMENT

AICTE supported this work under the scheme of AICTE Doctoral Fellowship to A. Ghosh, with Ref. No.2.2.1/Regis./Appt.(AG)/Ph.D(ADF)/ 2021 dated 01.02.2021. UGC Start-up Grant supported this work to S. Saha under the scheme of Basic Scientific Research, File No. F.30-449/2018(BSR) dated 21.11.2019 and the university research seed money to S. Saha, File No.: 9.6/Regis./SD/Mn. (SS)/2019 dated 19.06.2019.

REFERENCES

Abiodun, O. I., Jantan, A., Omolara, A. E., Dada, K. V., Umar, A. M., Linus, O. U., Arshad, H., Kaza-ure, A. A., Gana, U., & Kiru, M. U. (2019). Comprehensive review of artificial neural network applications to pattern recognition. *IEEE Access : Practical Innovations, Open Solutions, 7*, 158820–158846. doi:10.1109/ACCESS.2019.2945545

Aghaeeaval, M. (2021). Prediction of patient survival following postanoxic coma using EEG data and clinical features. In *2021 43rd Annual International Conference of the IEEE Engineering in Medicine & Biology Society (EMBC)*. IEEE. 10.1109/EMBC46164.2021.9629946

Almeida, L. B. (2020). Multilayer perceptrons. In *Handbook of Neural Computation* (pp. C1–C2). CRC Press.

Amin, S. U., Hossain, M. S., Muhammad, G., Alhussein, M., & Rahman, M. A. (2019). Cognitive Smart Healthcare for Pathology Detection and Monitoring. *IEEE Access : Practical Innovations, Open Solutions, 7*, 10745–10753. doi:10.1109/ACCESS.2019.2891390

Aqeel, K. H., Rahat, U. A., Mehmood, K. A., Tanveer, B. H., Saima, S., Wasim, A., Didier, S., & Faisal, S. (2022). The NMT Scalp EEG Dataset: An Open-Source Annotated Dataset of Healthy and Pathological EEG Recordings for Predictive Modeling. *Frontiers in Neuroscience, 15*, 755817. doi:10.3389/fnins.2021.755817 PMID:35069095

Arora, D., Garg, M., & Gupta, M. (2020). Diving deep in Deep Convolutional Neural Network. In *2020 2nd International Conference on Advances in Computing, Communication Control and Networking (ICACCCN)* (pp. 749-751). IEEE. 10.1109/ICACCCN51052.2020.9362907

Arpita, N. (2023). Incorporating Artificial Intelligence (AI) for Precision Medicine: A Narrative Analysis. In AI and IoT-Based Technologies for Precision Medicine (1st ed.). IGI Global Press. doi:10.4018/979-8-3693-0876-9.ch002

Bag, D., Ghosh, A., & Saha, S. (2023). An Automatic Approach to Control Wheelchair Movement for Rehabilitation Using Electroencephalogram. In *Design and Control Advances in Robotics* (pp. 105–126). IGI Global.

Bera, S., & Shrivastava, V. K. (2020). Analysis of various optimizers on deep convolutional neural network model in the application of hyperspectral remote sensing image classification. *International Journal of Remote Sensing, 41*(7), 2664–2683. doi:10.1080/01431161.2019.1694725

Biswas, A., Mitra, A., Ghosh, A., Das, N., Ghosh, N., & Ghosh, A. (2022). A Deep Learning Approach to Classify the Causes of Depression from Reddit Posts. In *Machine Vision for Industry 4.0* (pp. 141–168). CRC Press. doi:10.1201/9781003122401-7

Boden, M., & Hawkins, J. (2005, March). Improved access to sequential motifs: A note on the architectural bias of recurrent networks. *IEEE Transactions on Neural Networks, 16*(2), 491–494. doi:10.1109/TNN.2005.844086 PMID:15787155

Bolhasani, H., Mohseni, M., & Rahmani, A. M. (2021). Deep learning applications for IoT in health care: A systematic review. *Informatics in Medicine Unlocked, 23*. doi:10.1016/j.imu.2021.100550

Cai, L., Gao, J., & Zhao, D. (2020). A review of the application of deep Learning in medical image classification and segmentation. *Annals of Translational Medicine*, *8*(11), 713. doi:10.21037/atm.2020.02.44 PMID:32617333

Chakraborty, D., Ghosh, A., & Saha, S. (2020). A survey on Internet-of-Thing applications using electroencephalogram. In *Emergence of Pharmaceutical Industry Growth with Industrial IoT Approach* (pp. 21–47). Academic Press. doi:10.1016/B978-0-12-819593-2.00002-9

Chong, & Ali, S. (2021). Schema Ontology Model to Support Semantic Interoperability in Healthcare Applications: Use Case of Depressive Disorder. In *2021 Twelfth International Conference on Ubiquitous and Future Networks (ICUFN),* (pp. 409-412). IEEE. 10.1109/ICUFN49451.2021.9528708.s

Chowdhury, N. & Kashem, M. (2008). A comparative analysis of Feedforward neural network & Recurrent Neural network to detect intrusion. In *2008 International Conference on Electrical and Computer Engineering* (pp. 488-492). IEEE. . doi:10.1109/ICECE.2008.4769258

Das, S. & Bhattacharya, A. (2021). *ECG Assess Heartbeat rate. Classifying using BPNN while Watching Movie and send Movie Rating through Telegram.* Springer. . doi:10.1007/978-981-15-9774-9_43

Das, S., Das, J., Modak, S., & Mazumdar, K. (2022). *Internet of Things with Machine Learning based smart Cardiovascular disease classifier for Healthcare in Secure platform.* Taylor & Francis.

Das, S., & Ghosh, L., & Saha, S. (2020). *Analyzing Gaming Effects on Cognitive Load Using Artificial Intelligent Tools.* IEEE. . doi:10.1109/CONECCT50063.2020.9198662

Desai, S. J., Shoaib, M., & Raychowdhury, A. (2015). An ultra-low power, "always-on" camera front-end for posture detection in body worn cameras using restricted boltzman machines. *IEEE Transactions on Multi-Scale Computing Systems*, *1*(4), 187–194. doi:10.1109/TMSCS.2015.2513741

Eswaran, U. (2023). Applying Machine Learning for Medical Image Processing. AI and IoT-Based Technologies for Precision Medicine (1st ed.). IGI Global Press. doi:10.4018/979-8-3693-0876-9.ch009

Fan, Z.-C., Chan, T.-S. T., Yang, Y.-H., & Jang, J.-S. R. (2020, July). Backpropagation With N -D Vector-Valued Neurons Using Arbitrary Bilinear Products. *IEEE Transactions on Neural Networks and Learning Systems*, *31*(7), 2638–2652. doi:10.1109/TNNLS.2019.2933882 PMID:31502991

Flöck, A. N., & Walla, P. (2020). Think outside the box: small, enclosed spaces alter brain activity as measured with electroencephalography (EEG). In Information Systems and Neuroscience: NeuroIS Retreat 2020 (pp. 24-30). Springer International Publishing.

Gao, X., Wang, Y., Chen, X., & Gao, S. (2021). Interface, interaction, and intelligence in generalized brain–computer interfaces. *Trends in Cognitive Sciences*, *25*(8), 671–684. doi:10.1016/j.tics.2021.04.003 PMID:34116918

Gao, Z., Wang, X., Yang, Y., Li, Y., Ma, K., & Chen, G. (2021, December). A Channel-Fused Dense Convolutional Network for EEG-Based Emotion Recognition. *IEEE Transactions on Cognitive and Developmental Systems*, *13*(4), 945–954. doi:10.1109/TCDS.2020.2976112

Ghosh, A., & Saha, S. (2021, August). Recurrent neural network based cognitive ability analysis in mental arithmetic task using electroencephalogram. In *2021 8th International Conference on Signal Processing and Integrated Networks (SPIN)* (pp. 1165-1170). IEEE. 10.1109/SPIN52536.2021.9566099

Ghosh, A., & Saha, S. (2022). Suppression of positive emotions during pandemic era: A deep learning framework for rehabilitation. *International Journal of Modelling Identification and Control*, *41*(1-2), 143–154. doi:10.1504/IJMIC.2022.127101

Gong, M., Liu, J., Qin, A. K., Zhao, K., & Tan, K. C. (2021, January). Evolving Deep Neural Networks via Cooperative Coevolution With Backpropagation. *IEEE Transactions on Neural Networks and Learning Systems*, *32*(1), 420–434. doi:10.1109/TNNLS.2020.2978857 PMID:32217489

Goularas, D., & Kamis, S. (2019). Evaluation of Deep Learning Techniques in Sentiment Analysis from Twitter Data. In *2019 International Conference on Deep Learning and Machine Learning in Emerging Applications (Deep-ML)* (pp. 12-17). IEEE. 10.1109/Deep-ML.2019.00011

Jiang, Z., & Shen, G. (2019). Prediction of House Price Based on The Back Propagation Neural Network in The Keras Deep Learning Framework. In *2019 6th International Conference on Systems and Informatics (ICSAI)*. IEEE. 10.1109/ICSAI48974.2019.9010071

Kawala-Sterniuk, A., Podpora, M., Pelc, M., Blaszczyszyn, M., Gorzelanczyk, E. J., Martinek, R., & Ozana, S. (2020). Comparison of smoothing filters in analysis of EEG data for the medical diagnostics purposes. *Sensors (Basel)*, *20*(3), 807. doi:10.3390/s20030807 PMID:32024267

Keerthika, K., Kannan, M., & Khang, A. (2023). Medical Data Analytics: Roles, Challenges, and Analytical Tools. In AI and IoT-Based Technologies for Precision Medicine (1st ed.). IGI Global Press. doi:10.4018/979-8-3693-0876-9.ch001

Khang, A. (2023a). *AI and IoT-Based Technologies for Precision Medicine* (1st ed.). IGI Global Press. doi:10.4018/979-8-3693-0876-9

Khang, A. (2023b). Enabling the Future of Manufacturing: Integration of Robotics and IoT to Smart Factory Infrastructure in Industry 4.0. In AI-Based Technologies and Applications in the Era of the Metaverse. (1st Ed.). IGI Global Press. doi:10.4018/978-1-6684-8851-5.ch002

Khang, A., & Abdullayev, V. A. (2023). AI-Aided Data Analytics Tools and Applications for the Healthcare Sector. In AI and IoT-Based Technologies for Precision Medicine" (1st ed.). IGI Global Press. doi:10.4018/979-8-3693-0876-9.ch018

Khang, A., & Muthmainnah, M. (2023). AI-Aided Teaching Model for the Education 5.0 Ecosystem. AI-Based Technologies and Applications in the Era of the Metaverse. (1st Ed.) IGI Global Press. doi:10.4018/978-1-6684-8851-5.ch004

Khang, A., Shah, V., & Rani, S. (2023). *AI-Based Technologies and Applications in the Era of the Metaverse* (1st ed.). IGI Global Press. doi:10.4018/978-1-6684-8851-5

Liu, F., Xu, F., & Yang, S. (2017). A Flood Forecasting Model Based on Deep Learning Algorithm via Integrating Stacked Autoencoders with BP Neural Network. In *2017 IEEE Third International Conference on Multimedia Big Data (BigMM)* (pp. 58-61). IEEE. 10.1109/BigMM.2017.29

Lydia, A., & Francis, F. S. (2019). Convolutional Neural Network with an Optimized Backpropagation Technique. In *2019 IEEE International Conference on System, Computation, Automation and Networking (ICSCAN)* (pp. 1-5). IEEE. 10.1109/ICSCAN.2019.8878719

Mitra, A., Biswas, A., Chakraborty, K., Ghosh, A., Das, N., Ghosh, N., & Ghosh, A. (2022). A Machine Learning Approach to Identify Personality Traits from Social Media. In *Machine Learning and Deep Learning in Efficacy Improvement of Healthcare Systems* (pp. 31–60). CRC Press. doi:10.1201/9781003189053-2

Muhammad, G., Alshehri, F., Karray, F., El Saddik, A., Alsulaiman, M., & Falk, T. H. (2021). A comprehensive survey on multimodal medical signals fusion for smart healthcare systems. *Information Fusion*, *76*, 355–375. doi:10.1016/j.inffus.2021.06.007

Nahmias, D. O., Civillico, E. F., & Kontson, K. L. (2020). Deep learning and feature based medication classifications from EEG in a large clinical data set. *Scientific Reports*, *10*(1), 14206. doi:10.1038/s41598-020-70569-y PMID:32848165

Najdi, S., Gharbali, A. A., & Fonseca, J. M. (2017). Feature transformation based on stacked sparse autoencoders for sleep stage classification. In *Doctoral Conference on Computing, Electrical and Industrial Systems* (pp. 191-200). Springer. 10.1007/978-3-319-56077-9_18

Namita, P. (2023). Application of Machine Learning for Image Processing in the Healthcare Sector. AI and IoT-Based Technologies for Precision Medicine (1st ed.). IGI Global Press. doi:10.4018/979-8-3693-0876-9.ch004

Newell, M. E., Adhikari, S., & Halden, R. U. (2022). Systematic and state-of the science review of the role of environmental factors in Amyotrophic Lateral Sclerosis (ALS) or Lou Gehrig's Disease. *The Science of the Total Environment*, *817*, 152504. doi:10.1016/j.scitotenv.2021.152504 PMID:34971691

Newson, J. J., & Thiagarajan, T. C. (2019). EEG frequency bands in psychiatric disorders: A review of resting state studies. *Frontiers in Human Neuroscience*, *12*, 521. doi:10.3389/fnhum.2018.00521 PMID:30687041

Nguyen, K., Fookes, C., & Sridharan, S. (2015). Improving deep convolutional neural networks with unsupervised feature learning. *2015 IEEE International Conference on Image Processing (ICIP)*, (pp. 2270-2274). IEEE. 10.1109/ICIP.2015.7351206

Nguyen, M., Sun, N., Alexander, D. C., Feng, J., & Yeo, B. T. (2018). Modeling Alzheimer's disease progression using deep recurrent neural networks. In *2018 International Workshop on Pattern Recognition in Neuroimaging (PRNI)* (pp. 1-4). IEEE. 10.1109/PRNI.2018.8423955

Olichney, J., Xia, J., Church, K. J., & Moebius, H. J. (2022). Predictive power of cognitive biomarkers in neurodegenerative disease drug development: Utility of the P300 event-related potential. *Neural Plasticity*, *2022*, 2022. doi:10.1155/2022/2104880 PMID:36398135

Park, S. U., Park, J. H., Al-Masni, M. A., Al-Antari, M. A., Uddin, M. Z., & Kim, T. S. (2016). A depth camera-based human activity recognition via deep learning recurrent neural network for health and social care services. *Procedia Computer Science*, *100*, 78–84. doi:10.1016/j.procs.2016.09.126

Račić, L., & Popović, T. S. (2021). Pneumonia Detection Using Deep Learning Based on Convolutional Neural Network. *2021 25th International Conference on Information Technology (IT),* (pp. 1-4). IEEE. 10.1109/IT51528.2021.9390137

Rasamoelina, A. D., Adjailia, F., & Sinčák, P. (2020). A review of activation function for artificial neural network. In *2020 IEEE 18th World Symposium on Applied Machine Intelligence and Informatics (SAMI)* (pp. 281-286). IEEE. 10.1109/SAMI48414.2020.9108717

Ren, F., & Bao, Y. (2020). A review on human-computer interaction and intelligent robots. *International Journal of Information Technology & Decision Making, 19*(01), 5–47. doi:10.1142/S0219622019300052

Riccio, A., Simione, L., Schettini, F., Pizzimenti, A., Inghilleri, M., Belardinelli, M. O., Mattia, D., & Cincotti, F. (2013). Attention and P300-based BCI performance in people with amyotrophic lateral sclerosis. *Frontiers in Human Neuroscience, 7,* 732. doi:10.3389/fnhum.2013.00732 PMID:24282396

Ryeu, J. K., Tak, H. Y., Heo, N. W., & Chung, H. S. (1993). Recognition of Korean spoken digit using single layer recurrent neural networks. *Proceedings of 1993 International Conference on Neural Networks (IJCNN-93-Nagoya, Japan).* IEEE. 10.1109/IJCNN.1993.713908

Sampath, B. (2023). AI-Integrated Technology for a Secure and Ethical Healthcare Ecosystem. AI and IoT-Based Technologies for Precision Medicine (1st ed.). IGI Global Press. doi:10.4018/979-8-3693-0876-9.ch003

Shao, H. (2008, September). Delay-Dependent Stability for Recurrent Neural Networks With Time-Varying Delays. *IEEE Transactions on Neural Networks, 19*(9), 1647–1651. doi:10.1109/TNN.2008.2001265 PMID:18779095

Sharma, A. (2016). Univariate short term forecasting of solar irradiance using modified online back-propagation through time. *2016 International Computer Science and Engineering Conference (ICSEC),* (pp. 1-6). IEEE. 10.1109/ICSEC.2016.7859922

Sharma, G., & Joshi, A. M. (2021). Novel EEG based Schizophrenia Detection with IoMT Framework for Smart Healthcare. *arXiv preprint arXiv:2111.11298.*

Shen, Y., & Wang, J. (2008, March). An Improved Algebraic Criterion for Global Exponential Stability of Recurrent Neural Networks With Time-Varying Delays. *IEEE Transactions on Neural Networks, 19*(3), 528–531. doi:10.1109/TNN.2007.911751 PMID:18334371

Suganthan, P. N., & Katuwal, R. (2021). On the origins of randomization-based feedforward neural networks. *Applied Soft Computing, 105,* 107239. doi:10.1016/j.asoc.2021.107239

Takase, H., Gouhara, K., & Uchikawa, Y. (1993). Time sequential pattern transformation and attractors of recurrent neural networks. *Proceedings of 1993 International Conference on Neural Networks (IJCNN-93-Nagoya, Japan)* (pp. 2319-2322). IEEE. 10.1109/IJCNN.1993.714189

Tharwat, A. (2021). Independent component analysis: An introduction. *Applied Computing and Informatics, 17*(2), 222–249. doi:10.1016/j.aci.2018.08.006

Uçkun, F. A., Özer, H., Nurbaş, E., & Onat, E. (2020). Direction Finding Using Convolutional Neural Networks and Convolutional Recurrent Neural Networks. *2020 28th Signal Processing and Communications Applications Conference (SIU)*, 1-4. 10.1109/SIU49456.2020.9302448

Wang, A., Chen, G., Shang, C., Zhang, M., & Liu, L. (2016). Human activity recognition in a smart home environment with stacked denoising autoencoders. In *International conference on web-age information management* (pp. 29-40). Springer. 10.1007/978-3-319-47121-1_3

Wardana, A. A., Rakhmatsyah, A., Minarno, A. E., & Anbiya, D. R. (2019). *Internet of things platform for manage multiple message queuing telemetry transport broker server. Kinetik: Game Technology.* Information System, Computer Network, Computing, Electronics, and Control.

Wright, L. G., Onodera, T., Stein, M. M., Wang, T., Schachter, D. T., Hu, Z., & McMahon, P. L. (2022). Deep physical neural networks trained with backpropagation. *Nature*, *601*(7894), 549–555. doi:10.1038/s41586-021-04223-6 PMID:35082422

Xue, Q., Wang, X., Meehan, S., Kuang, J., Gao, J. A., & Chuah, M. C. (2018). Recurrent neural networks based obesity status prediction using activity data. In *2018 17th IEEE International Conference on Machine Learning and Applications (ICMLA)* (pp. 865-870). IEEE. 10.1109/ICMLA.2018.00139

Yaxue, Q. (2020). Convolutional Neural Networks for Literature Retrieval. *2020 International Conference on Computer Vision, Image and Deep Learning (CVIDL)*, (pp. 393-397). IEEE. 10.1109/CVIDL51233.2020.00-64

Yu, J., Yi, Z., & Zhou, J. (2010, October). Continuous Attractors of Lotka–Volterra Recurrent Neural Networks With Infinite Neurons. *IEEE Transactions on Neural Networks*, *21*(10), 1690–1695. doi:10.1109/TNN.2010.2067224 PMID:20813637

Zhang, R., & Cui, J. (2020). Application of Convolutional Neural Network in multi-channel Scenario D2D Communication Transmitting Power Control. *2020 International Conference on Computer Vision, Image and Deep Learning (CVIDL)*, (pp. 668-672). IEEE. 10.1109/CVIDL51233.2020.000-3

Zheng, S. (2021). Network Intrusion Detection Model Based on Convolutional Neural Network. *2021 IEEE 5th Advanced Information Technology, Electronic and Automation Control Conference (IAEAC)*, 634-637. 10.1109/IAEAC50856.2021.9390930

Zhong, R., Li, M., Chen, Q., Li, J., Li, G., & Lin, W. (2019). The P300 event-related potential component and cognitive impairment in epilepsy: A systematic review and meta-analysis. *Frontiers in Neurology*, *10*, 943. doi:10.3389/fneur.2019.00943 PMID:31543861

Chapter 12
Investigation on Identification of Three–Compartment Model for the Benchmark Pharmacokinetic System

V. Sujatha

SRM Institute of Science and Technology, India

Alex Khang

ⓘ https://orcid.org/0000-0001-8379-4659

Global Research Institute of Technology and Engineering, USA

ABSTRACT

This chapter investigates identification of blood concentration in three compartment model of pharmacokinetic system. The dynamic behaviour of blood concentration in blood tissues are described using the compartmental models. The model is derived using first-principles method for the benchmark pharmacokinetic system. Using MATLab, the concentrations in all the three-compartments are estimated and validated with the experimental value. The quality of estimation has been verified based on the validation of experimental values with the estimated concentration values in all the three compartments. Quantitative comparison also done based on the computation and comparison of square relative error. Both the qualitative and quantitative measurements are done for benchmark pharmacokinetic system.

1. INTRODUCTION

Pharmacokinetics is defined as the study of dynamic behaviour of drug concentrations in blood tissues of human body. The pharmacokinetics is described using the compartmental models. In this chapter, the common 3-compartment model is used. The drug is infused directly in Compartment 1 representing blood plasma. Well-perfused tissues and residual tissues are represented by Compartment 2 and compartment 3 respectively. Assuming that the drug can be diffused between compartment 1 and 2, compartments 2

DOI: 10.4018/979-8-3693-3679-3.ch012

and 3. The transfer parameters are K10, K12, K13, K21, K31 for three compartment model. It is difficult to achieve desired concentration with intravenous drug delivery in the compartment model. Physicians recommend the intravenous delivery of drugs dose per kilogram of body weight by manually controlled infusion pumps in practice. The concentration in compartment 1, 2 and 3 are estimated for all the five pharmacokinetic model in this chapter. This estimation will enable the clinician not only to explore about the drug concentration in blood but also to administer the intravenous delivery of drugs based on pharmacokinetic models. With the help of computer simulation, the blood-drug concentration can be estimated thereby allowing the anaesthesiologist to deliver the intravenous drugs to a subject (Khang & Abdullayev et al., 2023).

A comparison sets of propofol pharmacokinetic parameter is presented in Jaap Vuyk et al (1995) where the performance of the computer-controlled infusion of propofol in female patients are analysed. The modelling equations in this paper are taken from the pharmacokinetic three compartment model cited in Wayne Bequette (2002). By using three compartment modelling approach for pharmacokinetics of remifentanil, a simple model was developed and validated to evaluate the plasma concentration in the work done in Sara Cascone et al. (2013). Rifai et al (2016) proposed that for pharmacokinetics model inter-individual variability represents a challenging aspect in Total I.V. Anaesthesia, hence care must be taken to ensure that the expected clinical response is actually obtained. Kartono et al (2020) estimated the parameters of the pharmacokinetic model using particle swarm optimization (PSO) algorithm.

An approach that help pharmacometricians to determine a theoretical method to establish compatibility between the models in Hyo Jeong Ryu et al, 2022. Presently there is no best model available for propofol infusion. This chapter aims to make the clinicians should become familiar with the model which matches the characteristics of the patient among the usual patient population. However, all the existing pharmacokinetic models are having inherent assumptions which lead to inaccuracy in the estimated model. Hence, the role of anaesthetist is to have the close clinical monitoring of the patient under treatment. This chapter focusses on the mathematical modelling of pharmacokinetic models with no assumptions (Anh et al., 2024).

The aim of this article is to analysis the pharmacokinetic model using three compartments. The rest of the article is carried out as follows: section 2 discusses benchmark pharmacokinetic model. The proposed modelling of pharmacokinetics is explained in section 3. Investigation of the concentration in all the three compartments are given in section 4. At the end, conclusion is drawn.

2. PHARMACOKINETIC MODEL: THREE-COMPARTMENT MODEL

For examining the behaviour of intravenous delivery of drugs to the subject, the pharmacokinetic model is used. The same model are used to estimate the blood concentration in all the compartments. The benchmark three-compartment model is shown in Figure 1.

The commonly used models are five pharmacokinetic models are taken for study.

Let I be the Mass infusion rate of the drug (mass/unit time), then the mass balance equations are represented as:

$$\frac{dM_1}{dt} = -\left(K_{12} + K_{13} + K_{10}\right)M_1 + K_{21}M_2 + K_{31}M_3 + I \tag{1}$$

Figure 1. Three compartment model

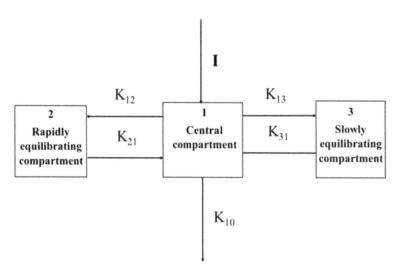

$$\frac{dM_2}{dt} = K_{12}M_1 - K_{21}M_2 \tag{2}$$

$$\frac{dM_3}{dt} = K_{13}M_1 - K_{31}M_3 \tag{3}$$

It is required to concern more about drug concentrations, rather than the total amount of drug. Thus, the blood plasma concentration can also be related by $C_1 = M_1/V_1$. The mass balance equation of three-compartment model whose parameters are described in table 1 can also be represented in terms of blood plasma concentration:

$$\frac{dC_1}{dt} = -\left(K_{12} + K_{13} + K_{10}\right)C_1 + K_{21}C_2 + K_{31}C_3 + \frac{1}{V_1}I \tag{4}$$

$$\frac{dC_2}{dt} = K_{12}C_1 - K_{21}C_2 \tag{5}$$

$$\frac{dC_3}{dt} = K_{13}C_1 - K_{31}C_3 \tag{6}$$

$$C_1 = C_1 \tag{7}$$

Table 1. Description of parameters in Bergman minimal model

Symbol	Description	Unit
I	Mass infusion rate	Mass/time
C_1	Blood plasma concentration in compartment 1	µg/ml
C_2	Blood plasma concentration in compartment 2	µg/ml
C_3	Blood plasma concentration in compartment 3	µg/ml
K_{10}	Rate constant for drug elimination from central compartment	min^{-1}
K_{12}	Rate constant between 1 and 2	min^{-1}
K_{21}	Rate constant between 2 and 1	min^{-1}
K_{13}	Rate constant between 1 and 3	min^{-1}
K_{31} V_1	Rate constant between 3 and 1 volume of the blood plasma compartment	min^{-1} litres

Table 2. Parameter values of five Pharmacokinetic model for propofol infusion

Parameters	Gepts et al. (1987)
I	3
K_{10}	0.1190
K_{12}	0.1140
K_{21}	0.0550
K_{13}	0.0419
K_{31}	0.0033
V_1	16.2

3. MODELLING OF PHARMACOKINETIC MODELS

The minimal model of pharmacokinetic models were implemented using Simulink. Using ODE solver in MATLAB, the blood plasma concentration in three compartments is estimated for the normal individual.

3.1 Model of Gepts et al. (1987)

The pharmacokinetic model proposed by Gepts et al. (1987) has been taken for study.

3.2 Simulation of Gepts et al. (1987)

It is clear that both the simulated concentration is close to the estimated concentration value as shown in the figure 2, 3 and 4. It is required to compute the relative error using the following in order to justify how the estimated value close to the true or actual value:

Figure 2. Plot of concentration C1 for Gepts et al. (1987) pharmacokinetic models

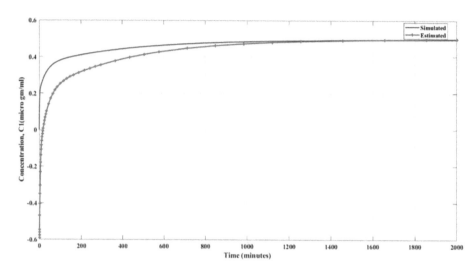

Figure 3. Plot of concentration C2 for Gepts et al pharmacokinetic models

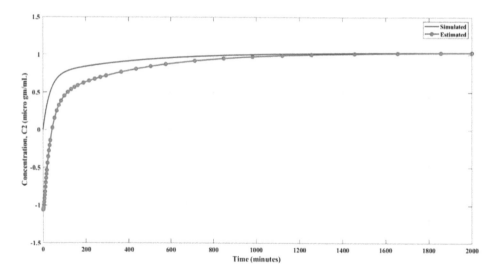

$$\text{Relative error} = \frac{C - \hat{C}}{C}$$

where C is the actual concentration value obtained through simulation and $\hat{C}$ is the estimated concentration value obtained using solver.

Table 3 presents both the simulated and estimated concentration values in all the three compartments along with the relative error. It was found from the relative square error that the estimated concentration is closer to the true value.

Figure 4. Plot of concentration C3 for Gepts et al. (1987) pharmacokinetic models

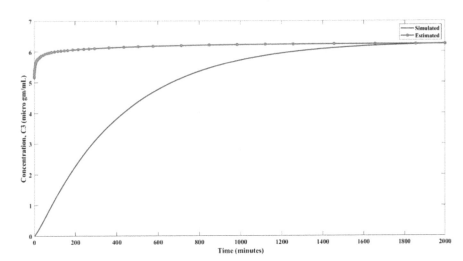

Table 3. Simulated and estimated values of concentration for Gepts et al. (1987)

C_1	$\widehat{C}_1$	Square Relative error	C_2	$\widehat{C}_2$	Square Relative error	C_3	$\widehat{C}_3$	Square Relative error
0.33	0.011	0.966667	0.6	0.07	0.883333	0.24	4.54	-17.9167
0.41	0.196	0.521951	0.9	0.52	0.422222	1.52	4.58	-2.01316
0.46	0.347	0.245652	1.0	0.7	0.3	2.9	4.57	-0.57586
0.48	0.397	0.172917	1.03	0.8	0.223301	4.09	4.56	-0.11491
0.51	0.46	0.098039	1.08	0.97	0.101852	4.15	4.56	-0.0988
0.53	0.50	0.056604	1.16	1.08	0.068966	4.3	4.56	-0.06047
0.54	0.52	0.037037	1.19	1.15	0.033613	4.34	4.56	-0.05069
0.546	0.536	0.018315	1.21	1.20	0.008264	4.50	4.55	-0.01111
0.547	0.537	0.018282	1.229	1.22	0.007323	4.48	4.55	-0.01562
0.547	0.547	0	1.23	1.23	0	4.55	4.55	0

4. RESULTS AND DISCUSSIONS

Figure 5, 6, 7 represents the concentration in all the three compartments is analysed for pharmacokinetic models. From the response, it is clear that the concentration C_1 is low compared to C_2 and C_3. Similarly, the concentration in compartment C_2 is lesser than C_3. Figure 5, 6, 7 shown the Comparison of Concentration in all three compartments for Gepts et al. (1987).

Figure 5. Concentration C₁ in compartment 1

Alt-text: Figure 5 shown the Comparison of Concentration in compartment 1 for Gepts et al. (1987)

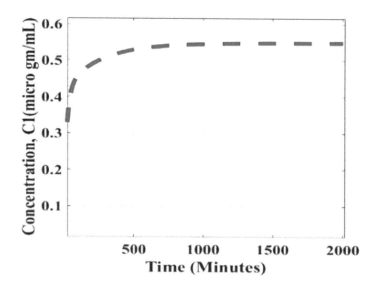

Figure 6. Concentration C₂ in compartment 2

Alt-text: Figure 6 shown the Comparison of Concentration in compartment 2 for Gepts et al. (1987)

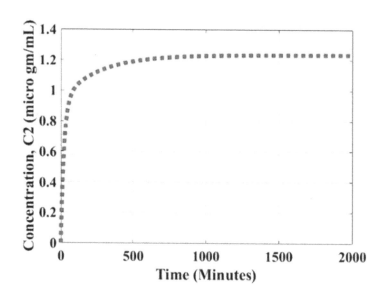

5. CONCLUSION

Three compartment models are used to estimate the concentration in Pharmacokinetic model. This non-linear system having mass infusion rate as single input and blood concentration in compartment 1, 2 and 3 as three outputs variable. Hence this biological system can be modelled as non-square systems. This

Figure 7. Concentration C_3 in compartment 3
Alt-text: Figure 7 shown the Comparison of Concentration in compartment 3 for Gepts et al. (1987)

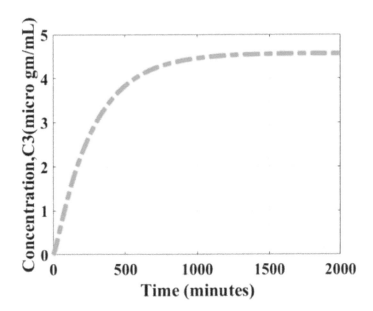

non-linear system has been modelled as non-square system having one input and three output system. Modelling can be done using first principles method and its parameters are estimated using ODE solver.

The concentration values in all the three compartment models are estimated and the same values are compared with the simulated values by calculating relative square error. The enhanced performance is ensured based on minimum relative square error for the pharmacokinetic models (Khang & Medicine, 2023). Overall this chapter can be concluded based on computer simulation, will help both the clinician and anaesthesiologist not only to estimate the drug concentration in blood but also to administer the intravenous delivery of drugs to the subjects (Khang & Hajimahmud et al., 2024).

REFERENCES

Al Rifai, Z., & Mulvey, D. (2016). Principles of total intravenous anaesthesia: Basic pharmacokinetics and model descriptions. *BJA Education*, *16*(3), 92–97. doi:10.1093/bjaceaccp/mkv021

Anh, P. T. N. (2024). AI Models for Disease Diagnosis and Prediction of Heart Disease with Artificial Neural Networks. Computer Vision and AI-integrated IoT Technologies in Medical Ecosystem (1st ed.). CRC Press. doi:10.1201/9781003429609-9

Cascone, S., Lamberti, G., Titomanlio, G., & Piazza, O. (2013). Pharmacokinetics of Remifentanil: A three-compartmental modeling approach. *Translational Medicine @ UniSa*, 18–22. PMID:24251247

Cockshott, I. D., Douglas, E. J., & Prys-Roberts, C. (1987). Pharmacokinetics of propofol during and after intravenous infusion in man. *British Journal of Anaesthesia*, *59*, 941.

Gepts, E., Camu, F., Cockshott, I. D., & Douglas, E. J. (1987). Disposition of propofol administered as constant rate infusions in humans. *Anesthesia and Analgesia, 66*(12), 1256–1263. doi:10.1213/00000539-198712000-00010 PMID:3500657

Kartono, A., Anggraini, D., Wahyudi, S. T., Setiawan, A. A., & Irmansyah. (2021). Study of Parameters Estimation of The Three-Compartment Pharmacokinetic Model using Particle Swarm Optimization Algorithm. *Journal of Physics: Conference Series, 1805*(1), 012032. doi:10.1088/1742-6596/1805/1/012032

Khang, A. (2023). *AI and IoT-Based Technologies for Precision Medicine* (1st ed.). IGI Global Press. doi:10.4018/979-8-3693-0876-9

Khang, A., & Abdullayev, V. A. (2023). AI-Aided Data Analytics Tools and Applications for the Healthcare Sector. AI and IoT-Based Technologies for Precision Medicine (1st ed.). IGI Global Press. doi:10.4018/979-8-3693-0876-9.ch018

Khang, A., & Hajimahmud, V. A. (2024). Application of Computer Vision in the Healthcare Ecosystem. Computer Vision and AI-integrated IoT Technologies in Medical Ecosystem (1st ed.). CRC Press. doi:10.1201/9781003429609-1

Kirkpatrick, T., Cockshott, I. D., Douglas, E. J., & Nimmo, W. S. (1988). Pharmacokinetics of propofol (Diprivan) in elderly patients. *British Journal of Anaesthesia, 60*, i46–i150. PMID:3257879

Shafer, A., Doze, V. A., Shafer, S. L., & White, P. F. (1988). Pharmacokinetics and pharmacodynamics of propofol infusions during general anesthesia. *Anesthesiology, 69*(3), 348–356. doi:10.1097/00000542-198809000-00011 PMID:3261954

Tackley, R. M., Lewis, G. T. R., Prys-Roberts, C., Boaden, R. W., Dixon, J., & Harvey, J. T. (1989). Computer-controlled infusion of propofol. *British Journal of Anaesthesia, 62*(1), 46–53. doi:10.1093/bja/62.1.46 PMID:2783854

Vuyk, J., Engbers, F. H. M., Bum, A. G. L., Vletter, A. A., & Bovill, J. G. (1995). Performance of Computer-Controlled Infusion of Propofol: An Evaluation of Five Pharmacokinetic Parameter Sets. *Anesthesia and Analgesia, 81*, 1275–1282. PMID:7486116

Wayne, B. (2002). *Process Control: Modeling, Design, and Simulation*. Prentice Hall PTR.

Chapter 13
Implementation of Machine Learning for Smart Wearables in the Healthcare Sector

Harishchander Anandaram
https://orcid.org/0000-0003-2993-5304
Amrita Vishwa Vidyapeetham, India

Deepa Gupta
https://orcid.org/0000-0002-5524-6898
Amity University, Noida, India

Ch. Indira Priyadarsini
Chaitanya Bharathi Institute of Technology, Hyderabad, India

Benita Christopher
Westford University College, Sharjah, UAE

ABSTRACT

Artificial intelligence (AI) and the internet of things (IoT) are two of the world's most rapidly expanding technologies. More and more people are settling in urban areas, and the notion of a "smart city" centres on improved access to high-quality medical services. An exhaustive knowledge of the different brilliant city structures is vital for carrying out IoT and man-made intelligence for remote health monitoring (RHM) frameworks. The advancements, devices, frameworks, models, plans, use cases, and software programmes that comprise the backbone of these frameworks are all essential components. Clinical decision support systems and other variants of healthcare delivery also make use of ML techniques for creating analytic representations. After each component has been thoroughly examined, clinical decision support systems provide personalized recommendations for therapy, lifestyle changes, and care plans to patients. Medical care applications benefit from wearable innovation's ability to monitor and analyse data from the user's activities, temperature, heart rate, blood sugar, etc.

DOI: 10.4018/979-8-3693-3679-3.ch013

1. INTRODUCTION

The Internet of Things (IoT) is a vital part of the next generation of computing infrastructure. In order to identify progressively anything or cycle that should be checked, IoT employs a wide range of information sensing devices and connects them all together through the internet to build a massive, interconnected network. Its goal is to unite disparate things and people with the goal that they might be all the more effectively recognized, made due, and controlled. The web stays the backbone and cornerstone of IoT, allowing the client and his or her linked network to grow to include numerous things and exchange and share information (Alkhatib et al., 2014; Madakam et al., 2015).

Sensor networks, RFID, and QR codes are only a couple of the innovations that contribute to the Internet of Things and enable devices to collect data about the real world. Technologies like Bluetooth, WLANs, and the internet all serve as routes for data transfer. There are three basic layers of technology used in IoT implementation, application, and study: the discernment layer, the organization layer, and the application layer. The information obtained by IoT is then used by the application layer. Perception and networking technologies are the foundation of the Internet of Things.

In this context, technologies like QR codes, RFID, sensors, etc., make up the sensing layer. Wi-Fi, Narrow Band Internet of Things (NB-IoT), Zigbee, Portable Correspondence Innovation (4G/5G, and so forth), Low Power Remote Individual Region Organization (LoWPAN), Machine-to-Machine (M2M) Innovation, and so on are instances of wide organization layer technologies (Gubbi et al., 2013). 5G is an up and coming age of portable correspondence networks that utilizes a low-postpone Dalian connect to achieve its high speeds. As a result, 5G considerably aids in the expansion of the Internet of Things and more adequately satisfies the requirements of IoT applications, for example, portable clinical and crisis requirements (Haider, 2014).

Medical professionals, patients, and hospital administrators may all benefit greatly from IoT because of how 5G is enhancing the current medical care system. Telemedicine, emergency care, and first aid are just a few examples of how this facilitates quick progress towards mobile, intelligent, and visualised ways of clinical care while also enhancing service capacities and management efficiency. Collaboration in diagnosis and treatment, as well as critical care using 5G convergent networks, are two examples of the novel application possibilities made possible by IoT (Joyia et al., 2017).

1.1 Computing on the Cloud

Distributed computing is a sort of circulated figuring that utilizes an organization called the "cloud" to separate huge information handling programs into a large number of smaller ones. The cloud then runs these little programmes over a network of computers to analyse the data and provide the findings to the consumers. Distributed computing is another registering worldview that looks to give clients a protected, versatile, and excellent figuring experience on the cloud. Framework as a help (IaaS), stage as a help (PaaS), and programming as an assistance (SaaS) are the three broad categories into which cloud computing services fall (Hingmire et al., 2017; Sultan, 2014). Multiple technologies are needed for cloud computing to be implemented (Wang et al., 2010). By creating an on-demand virtualized IT infrastructure, virtualization technology provides users access to cloud services through a personalised network setting.

Cloud computing relies on this because it allows for highly adaptable and scalable hardware services. By offering a comprehensive collection of service templates, administration cycle and work process innovation organizes administrations from many sources and sorts naturally to create a reasonable and dynamic help stream or work process. Web administrations are the run of the mill way that SOA innovation and distributed computing administrations are made available to users, and these services must adhere to industry standards like WSDL and UDDI.

With the help of network storage technologies, users may rent out storage space, and users can utilise straightforward cloud programming models to acclimate to the cloud's architecture. High efficiency and low cost medical services are now available thanks to cloud computing, which also assists with improving the nature of patient consideration. Distributed computing, for example, may work with between framework information sharing, common acknowledgment of test discoveries, hearty help for far off discussion, development of excellent clinical assets, and reduction of the burden of getting an appointment with a doctor (Ahuja et al., 2012).

1.2 Analysis of Massive Data Sets

The objective of enormous information examination is to draw conclusions, aid in forecasting, spot patterns, unearth previously unknown facts, and guide decision-making (Marjani et al., 2017). Bunch investigation, arrangement mining calculations, text mining calculations, and information visualisation methods are the backbone of the data mining technology stack. Data is clustered using some metric of similarity and then examined for patterns. This kind of exploratory research may beforehand categorise data samples based on a predetermined rule. An essential objective of the grouping mining calculation is to make a planning between the crude information and the last names. Choice trees (Kufrin, 1997), Bayesian inference (Gondy et al., 1993), and ANNs (Chen et al., 2016) are the most well-known order mining strategies. Choice tree learning is an inductive learning procedure that uses examples to gather the grouping rules written as a choice tree. Bayesian deduction offers a characteristic method for communicating causal data to uncover the likely connection between information, since it is a graphical example approach used to portray the association likelihood between factors.

An ANN is a numerical model for data handling that copies the synaptic associations in the cerebrum by utilizing an equal nonlinear powerful framework. The objective of the text mining algorithm (Judith & James, 2001) is to find interesting or relevant patterns in vast amounts of unstructured text data and to make this information accessible to consumers. Text pre-processing, text word division, text mining, semantic examination, and so on, are the backbones of this strategy. Information representation technology (Krallinger et al., 2014) is the way of thinking, method, and innovation of changing information into visuals or pictures and showing and handling them in an intuitive way using PC illustrations and picture handling innovation. Sickness anticipation, finding, treatment, clinical exploration, and comparing the effects of medicinal applications may all benefit greatly from big data analytic technology (Hua et al., 2015; Quan et al., 2021).

1.3 Artificial Intelligence

In order to discover statistical patterns in high-dimensional and multivariate data sets, machine learning is a specialised data-driven analytical tool that can automatically construct models. Pattern recognition is fundamental to machine learning, which aids in the prognosis and decision-making stages of healthcare planning (Bhardwaj et al., 2017; Dash et al., 2019). Both supervised and unsupervised machine learning are common. Supervised learning is the first approach, and it involves teaching algorithms by observation of labelled data. By comparing empirical findings with the proper outputs, the machine learns to recognise mistakes given a certain amount of inputs and accurate outputs.

Classification and regression are the primary areas of attention in this kind of learning, which is used when past occurrences may be utilised to make predictions about the future. Conversely, unaided learning requires the machine to effectively research information utilizing a preparation model to uncover dormant examples in the information without being given any sign of the legitimate result. This strategy relies heavily on clustering techniques in order to detect and categorise anomalies (Abramson et al., 2006). Current electronic medical records only include around 20% structured data, while the remaining 80% consists of unstructured data. Because of medicine's narrative character, machine learning applications in healthcare should pay special attention to the challenges of working with and making sense of massive amounts of unstructured raw data. There might be far-reaching ramifications for the medical industry as a result of this (Abramson et al., 2006).

2. ALGORITHMS AND METHODS

Movement ID, conduct acknowledgment, irregularity discovery, assistant direction, anonymization, security assurance, and other mechanical spaces are essential to the utilization of computer based intelligence and IoT in clinical practice. What follows is a condensed explanation of the fundamental algorithms and techniques used in a wide range of technological disciplines.

2.1 Detecting Actions

In clinical medicine, inertial sensors are often used for activity recognition monitoring of patients. Preprocessing, segmenting, feature extraction, reduction, and classification are the key processing phases. Separate algorithms and approaches are required for each stage (Avci et al., 2010).

2.1.1 In-Phase Preparation

Before using sensor data, it must be pre-processed to get rid of the high-frequency noise. Nonlinear, low-pass middle, Laplace, and Gaussian channels, among others, are among the tools at your disposal. Although relevant details are preserved, the authentic facts must still be shown. Some common techniques for doing so include the Piecewise Linear Representation (PLR), the Fourier Transform (FT), and the Wavelet Transform (WT), all of which improve the representation of functions with discontinuities and spikes, respectively. Discrete-WT (DWT) is a strong technique for recognising the transition between movements and filtering out background noise during activities like walking and running by discretely sampling the wavelet.

2.1.2 Classification

Extracting relevant and actionable data from ceaseless surges of sensor information is difficult for constant movement discovery. Therefore, a time series data segmentation approach, for example, a sliding window, hierarchical, base up, or sliding window and base up, is required. The sliding window method stands out among these choices because it is easy to use, can be accessed online, and is widely used in the medical community. In this technique, a brief time frame series is utilized as a starting point, and further data points are added until the fitting blunder of the potential section surpasses a client determined edge.

2.1.3 Extracting Features

Time space highlights, recurrence area highlights, and time-recurrence area highlights, heuristic elements, space explicit capabilities, and so forth are the most common feature types that may be retrieved. Simple waveform characteristics and signal statistics are examples of what may be derived directly from a data segment using time domain features. The periodic nature of the signal is highlighted by the frequency domain features, allowing the periodicity of acceleration data to be captured and utilised to differentiate between light and heavy activity. Studying the time-frequency properties of signals is often done using wavelet technology, and it is mostly used to identify the change from one activity to another. Time-Domain Gait identification is an example of an application-specific function that makes use of a time domain technique for step distinguishing proof notwithstanding the Quick Fourier Change (FFT). This allows for a detection accuracy of up to 95% for step sizes.

2.1.4 Diminutive Reduction of Dimensions

Include determination and element change are regular instances of dimensionality decrease strategies. The objective of element determination is to pick the highlights that will work on the classifier's presentation by the most. Strategies like help vector machine-based include choice, k-implies bunching, Forward-In reverse consecutive pursuit, and so forth, may be used to find this method, which will generate a subset of the current features. The objective of element change innovation is to lessen the quantity of special component mixes by planning high-layered include space to a lower aspect. This may be accomplished with the use of several statistical approaches such as principal component analysis (PCA), independent component analysis (ICA), local discriminant analysis (LDA), etc.

2.1.5 Recognition and Categorization

Methods in light of edges are frequently utilized for this purpose. In contrast, examples of pattern recognition technologies range from decision tables and trees through Nearest Neighbour and Naive Bayes algorithms, Support Vector Machines and Hidden Markov and Gaussian Mixture Models, and so on.

2.2 Recognising Behaviour

Both in the realm of computer vision research and in the realm of therapeutic applications, behaviour recognition has been and continues to be an important technological component. Through remote video recording, it is possible to keep tabs on patients' activities in situations such as critical care, emergency rescue, rehabilitation, and assessment. Convolution neural networks (CNNs) and recurrent neural networks (RNNs) are now the most popular tools for behaviour recognition. AlexNet and VGG16 are two examples of conventional convolutional neural networks (CNNs) that use convolution, pooling, and fully connected layers to extract a variety of features (Ijjina & Mohan, 2016). Input sequence data is fed into an RNN, which then recurses the other way of the succession and passes the unit around in a chain (Goodfellow et al., 2016). Most current deep learning-based behaviour recognition algorithms are built upon double-stream networks, 3D CNNs, and RNNs — specifically, long momentary memory (LSTM) organizations.

The point of conduct acknowledgment for the profound learning calculation of twofold stream network-based behaviour identification is additional video. This approach requires more time series data as compared to a single image. Subsequently, the twofold stream convolution organization is trained independently on spatial flow and temporal flow features before combining them to provide a recognition output. This technique compensates for the absence of time flow features in more conventional approaches. Simultaneously, the time stream might be additionally partitioned into nearby time stream and worldwide time stream inside the twofold stream organization, bringing about a three-stream network that can upgrade the versatility of spatio-fleeting data and the precision of identification outcomes (Liu & Yang, 2018; Wang et al., 2017).

The RNN's cyclic network module, which is used in the LSTM network-based conduct acknowledgment strategy, it is able to both learn new information and retain historical time series data. However, a RNN is helpless against the issue of slope vanishing when contrasted with data with longer time series. Presently, an LSTM network may be utilised to address this issue by acting as a memory unit and utilizing cell states in lieu of the secret layer hubs in the first RNN model. The condition of the cell might be changed or taken out utilizing a sigmoid capability and a point-by-point item activity, which are implemented in three separate gate structures (Du et al., 2017; Ng et al., 2015).

2.3 Detection of Abnormalities

The goal of abnormality detection is to distinguish anomalies, or information focuses that don't fit the overall pattern or display unexpected behaviour (Ren et al., 2017). The ability to detect anomalies is crucial for ensuring the integrity of medical procedures. Directed learning and unaided learning are two of the most utilized anomaly discovery strategies. To find lasting success, directed learning requires marked information to fabricate a preparation set, which is then investigated by a help vector machine or comparative classifier. Nonetheless, as a general rule, the labelled information used for unusual discovery is rarely open, and difficult to cover all possible special cases might happen in a space.

For this reason solo learning is so popular for solving anomaly detection issues. Disease detection, medicine development, and problem identification are just a few areas where unsupervised learning has proven invaluable. Circulation based, profundity based, distance-based, grouping based, and thickness based calculations are all examples of unsupervised learning approaches to abnormality identification. Clustering algorithms provide a straightforward unsupervised approach to finding out which items belong to which clusters and which do not. Some unsupervised methods use the distance between the instance and its closest neighbour on the assumption that outliers tend to be concentrated in sparse areas. The inexact K-closest neighbours (AKNN) procedure, the opposite K-closest neighbour (KNN), and the nearby anomaly factor are the most used proximity algorithms. Statistical and probabilistic analysis are two other common approaches. Outlier analysis, as well as the allocation and transfer of scores (Ren et al., 2017; Wsy & Syh, 2006), are components of the abnormality detection approach.

2.4 Determination Helpers

The diagnostic process may be sped up and improved with the use of auxiliary decision-making tools. In order to diagnose a new patient, it employs information mining procedures to make an order model utilizing clinical multi-faceted information (Alabdulkarim et al., 2019). Auxiliary decision-making's prediction tasks may be broken down into two classifications: prescient and clear. Prescient displaying includes planning information tests as per both info and result (managed learning) to get a capability from an assortment of marked preparing tests. Regulated learning methods incorporate things like brain organizations, order trees, and backing vector machines capable of regression and classification. In contrast, descriptive tasks, including grouping and association algorithms, make inferences from untagged input data. They cluster items or discover novel relationships between database variables. K-implies grouping, various levelled bunching, and the continuous item set rule extractor are all examples of such methods.

Classification of clinical data is important to these strategies, and a variety of classifiers, including group, choice tree, rule-based, Bayesian, and brain network classifiers, must be considered (Tama & Lim, 2020). The primary purpose of the widely used C4.5 classification method is to construct a decision tree from given samples and associated data. Each iteration of the method uses entropy and information gain calculations to try to determine which attributes will provide the greatest results when used to partition the data set. Heart disease, diabetes, lung cancer, etc. have all been diagnosed with the use of data mining tools. The maximum accuracy is shown by C4.5 in SVMs, KNNs, and neural networks. Additionally, J48 shows better performance accuracy than Bayesian networks. Accordingly, the decision tree is the most reliable classifier for use in the medical field (Chen et al., 2016).

3. EMERGENCY AND FIRST AID PRACTISES BASED ON SCENARIOS

The unequal degree of analysis and therapy of clinical professionals has long been a problem in emergency care, as has the necessity for prompt emergency and therapy of crisis and fundamentally wiped out patients. This exhibits the basic need of utilizing computerized reasoning and the web of things to process and interpret enormous amounts of data relating to emergency diagnosis and treatment. Pre-hospital first aid is a significant part of the crisis clinical framework, and assumes a pivotal part in saving the existences of crisis and fundamentally wiped out patients. This indicates the critical need of using cutting-edge technology to provide early admonition and mediation in pre-clinic emergency treatment, which improves their prognosis and boosts their chances of recovery.

Combining machine learning methods with geographic information systems (GIS), Chen et al. (2016) anticipated and envisioned pre-clinic crisis clinical consideration requests. We are additionally exploring the utilization of IoT to accumulate information on patients' important bodily functions, which can then be combined with EMRs and different information to make a keen early-cautioning model for performing critical-degree grading in real-time during ambulance transport. Due to the high volume of emergency cases in the past, one of the most critical responsibilities of the emergency room has been the prediction of early illness diagnosis and the correct identification of the diagnostic and therapeutic intervention at an early stage. Artificial intelligence (AI) and other methods have made it possible to perform early supplemental diagnosis, increase the effectiveness of finding and treatment, and reduction the quantity of undiscovered cases. Tsien et al. (1998) utilized ML and other methods to detect AMI in individuals presenting to emergency rooms complaining of chest discomfort. A neural network model for predicting emergency cases of acute coronary syndrome was built by Green et al. (2006).

The ability to foretell the course of a disease is crucial in both routine clinical practise and emergency situations. In a study predicting cerebral haemorrhage following thrombolysis, Bentley et al. (2014) used artificial intelligence to analyse head CTs of patients suffering from ischemic stroke. It is vital to set up a process for checking and early admonition for general wellbeing emergencies to adapt to the development of public crises like the Coronavirus pandemic. To additional improve the early admonition component for serious fiascoes, reinforce the clinical treatment security framework, and build an astute dynamic framework, we should likewise utilize the blend of IoT, computer based intelligence, and crisis salvage.

In a similar vein, Toltzis et al. (2015) employed AI to construct a model that could quickly determine which children among victims of mass casualties would need to be owned up to the basic consideration unit. Using computer simulation technologies and other tools, France et al. (2015) were able to infer the quantitative markers and streamlining strategies of the medical clinic's capacity to manage the surge of patients following catastrophes, therefore improving the hospital's disaster emergency management capacity.

4. THE OBSTACLES

Intelligent medical IoT has many novel attributes because of the union of computer based intelligence, the Web of Things, and the healthcare sector. Data modalities for IoT connection terminals are many, heterogeneous, and show cross-domain fusion properties. Therefore, interdisciplinary knowledge fusion is required, drawing from fields as varied as medicine, artificial intelligence, big data, information engineering, etc. However, with the addition of new capabilities come new dangers and difficulties, and the Internet of Medical Things is no exception.

4.1 Threats to Information Security

There are a plethora of smart medical IoT terminals, and they are often installed in groups. Distributed denial of service attacks may be launched quickly and simply by brute-force cracking and the transmission of malicious data packets. Congestion, paralysis, and service disruption caused by these assaults pose a danger to patient safety and the ability to provide accurate diagnoses. The infrastructure of intelligent medical IoT consists of virtual machines, cloud stages, information bases, middleware, web applications, and so forth, and gathers a vast quantity of data on the lives and health of groups of people. Security threats for example, confirmation sidestep, unapproved access, information control, controller, administration disturbance, and more exist because of blemishes in programming configuration, process plan, and different variables. Services and apps accessed over the internet pose a threat to users' privacy and security, as proven by AbdallahSoualmi et al. (2020), since third parties may gain access to, misuse, edit, or delete personal information.

4.2 There is a Deficit in IoT Data Standards

It is difficult to effectively ensure the quality of IoT terminal goods because of the immense number of makers of keen clinical IoT hardware, which in turn poses the difficulty of assuring the dependability and quality of data (Tuli et al., 2020). However, the efficacy of AI algorithms like machine learning relies heavily on the enormous preparing set delivered by IoT hardware based bunch life and wellbeing information. Informational collections produced by IoT terminals might be one-sided and may not completely cover every single clinical situation, as noted by FarhadAhamed et al. (2018). This can have serious consequences for the precision and efficacy of intelligent diagnosis, and may even cause "personalised medical care" to veer off course.

IoT standardisation has come a long way, however right now the primary areas of interest are in architecture and security technologies such lightweight encryption, authentication, privacy management, etc. In spite of the fact that HL7 and other clinical normalization associations have given reference data models like Reference Data Model (Edge), V2.X, V3.0, Guaranteed Information Expert (CDA), and so forth., in the context of traditional medical informatization, their applications principally center around ordinary clinical data and are not conducive to the incorporation of IoT data like medical images, multi-text records, waveforms, etc.

4.3 Dangers Associated With the Growth of Specialisation

One distinguishing aspect of contemporary medical practise is the development of ever-more-precise subspecialties. Although illness or medical field-specific research might increase the pace of diagnosis and therapy, if a specialised becomes too focused, clinicians lose the big picture. Misdiagnosis is a real possibility in such a situation. Currently, studies and practical applications of medical AI are generally tailored to a specific condition. This method perfectly initailizes the present medical subfield inside the realm of AI, hence affecting the diagnostic accuracy of such systems. In order to reach a precise medical aim, medical AI should be designed with a holistic perspective that takes into consideration the whole range of diagnostic and therapeutic options available.

4.4 The Influence of AI on Morality

Traditional medical ethics have been altered somewhat by the advent of AI in medicine. Patients may have a hard time trusting a machine to replace their doctor when it comes to matters of health and wellness. Patients lose faith in their physicians as a consequence, which may spark a chain reaction of arguments and perhaps legal action. However, medical decision-making has become increasingly complex, and the outcome of simulated intelligence applications relies upon the extensiveness and precision of training data as well as the sophistication of AI algorithms. Economic accessibility, mental resistance of determination and treatment plans, and provincial contrasts in friendly behaviours are examples of intangibles that might be difficult to account for. Therefore, it's possible that, after considering all of the relevant data, the AI's choice won't be the best option for patients. In contrast, AI's decision-making process necessitates the participation of medical specialists, and it is one-sided (Khang, Shah, & Rani, 2023).

5. THE AGE OF AIoT: A TIME OF EXPLOSIVE GROWTH

As a natural progression of the two technologies, AIoT (also written as "AI+IoT") represents the pinnacle of IoT's intelligent evolution. Together, AI and IoT can gather, transmit, and interpret data from the physical world in unprecedented ways. By mining and examining this information, man-made intelligence upgrades the worth of the Web of Things. As of late, the most immediate application situations and information hotspots for AIoT have come from the improvement of shrewd medication, on account of the forward leap of computer based intelligence innovation in the clinical business. During the Coronavirus pandemic, AIoT and large information innovation were important in monitoring the spread of the disease and developing effective countermeasures, leading to the quick integration of several AIoT use cases (Bangui et al., 2018).

5.1 AI is Proliferating on Peripheral Devices

Since medical IoT technology is still developing, most AI-powered IoT applications must be built on the cloud at this time (Alaybeyi & Lheureux, 2019; Zhou et al., 2019). Connected to IoT terminals in the future will be a plethora of medical equipment from the exam and imaging rooms to the intensive care units, emergency rooms, wards, and, surprisingly, wearable local area and family wellbeing gadgets. Edge registering is consolidated in the IoT access terminal of clinical hardware for limited information calculation, stockpiling, and edge wise administrations on the grounds that to its brilliant reasonableness, convenience, and deployability. Clinical gadgets with edge registering capacities are a sort of IoT terminal item that will before long arrive at development. Remote checking, clinical imaging, telemedicine, and different administrations will also benefit from the proliferation of such devices in medical clinic diagnostics and therapy plans, post-medical clinic restoration, and everyday wellbeing the board. Cloud and edge device fusion might be used in healthcare settings (Ferdinand et al., 2021).

5.2 Smart Systems for Real-Time Tracking, Detection, and Intelligent Diagnosis

5.2.1 Application of Technology to the Study of Infectious Diseases

Microorganism and genome data mix for irresistible sickness checking and early admonition is now being investigated by certain industrialised countries (European Centre for Disease Prevention and Control, 2018; Qiu et al., 2018). Multivariate man-made intelligence the board investigation and early pandemic admonition are performed by utilizing the etiology, climate, and human science associated with the spread of enormous irresistible illness information. Artificial intelligence (AI) diagnostic technologies and equipment have significantly increased the effectiveness of clinical infectious disease diagnosis (World Robotics, 2020). Programmed test handling innovation, as well as fast, delicate, explicit, and high-throughput microorganism identification innovation, will all see huge headways on account of the utilization of artificial intelligence in irresistible ailment diagnostics later on. These developments will aid in the identification and detection technologies of host-based biomarkers.

5.2.2 The Medical Robot Industry Will Expand

As the global population ages, there will be a greater need for medical robots, making this a key area of AI's potential impact on healthcare. Medical procedure robots, nursing robots, administration robots, guide robots, coordinated factors robots, recovery robots, prescription apportioning robots, and so on are just a few examples of the many types of medical robots now in use. Medical robots will undergo significant advancements because of the application and reconciliation of man-made consciousness, 5G, and other state-of-the-art technology. The widespread implementation of clinical robots will become ordinary sooner rather than later. Figure 8 depicts the worldwide sales and projected growth of medical robots from 2018–2019 to 2020–2023.

5.2.3 Intelligent Decision Support Systems in the Field of Medicine in the Future

It's going to Happen Gene detection technology and smart wearable gadgets are becoming more widely used, which will lead to more comprehensive real-world data. Future treatment planning will be individualised based on patient data, which will significantly alter the current clinical medicine paradigm. The future of medicine will be greatly aided by the insightful choice emotionally supportive network that utilizes IoT, huge information, man-made intelligence, and different advancements. From in-hospital to out-of-hospital, medical group to regional medical, the next generation of intelligent decision support systems will have numerous potential applications. The integration of the application forms with the medical information system will eventually be utilized by auxiliary diagnosis and treatment, in addition to other specific clinical applications like medical and health. Individual wellbeing the board, clinical benefits, clinical quality administration, activity and upkeep, clinical logical exploration, and drug hardware R&D will all benefit from the widespread dissemination of these software programmes (Khang, 2023).

6. CONCLUSION

With the help of IoT, this chapter's data was gathered and uploaded to the cloud or another location, where it could be processed by algorithms and methods like artificial intelligence (AI) movement ID, conduct ID, strange discovery, and helped decision-production to yield valuable bits of knowledge. In clinical medicine, the combination of AI and IoT is already being utilised to improve health care via increased intelligence. Collaborations in remote diagnosis and treatment have the potential to hasten the standardisation of diagnostic and therapeutic services for all patients. The combination of medical IoT and AI model algorithms allows for early risk identification for patients in the NICU and CCU, as well as the recommendation of treatment strategies and the prediction of treatment outcomes (Khang & Muthmainnah, 2023).

AI and IoT have the potential to revolutionise emergency care by providing timely and precise diagnosis and treatment, hence extending survival time till rescue personnel arrive. The incidence of VTE may be decreased and patients' quality of life improved via early detection of those at high risk and prompt care. The monitoring level and patient safety may both be significantly increased with the use of ongoing showcase of imperative sign information and savvy alarms by perceiving anomalies. Man-made brainpower works on the productivity and accuracy of medical picture detection and diagnosis (Khang, Rana, Tailor et al, 2023).

REFERENCES

Abramson, N., Braverman, D. J., & Sebestyen, G. S. (2006). Pattern Recognition and Machine Learning. *Publications of the American Statistical Association*, *103*(4), 886–887.

Ahamed, F., & Farid, F. (2018). Applying Internet of Things and Machine-Learning for Personalized Healthcare: Issues and Challenges. *2018 International Conference on Machine Learning and Data Engineering (iCMLDE)*. IEEE.

Ahuja, S. P., Sindhu, M., & Jesus, Z. (2012). A Survey of the State of Cloud Computing in Healthcare. *Network CommunTechnol*, *1*(2), 12–19. doi:10.5539/nct.v1n2p12

Alabdulkarim, A., Al-Rodhaan, M., & Al-Dhelaan, T. A. (2019). A Privacy-Preserving Algorithm for Clinical DecisionSupport Systems Using Random Forest. *Computers, Materials & Continua*, *58*(3), 585–601. doi:10.32604/cmc.2019.05637

Alaybeyi, S., & Lheureux, B. (2019). *Survey Analysis: Artificial Intelligence Establishes a Foothold in IoT Projects*. Gartner. https://www. gartner.com/en/documents/3968034/survey-analysisartificial-intelligence-establishes-a-fo

Alkhatib, H., Faraboschi, P., & Frachtenberg, E. (2014). *IEEE CS 2022 Report*. IEEE Computer Society.

Avci, A., Bosch, S., & Marin-Perianu, M. (2010). *Activity Recognition Using Inertial Sensing for Health-care, Wellbeing and Sports Applications: A Survey*. 23th International Conference on Architecture of Computing Systens 2010, Hannover, Germany.

Bangui, H., Rakrak, S., Raghay, S., & Buhnova, B. (2018). Moving to the Edge-Cloud-of-Things: Recent Advances and Future Research Directions. *Electronics (Basel)*, *7*(11), 309. doi:10.3390/electronics7110309

Bentley, P., Ganesalingam, J., Carlton Jones, A. L., Mahady, K., Epton, S., Rinne, P., Sharma, P., Halse, O., Mehta, A., & Rueckert, D. (2014). Prediction of stroke thrombolysis outcome using CT brain machine learning. *NeuroImage. Clinical*, *4*, 635–640. doi:10.1016/j.nicl.2014.02.003 PMID:24936414

Bhardwaj, R., Nambiar, A. R., & Dutta, D. (2017). A Study of Machine Learning in Healthcare. *2017 IEEE 41st Annual Computer Software and Applications Conference (COMPSAC)*. IEEE.

Chen, A. Y., Lu, T. Y., Ma, M. H., & Sun, W.-Z. (2016). Demand Forecast Using Data Analytics for the Preallocation of Ambulances. *IEEE Journal of Biomedical and Health Informatics*, *20*(4), 1178–1187. doi:10.1109/JBHI.2015.2443799 PMID:26087507

Dash, S., Shakyawar, S. K., Sharma, M., & Kaushik, S. (2019). Big data in healthcare: Management, analysis and future prospects. *Journal of Big Data*, *6*(1), 54. doi:10.1186/s40537-019-0217-0

Du, W., Wang, Y., & Yu, Q. (2017). RPAN: An End-to-End Recurrent Pose-Attention Network for Action Recognition in Videos. *2017 IEEE International Conference on Computer Vision (ICCV)*. IEEE. 10.1109/ICCV.2017.402

European Centre for Disease Prevention and Control. (2018). *Monitoring the use of whole-genome sequencing in infectious disease surveillance in Europe*. ECDC.

Ferdinand, A. S., Kelaher, M., Lane, C. R., da Silva, A. G., Sherry, N. L., Ballard, S. A., Andersson, P., Hoang, T., Denholm, J. T., Easton, M., Howden, B. P., & Williamson, D. A. (2021). An implementation science approach to evaluating pathogen whole genome sequencing in public health. *Genome Medicine*, *13*(1), 121. doi:10.1186/s13073-021-00934-7 PMID:34321076

Franc, J. M., Ingrassia, P. L., Verde, M., Colombo, D., & Della Corte, F. (2015). A simple graphical method for quantification of disaster management surge capacity using computer simulation and process-control tools. *Prehospital and Disaster Medicine*, *30*(1), 9–15. doi:10.1017/S1049023X1400123X PMID:25407409

Gondy, L. A., Thomas, C., & Bayes, N. (1993). Programs for machine learning. *Advances in Neural Information Processing Systems*, *79*(2), 937–944.

Goodfellow, I., Bengio, Y., & Courville, A. (2016). *Deep learning*. MIT Press.

Green, M., Bjrk, J., & Forberg, J. (2006). Comparison between neural networks and multiple logistic regression to predict acute coronary syndrome in the emergency room. *Artificial Intelligence in Medicine*, *38*(3), 305–318. doi:10.1016/j.artmed.2006.07.006 PMID:16962295

Gubbi, J., Buyya, R., Marusic, S., & Palaniswami, M. (2013). Internet of Things (IoT): A Vision, Architectural Elements, and Future Directions. *Future Generation Computer Systems*, *29*(7), 1645–1660. doi:10.1016/j.future.2013.01.010

Haider, F. (2014). Cellular architecture and key technologies for 5G wireless communication networks. *J Chongqing Univ Posts Telecommun*, *52*(2), 122–130.

Hingmire, M., Bagjilewale, M., & Dakhole, M. (2017). What is Cloud Computing. *Springer VerlagNy*, *17*(1), 3–20.

Hua, X., Aldrich, M. C., & Chen, Q. (2015). Validating drug repurposing signals using electronic health records: A case study of metformin associated with reduced cancer mortality. *Journal of the American Medical Informatics Association : JAMIA*, (1), 179–191. PMID:25053577

Ijjina, E. P., & Mohan, C. K. (2016). Hybrid deep neural network model for human action recognition. *Applied Soft Computing*, *46*, 936–952. doi:10.1016/j.asoc.2015.08.025

Joyia, G. J., Liaqat, R. M., & Farooq, A. (2017). Internet of medical things (IOMT): Applications, benefits and future challenges in healthcare domain. *Journal of Communication*, *12*(4), 240–247.

Judith, E., & James, M. (2001). Artificial neural networks. *Cancer*, *91*(S8), 1615–1635. doi:10.1002/1097-0142(20010415)91:8+<1615::AID-CNCR1175>3.0.CO;2-L PMID:11309760

Khang, A. (2023). Enabling the Future of Manufacturing: Integration of Robotics and IoT to Smart Factory Infrastructure in Industry 4.0. AI-Based Technologies and Applications in the Era of the Metaverse. IGI Global Press. doi:10.4018/978-1-6684-8851-5.ch002

Khang, A., & Muthmainnah, M. (2023). AI-Aided Teaching Model for the Education 5.0 Ecosystem. AI-Based Technologies and Applications in the Era of the Metaverse. IGI Global Press. doi:10.4018/978-1-6684-8851-5.ch004

Khang, A., Rana, G., Tailor, R. K., & Hajimahmud, V. A. (2023). *Data-Centric AI Solutions and Emerging Technologies in the Healthcare Ecosystem* (1st ed.). CRC Press. doi:10.1201/9781003356189

Khang, A., Shah, V., & Rani, S. (2023). *AI-Based Technologies and Applications in the Era of the Metaverse* (1st ed.). IGI Global Press., doi:10.4018/978-1-6684-8851-5

Kosmatos, E. A., Tselikas, N. D., & Boucouvalas, A. C. (2011). Integrating RFIDs and Smart Objects into a UnifiedInternet of Things Architecture. *Adv Internet Things*, *1*(1), 5–12. doi:10.4236/ait.2011.11002

Krallinger, M., Leitner, F., Vazquez, M., & Valencia, A. (2014). Text Mining. *Compr Biomed Phys*, *6*(10, Supplement), 51–66. doi:10.1016/B978-0-444-53632-7.01107-2 PMID:15998455

Kufrin, R. (1997). Decision trees on parallel processors. *Machine Intelligence Pattern Recognition, 20,* 279–306.

Liu, X., & Yang, X. D. (2018). *Multi-stream with deep convolutional neural networks for human action recognition in videos.Neural Information Processing.* Springer International Publishing.

Madakam, S., Ramaswamy, R., & Tripathi, S. (2015). Internet of Things (IoT): A Literature Review. *J Comp Commun, 3*(3), 164–173. doi:10.4236/jcc.2015.35021

Marjani, M., Nasaruddin, F., & Gani, A. (2017). Big IoT Data Analytics: Architecture, Opportunities, and Open Research Challenges. *IEEE Access : Practical Innovations, Open Solutions, 5*(99), 5247–5261.

Ng, Y. H., Hausknecht, M., & Vijayanarasimhan, S. (2015). Beyond short snippets: Deep networks for video classification. *2015 IEEE Conference on Computer Vision and Pattern Recognition (CVPR).* IEEE.

Qiu, T., Yang, Y., Qiu, J., Huang, Y., Xu, T., Xiao, H., Wu, D., Zhang, Q., Zhou, C., Zhang, X., Tang, K., Xu, J., & Cao, Z. (2018). CE-BLAST makes it possible to compute antigenic similarity for newly emerging pathogens. *Nature Communications, 9*(1), 1772. doi:10.1038/s41467-018-04171-2 PMID:29720583

Quan, X.X., Yang, J. F., & Luo, Z. (2021). Models in digital business and economic forecasting based on big data IoT data visualization technology. *PersUbiquitComput, Current Medical Science, 41*(6), 1149 2021. doi:10.1007/s00779-021-01603-7

Ren, Z. H., Xu, H. Y., & Feng, S. L. (2017). Sequence labeling Chinese word segmentation method based on LSTM networks. *ComputAppl Res, 34*(5), 1321–1324.

Soualmi, A., Alti, A., & Laouamer, L. (2020). *Medical Data Protection Using BlindWatermarking Technique.* Enabl AI Appl Data Sci.

Sultan, N. (2014). Making use of cloud computing for healthcare provision: Opportunities and challenges. *International Journal of Information Management, 34*(2), 177–184. doi:10.1016/j.ijinfomgt.2013.12.011

Tama, B. A., & Lim, S. (2020). A Comparative Performance Evaluation of Classification Algorithms for Clinical Decision Support Systems. *Mathematics, 8*(8), 1814. doi:10.3390/math8101814

Toltzis, P., Soto-Campos, G., & Shelton, C. (2015). Evidence Based Pediatric Outcome Predictors to Guide the Allocation of Critical Care Resources in a Mass Casualty Event. *Pediatric Critical Care Medicine, 16*(7), e207–e216. doi:10.1097/PCC.0000000000000481 PMID:26121100

Tsien, C. L., Fraser, H. S., & Long, W. J. (1998). Using classification tree and logistic regression methods to diagnose myocardial infarction. *Studies in Health Technology and Informatics, 52*(1), 493–497. PMID:10384505

Tuli, S., Tuli, S., Wander, G., Wander, P., Gill, S. S., Dustdar, S., Sakellariou, R., & Rana, O. (2020). Next Generation Technologies for Smart Healthcare: Challenges, Vision, Model, Trends and Future Directions. *Internet Technology Letters, 3*(2), e145. doi:10.1002/itl2.145

Tuya Inc, & the Gartner Group. (2020). *2021 Global AIoT Developers Ecosystem White Paper.* Tech Show Developers Conference, Hangzhou, China

Wang, L., von Laszewski, G., Younge, A., He, X., Kunze, M., Tao, J., & Fu, C. (2010). Cloud Computing: A Perspective Study. *New Generation Computing*, *28*(2), 137–146. doi:10.1007/s00354-008-0081-5

Wang, L. L., Ge, L. Z., Li, R. F., & Fang, Y. (2017). Three-stream CNNs for action recognition. *Pattern Recognition Letters*, *92*, 33–40. doi:10.1016/j.patrec.2017.04.004

World Robotics. (2020). *Report* [DB/OL]. World Robotics. https://ifr.org/news/record-2.7-million-robots-work-infactories-around-the-globe

Wsy, A., & Syh, B. (2006). A process-mining framework for the detection of healthcare fraud and abuse. *ExpSystAppl*, *31*(1), 56–68.

Zhou, Z., Shuai, Y. U., & Chen, X. (2019). Edge intelligence:a new nexus of edge computing and artificial intelligence. *Big Data Res*, *5*(2), 53–63.

Chapter 14
Internet of Medical Laboratory Things (IoMLTs) in the High-Tech Healthcare Industry

Uchejeso Mark Obeta

ⓘ https://orcid.org/0000-0002-1382-6034

Federal College of Medical Laboratory Science and Technology, Jos, Nigeria

Alexander Lawrence

Prince Abubaka Audu University, Ayingba, Nigeria

Etukudoh

ⓘ https://orcid.org/0000-0002-5467-1665

Federal College of Medical Laboratory Science and Technology, Jos, Nigeria

Obiora Reginald Ejinaka

Federal College of Medical Laboratory Science and Technology, Jos, Nigeria

Imoh Etim Ibanga

ⓘ https://orcid.org/0000-0001-8242-3768

Federal College of Medical Laboratory Science and Technology, Jos, Nigeria

ABSTRACT

Internet of medical laboratory things (IoMLTs) is the use of internet and associated applications and package to carry out medical laboratory diagnosis, transmission, and storage of results for the sake of treatment, research and public health issues. Internet of medical laboratory things is a reality and has grown from the time of internet discovery to the extent that all stages of medical laboratory practice cannot be completed in this era. IoMLTs was multiplied during COVID-19 ranging from laboratory education to training and diagnosis. The internet of things started with other professional practices like banking and finance, production companies and healthcare in general. The associated characteristics of IoMLTs includes connectivity, dynamic changes, safety, heterogeneity, enormous scale, interconnectivity, and things-related services.

DOI: 10.4018/979-8-3693-3679-3.ch014

1. INTRODUCTION

There is little or no professional practice that do not use internet in this era. The use of internet spread like wide fire across the globe that has made it an inevitable necessity and its use in healthcare and medical laboratory in particular is vast ranging from information management system in medical laboratories (IMSML) (Obeta *et al.*, 2023), artificial intelligence, automation and robotics, data management system, result sharing and public health surveillance.

Internet of medical laboratory things has its root from internet of everything, internet of things and internet of medical things. Use of internet in laboratory cannot be complete without a well-equipped medical laboratory with internet of medical laboratory things (IoMLTs) compliant equipment. There is a rapid growth in IoMLTs across the globe but it is dependent on the strength and growth of networks and internet.

2. MEDICAL LABORATORY SCIENCE

Medical Laboratory Science (MLS) is a profession in medical practice that is responsible for the diagnosis of clients/patients of various ailments with the aid of medical samples like blood, urine, stool, cough, exudates, pus and other fluids.

Medical Laboratory Science is an aspect of medical practice that is applied science and technology in health, though it started like an Art (Ozuruoke, 2022). In Nigeria, the Medical Laboratory Science has been legalized as an independent profession not minding the interferences from the related professions like Medicine, Microbiology, Biochemistry, Physiology, and Science Laboratory Technology (Khang & Hajimahmud et al., 2024).

The profession has different nomenclature across the globe (Obeta *et al.*, 2021) like Biomedical Science, Clinical Laboratory Science, and Medical Technology etc. The profession started as low level man power just as many other healthcare professionals but currently a high level manpower as graduates of various universities followed by registration and licensing by regulatory bodies according to countries of practice or residence. The medical laboratory science grew from ancient / traditional parts to use of senses, local tools, automated machines and internet linked equipment improved and efficient services as shown in Figure 1.

Alt-text: Figure 1 depicts the growth of MLS from African point of view.

3. MEDICAL LABORATORY PRACTICE BEFORE THE INTERNET

Medical laboratory practice existed as early as possible in order to assist in human diseases discovery and solutions to same. During the ancient time like from 300 B. C till this internet age could be summarized following the literature works of Ozuruoke (2022). The Hippocrates provided a trace to the use of the mind and senses as diagnostic tools unlike the African practice where the "Igba Afa" was the order of the day. The use of mind and senses lead to diagnostic technique that led to looking and tasting the patients urine to note appearance and attraction of ants and insects when the urine is on the flow where bubbles on the surface of the urine specimen indicates to kidney disease and chronic illness, sweetness and attraction of ants showed high sugar and certain urinary sediments like blood and pus in urine were

Figure 1. The African perspective of growth in medical laboratory science practice

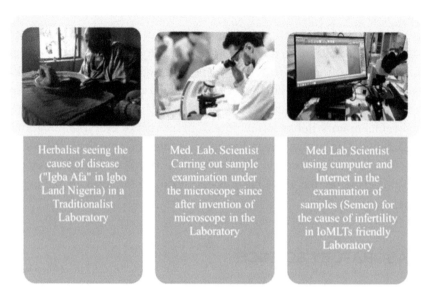

related to disease. This gave birth to Rufus of Ephesus discovery of haematuria around 500 A. D (Anh & Vladimir et al., 2024).

In middle ages, especially in 900 A.D, Isaac Judaeus introduced the guidelines for the use of urine (Uroscopy) as diagnostic aid making it popular by 1300 A.D in Europe. Around 17th and 18th Centuries, the development of the microscope (between and 1673) opened the door to the invisible world of medical laboratory diagnosis starting with the Galileo's telescope. Frederik Bekkers of Leiden in late 17th century (1694) observed protein in urine in form of a precipitate when boiled with acetic acid, while J.W. Tichy's observed sediments in the urine of febrile patients in 1774 leading to scientific urinalysis in diagnosis. The best quantitative analysis of urine at the time was pioneered by Thomas Willis (1621- 1675), due to his ability to notice the characteristic sweet taste of diabetic urine based on few quantities drinking of urine thereby establishing diabetes diagnosis. Mathew Dobson in 1776 proved that the sweetness of urine and serum in diabetes is caused by sugar leading to advent of chemical test for presence of sugar in urine by the observation of "colour change" rather than sugary taste is an example of early scientific discoveries that laid the foundation of Chemical pathology or Clinical chemistry specialty in Medical Laboratory Science.

In the 19th Century, there was emergence of sophistication in medical laboratory diagnosis and techniques. This was the onset of pathology laboratories where empiricism in medical practice was shown. From the 20th century upward, medical laboratory technicians were adequately considered for diagnosis in pathology laboratories in US and other parts of the world. From 1914 to 1918, there was an important factor in the growth of medical laboratory in the United States, both in the military and civilian hospitals and this resulted in giving medical training to both men and women. In 1915, there was a law that required all hospital to be equipped with adequate medical laboratories equipment and trained medical laboratory technicians employed. Trained Technicians advanced research on the medical laboratory improvement including automations tilled the arrival of internet.

4. INTERNET OF THINGS (IoTs)

Internet of Things (IoTs) is a network of things that are technologically connected according to standards using a compatible programs via the Internet. IoTs permit use of which are devices and assets that are well equipped with electronic components and softwares. IoTs also permits the reception, sorting, and sharing of data via the internet.

Internet of Things (IoTs) can be traced to Kevin Ashton who studied radio frequency identification (RFID) in the late 1990s. During the study, he used a technology that allows small items of radio frequency tags to be attached to various subjects, containing information and are readable at a distance. Kelvin can be quoted based on his suggestion "that every single thing, in the real physical world, in IoT would have a digital counterpart as its virtual representation". (Rayan *et al.*, 2021)

IoTs has been the talk of various researchers in various aspects of human life and practice of which the Internet of Medical Things (IoMTs) and Internet of Medical Laboratory Things (IoMLTs) could not be excluded.

5. INTERNET OF MEDICAL LABORATORY THINGS (IoMLTs)

Internet of Medical Laboratory Things (IoMLTs) is derived from Internet of Medical Things (IoMTs) traced from Internet of Things (IoTs) for the sake of Medical Laboratory Science practice. IoMLTs opens up all medical laboratory practice associated with use of computer and internet for smooth and improved Technological practice. Obeta and colleagues (2022) presented Internet of Medical Laboratory Things and its acceptability among female medical laboratory professionals with lots of hope in medical laboratory made easy both to professionals and to the patients.

Medical Laboratory Scientists therefore are professionals that deals with the testing of humans and animal samples like stool, urine, blood etc for the purpose of diagnosis and research. The Medical Laboratory Scientists are also involved in the production of biological including human vaccines, animals' vaccines and diagnostic reagents. They also fabricate and design medical laboratory equipment for the purpose of laboratory testing which are equally the part of the mandates for the practice of medical laboratory science profession in Nigeria (Obeta *et al.*, 2019; Etukudoh *et al* 2021).

There is no doubt that hospitals with a functional medical laboratory, manned by qualified and licensed Medical Laboratory Scientist provides quality results that contributes to 70-75% decisions on admissions and discharge of patients in such healthcare facility (Obeta *et al.*, 2019; Etukudoh *et al* 2021). It is true that the Medical Laboratory Scientists across the globe bears different names (Obeta et al., 2020) like Medical Laboratory Scientist, Medical Technologist, Biomedical Scientist, Clinical Laboratory Scientist Medical Laboratory Technologist, etc. but means same. Medical Laboratory Science practice and procedures lead to generation numerous medical results /data for adequate use in the management of the clients and patients in particular (Obeta *et al.*, 2019; Rehman *et al.*, 2021). There is an opportunity to manage the diseases with the aid of the results and of data analytics and the use of internet (Rehman *et al.*, 2021).

IoMLTs is referred to as object-based with medical laboratory equipment connected to networks where in real-time communication between physical (equipment or result) and cyber system is established. It is based on several information communication based technologies such as computers, smart sensors, mobile technologies and analytic platform. IoMLTs has a mutual intelligent relationship formation through sensing information, processing and networking among objects or equipment with the help of medical laboratory professionals (Maheshwari *et al.*, 2021). An IoMLTs' device is can be any device or laboratory equipment capable of communicating with any other devices with the aid of internet as shown in Figure 2.

Figure 2. Word cloud of internet of medical laboratory things
Source: Image created by Uchejeso Mark Obeta with the aid of Google WordCloud App

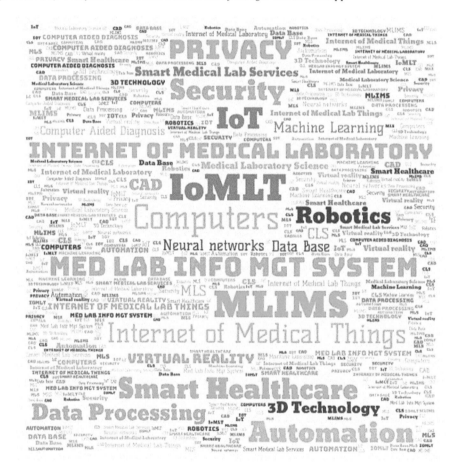

Alt-text: Figure 2 depicts the smart devices hold digital identities which allowed them to interact and communicate amongst themselves and with the environment while reacting autonomously to the physical world (Achituv *et al.*, 2016).

A medical device is an instrument, machine, implement, apparatus, in vitro reagent or other similar or related article including the component part or accessory which is recognize in the official national formulation or the United States pharmacopoeia or any supplement to them, intended for use in the diagnosis of disease or other conditions or in the care, mitigation, treatment or prevention of disease in men and other animals, or intended to affect the structure or any function of the body of Man or other animals and which does not achieve any of its primary intended purpose through chemical action within or on the body of Man or other animals which is not dependent upon human being metabolize for that achievement of any of its primary intended purpose (Achituv *et al.*, 2016).

Internet is one of the technologies that has changed every cycle of human endeavors that include; communication, science and technology, telecommunications, education and health among others. Technology has become part of human life and professional services. The internet of today makes human beings to express every bit of their emotions, the means and method by which human make use of technology today makes things very easy for them in all aspects ranging from passing of information, health care system, businesses and other activities (Rehman *et al.*, 2021).

The amount of online resources is constantly growing and this implies that there is an exponential growth of influence of the internet on professionals from all spheres of life, including health care professional. Emmanuel and Dan-Muhammadu (2017) describes the internet as one of the most versatile technologies in the human history and then versatility indicates that it is relevant to virtually all aspects of human life including health internet of things. The term was coined by Kevin Ashton in 1999 as a network of physical devices communicating with each other via the internet Kanakaradi *et al.*, (2021), today it is impossible to practice anything without internet. One of the most prominent Industries that have adopted and implemented IoT technologies is the Healthcare sector especially the medical laboratory science which is still benefiting from the internet (Khang & Hahanov et al., 2022).

IoTs is useful in medical laboratory science when new and advanced technological method of estimation and analysis are done. Several terms associated with Internet of Medical Laboratory Things (IoMLTs) are displayed in Figure 2. Predhan *et al* (2021) highlighted that IoTs/IoMLTs are transforming the current day healthcare services and medical laboratory services cannot be an exception. No wonder Jia (2015) said that medical laboratory management is better done with improved technologies backed by IoMLT. The Medical Laboratory services adoption of IoTs was a fulfilment of "the internet of things- promise of the future" as put by Coetzee & Eksteen (2011). This is because IoMLT is currently connecting professionals and clients in a sensory and intelligent manner across the globe. No wonder Nigeria medical laboratory services moved from grass to grace (Obeta et al., 2021) during COVID-19.

IoMLTs have been proven to provide succor to the testing and monitoring of some medical laboratory services for tests like blood sugar, Cholesterol, Haemoglobin, equipment and environmental temperature monitoring, sample storage and management, and certain local diseases burden for testing and monitoring (Pradhan *et al.*, 2021; WHO 2010; Ahmadi *et al* 2018; DCHS, 2018). IoMLTs also aids in data collection, data analytics, and data mining, medical laboratory information management system and result transmissions. IoMLTs shall encompass Tele-Medical Laboratory Science, where examination of samples, Slides and various medical laboratory procedures can be displayed using video calls for specialists and Consultant Medical Laboratory Scientists towards making in input in the procedures and results (Khang & Hajimahmud et al., 2024).

The IoMLT can harness the practice of Medical Laboratory Services either within the Departments/ Faculties within an institution and or with an outside organization and their experts to be easily carried out as illustrated with Figure 3.

Internet of medical laboratory things can be adequately applied in medical laboratory testing and diseases surveillance, medical laboratory clients' data management and medical laboratory associated research. Cancer care (CC) and diagnosis, diabetics testing and care, TB/Asthma testing and care and other diseases could be well handled by IoMLTs.

Diabetes is a model disease for assessing self-monitoring and adherence to treatment in various contexts including oral pharmacotherapy, injected insulin, blood glucose measurement, and blood pressure

Figure 3. IoMLTs service with medical laboratory sections linked to hospitals and external experts

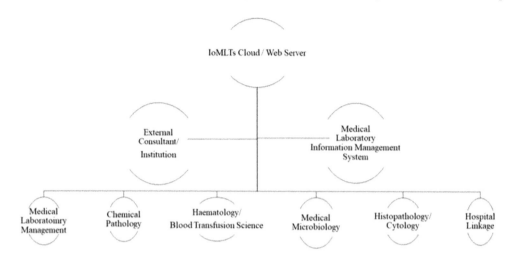

monitoring among others with the aid of IoMLT in addition to existing devices such as Android phones and some point of care testing (POCT) devices.

IoMLTs era is bridging the gap of gender and age (OECD, 2018). It makes "connectivity from any-time, any-place for any-one into any-time, any-place for anything" Bosley, 2018). This shall make any gender or age barrier for time and place a past story and any appointment about medical laboratory services is achieved through internet with ease. This era supports gender equality (Moloney *et al.*, 2020) including in medical laboratory services. The elderly and the fragile people was described by Zanella *et al* [2020] that IoMLT helped for their management in remove areas. Though numerous challenges exists with IoMLTs (Calvillo-Arbizu *et al* 2021; Amadin *et al.*, 2021; Kelly *et al.*, 2020;Singh *et al.*, 2019), the IoTs create many ways to tackle them and they are applicable to IoMLTs provided that the clients are satisfied with adequate quality improvement (Etukudoh *et al.*, 2021).

Obeta *et al* (2022) in a bid to describe the role of IoMLTs in the medical laboratory emphasized that: it streamlines diagnosis, aid self-maintenance of equipment, improved communication and connectivity among professionals and change from primitive way of practice to Tele-medical laboratory service and mobile-medical laboratory service.

6. ASSOCIATED CHARACTERISTICS OF IoMLTs

The characteristics of IoMLTs are related to the characters put by Parteek (2019), Rayan *et al* (2021), and Munir *et al* (2022) and are as follows:

6.1 Connectivity

Connectivity is germane in internet of medical laboratory things. This is because IoMLTs devices, hardware, sensors and other inbuilt electronics, hardware and applications including automated systems are usually connected to control systems and internet. The connectivity creates opportunities for medical laboratory clients to have access to their results with their access information.

6.2 Dynamic Changes

IoMLTs creates opportunities for dynamic changes with regards to gathering data and storage. Processes can easily be changed or improved by required connections or disconnections. Some required applications can be added or updated depending on the needs like location, temperature, etc as the case may be for dynamic changes depending on the time, place and person.

6.3 Safety

Knowing fully well that all IoT devices and applications are threatened by security, IoMLTs employs a very high level of privacy issue and transparency. IoMLTs is securing data between endpoints and networks.

6.4 Heterogeneity

IoMLTs equipment, devices and applications work on networks and hardware platforms and can interact with other devices through different networks. The heterogeneous networks requires modularity, scalabilities, extensibility, and interoperability.

6.5 Enormous Scale

Devices that can communicate with each other are much larger than the devices connected to the available internet. IoMLTs provides internet and control facilities very effectively no matter the number involved in the connectivity with devices and needed interpretation for applications.

6.6 Interconnectivity

The interconnectivity of IoMLTs devices is helpful for the development of a connected medical laboratory clients. Systems and patients' laboratory data are shared among all that have access through various gadgets like android, laptops, etc tat is compatible and approved for connection.

6.7 Things-Related Services

IoMLTs accepts carrying out things-related services within the acceptable limits, for example, semantic consistency and confidentiality protection between physical things and their related virtual things are possible.

7. ADVANTAGES AND DISADVANTAGES OF IoMLTs

The technological advancement in Medical Laboratory practice is encouraged especially in this era. However, this Chapter shall not fail to highlight basic advantages and disadvantages associated with IoTs and IoMLTs as earlier enumerated by Parteek (2019), Rayan *et al* (2021), and Munir *et al* (2022)

7.1 Associated Advantages of IoMLTs

The advantages of IoMLTs are listed but not limited to the following:

- **Good turn-around time**: IoMLTs saves time in medical laboratory services. This is because, the time meant for working around, writing out results and delivery to the needed points are taken care of by connectivity and internet.
- **More data in use**: In IoMLTs, data collection is enhanced thereby making information easily accessible not minding the location. Data are easily uploaded and updated without stress including real time practices.
- **Several devices connectivity**: IoMLTs makes it possible to connect various devices no matter the area of diagnosis, sample involved and result distribution to laboratory clients.
- **Guaranteed tracking and monitoring**: The IoMLTs helps to monitor and track all data in the system and was able to detect changes, corrections and access.
- **Research made easy**: Research is very easy with surplus data thereby aiding the diseases surveillance and future studies.
- **Good equipment, reagents and consumable management**: Medical laboratory logistics are also art of IoMLTs in the laboratory.
- **Medical Laboratory Automation**: IoMLTs encourages Automation and Robotics with very good medical laboratory information management systems
- **Preventive and surveillance diagnosis**: While IoMLTs minimizes the human effort, communication and interaction within the network in addition to some studies provides preventive and surveillance diagnosis.
- **Improved patience experience**: The IoMLTs is perfect tool that improves patience experience because of good turn-around time, and reduction in movement processes involving physical activities of the patient especially when the laboratory facilities are staggered
- **Improved security and little devices**: IoMLTs enhances security and offers some personal protection among patients with system connections and most importantly employs smarter systems and Android / mobile phones.
- **Use in traffic systems**: Medical laboratory commodities delivery, Asset tracking, traffic, surveillance, or transportation tracking, individual order tracking, inventory control, and customer management can be cost-effective with the right tracking using IoMLTs in medical laboratory science and technology.
- **Useful for safety concerns**: IoMLTs helps laboartories to detect potential dangers and provides warning signals to users.

7.2 Associated Disadvantages of IoMLTs

The disadvantages are listed but not limited to the following:

- **Privacy of data queries**: This involves all security issues where the existence of interconnectivity of medical laboratory data over various networks are at the risk of hackers and uninvited network attacks.

- **Security queries:** Though there are some security measures in place network Engineers and network breakers who show interest in destabilizing other networks may gain entry through dubious means. This makes data safety imperative in IoMLTs.

- **High cost of starting and maintenance**: The commencement of IoMLTs especially in poor resource certain is very expensive. This is because the existing laboratory structures are to be renovated and maintained to suit the new system. The cost of purchase and contract for such new facility including training may be huge.

- **Accuracy queries**: There would be very high queries on whether there is accuracy in data generated at the initial levels which may be dependent on the level of training of involved staff. There are also chances of IoMLTs system getting corrupted as a result of bug in the devices.

- **Data overload**: For the fact that IoMLTs is in place, staff may not consider that there is capacity of every system. This may lead to system over load with connections and storage of data arising from diagnostic machines.

- **Ethical matters**: Ethical matters arises because of those who may be doing various studies with available data on the network without prior ethical clearance and informed consent on the use of such data.

- **Increased unemployment**: IoMLTs surely would increase unemployment as non-professionals who are internet experts would have place in the laboratories more than the core professionals. The Automated machines and Robots, Smart surveillance cameras, Smart laboratory washing machines, smart heating systems, and IoMLTs compliant systems and applications would be on the increase to replace trained professionals on the bench.

- **System complexity**: The IoMLTs systems may be highly complex to comprehend by laboiartory professionals in terms of design, development, maintenance, and other linked technologies.

- **Lack of international standardizations**: IoT and IoMLTs have no standard organization and controls currently. There is lack of compatibility and cooperation among consumers and manufacturers due to an effective competition.

- **Over dependence on the internet**: This affects those medical laboratories in poor resource certain where internet is poor or not available.

- **Reduced mental and physical activity**: Medical laboratory professionals loses a lot of mental and physical activities involved in laboratory diagnosis because of IoMLTs leading to inactive and lethargic professionals.

The figure 4 provides the advantages and disadvantages of IoMLTs, however, the advantages outways the disadvantages which can also be tackled with the aid of IoMLTs.

8. CHALLENGES OF USING IoMLTs

The challenges of using IoMLTs in medical laboratory services about especially in underdeveloped and developing countries where there is less wide spread of use and 24 hours internet services challenges. Mostly internet use are private in nature and there is urgent use for government to provide internet across the length and breadth of the poor countries. The challenges could be broadly classified into ethical, financial, and technical challenges according to Rayan *et al* (2021).

Figure 4. Advantages and disadvantages of IoMLTs in medical laboratory service

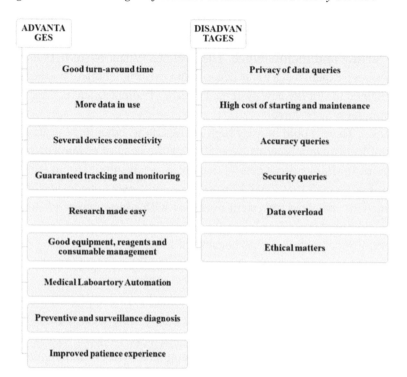

The Medical laboratory Scientists in Nigeria are interested IoMLTs as they have accepted Obeta *et al* (2022); Moloney *et al.* (2020) and Solangi *et al* (2017) not minding their marriage status, certificate possessed and age differences. However, they are challenged by IoMLT compliant equipment, unavailable new technologies, poor installations, unavailable internet services in their facilities for 24 hours

9. SOLUTIONS TO CHALLENGES MILITATING AGAINST IoMLTs

Dauwed *et al* (2018) enlisted network capacity and poor network as a challenge to IoTs and IoMLTs in healthcare. Obeta etal (2022) posited that Nigerian internet sources are mostly personal, private and institutional from Service providers. The Government and Medical Laboratory institutions is encouraged to do better with provision of internet so as to enjoy IoMLTs.

Adequate procurement and installation of IoMLTs equipment, tools and applications at various medical laboratory service levels would make that difference. There is an urgent need to reduce cost or subsidize cost for the sake of developing countries for the IoMLTs compliant equipment and applications for medical laboratory services that is IoMLTs in operation. The cost of commencement should be reduced to attract more facility users and the government is in the best position to lift the burden of financial challenges. There is need for more training among professionals and facilities.

10. COMPARATIVE ANALYSIS OF IoMLTs USAGE AMONG DEVELOPED AND DEVELOPING COUNTRIES

IoMLTs is evolving across the globe. The special reference to WHO member countries, indicates that the developing and underdeveloped member countries have more challenges and less use of IoTs and IoMLTs.

ITU (nd) in their contribution to the UN broadband commission for sustainable development with regards to Health, Water & Sanitation opined that area of IoTs to MDG 4, (Child Health); MDG 5, (Maternal health), MDG 6, (Combat HIV/ AIDS, malaria and other diseases); SDG 3, (Ensure healthy lives and promote well-being for all at all ages and SDG 6, (Ensure availability and sustainable management of water and sanitation for all) has a lot of instances at the moment including Sensor- and SMS-enabled village water pumps as seen in Rwanda & Kenya; GSM- connected refrigeration for vaccine delivery in the 'cold chain' as seen Globally; sensor-enabled 'band aid' to monitor Ebola patients' ECG, heart rate, oxygen saturation, body temperature, respiratory rate and position, all remotely as seen in West African countries; water stream gauge with sonar range sensor to monitor river flow and depth as seen in Honduras; water flow sensors and motion detectors in latrines to monitor efficacy of hygiene training and intervention as seen in Indonesia.

The usage of IoMLT/IoTs in various countries depends on the acceptability and use of Wireless Local Area Network (WLAN). Wireless Sensor Network (WSN), Wireless Wide Area Network (WWAN), Fourth-generation mobile (4G) and Fifth-generation mobile (5G). Edquist *et al.* (2019) pointed out that IoT including IoMLTs connections have been growing more rapidly in China when compared to the US in absolute figures, though the level, in terms of IoT per 100 inhabitants, was still higher in the US as at 2017. "Nevertheless, the rapid growth in Chinese IoT investments mean that the Chinese level in 2017 was higher than in many OECD-countries". Their study still showed that Sweden had exceptionally high levels of IoTs including IoMLTs connections per inhabitant. The study added that, the annual growth rate in non-OECD countries would have been approximately 23 percentage points higher during the investigated period, they would have reached the same level as OECD-countries in 2017. There is no doubt that Africa is still lagging in the aspect of IoTs/IoMLTs and needs more approach and interventions

11. CONCLUSION

Internet of Medical Laboratory Things (IoMLTs) in Nigeria and the world at large is a reality. Medical Laboratory Scientists as seen in this study have declared support for Internet of Medical Laboratory Things (IoMLTs), use of internet to transmit result to clients, use of IoMLT compliant equipment in medical laboratories no matter the level of operation such as Federal, State, and Local governments, including Faith Based Organizations (FBOs), Non-governmental organizations (NGOs) and private establishments.

It is therefore imperative for all medical laboratories to upgrade to the new era of practice where sample management and diagnosis are carried out with the aid of internet including the transmission of result to the clients. The acceptability, and use of IoMLTs is an eye opener to equipment producers and vendors to ensure the provision of IoMLT compliant equipment to Medical laboratory organizations in Nigeria (Khang & Kali et al., 2023).

This chapter is an improved review to put Internet of Medical Laboratory Things (IoMLTs) in proper perspective across the nations. The government and various medical laboratory institutions are encouraged to provide internet services for 24 hours as a way to motivate Medical Laboratory Scientists using Internet of Medical Laboratory Things in their services (Khang & Muthmainnah et al., 2023).

12. ACKNOWLEDGEMENT

We acknowledge Obeta, MU, Umar, IA, Ibanga, IE, Okey-Orji, VN, Ezeama, CJ, Ejinaka OR. Of the Federal College of Medical Laboratory Science & Technology, Jos who initially presented the related paper to the Fifth International Conference for Women in Data Science (WiDS) Prince Sultan University, Riyadh; from 28-29 March, 2022.

REFERENCES

Achituv, D.B. & Haiman, L. (2016). Physicians' attitudes toward the use of IoT medical devices as part of their practice. *Online Journal of Applied Knowledge Management. 4*(2).

Ahmadi, H. (2018). · Arji G, Shahmoradi L, Safdari R, Nilashi M, Alizadeh M. The application of internet of things in healthcare: A systematic literature review and classification. *Universal Access in the Information Society.* doi:10.1007/s10209-018-0618-4

Amadin, F. I., Egwuatu, J. O., Obienu, A. C., & Osazuwa, W. A. (2017). Internet of Things (IoT): Implications of a Wide Scale Use in Nigeria. *Computing, Information Systems, Development Informatics & Allied Research Journal, 8*(1), 95-102. www.cisdijournal.net

Anh, P. T. N. (2024). AI Models for Disease Diagnosis and Prediction of Heart Disease with Artificial Neural Networks. Computer Vision and AI-integrated IoT Technologies in Medical Ecosystem (1st ed.). CRC Press. doi:10.1201/9781003429609-9

Bosley M. (2018). *The Internet of Laboratory Equipment. Laboratory Products.* Labmate UK & Ireland.

Calvillo-Arbizu, J., Román-Martínez, I., & Reina-Tosina, J. (2021). Internet of things in health: Requirements, issues, and gaps. *Computer Methods and Programs in Biomedicine, 208,* 106231. Advance online publication. doi:10.1016/j.cmpb.2021.106231 PMID:34186337

Coetzee, L., & Eksteen, J. (2011). The Internet of Things – Promise for the Future? An Introduction. *IST-Africa 2011 Conference Proceedings.* IIMC International Information Management Corporation.

Dauwed, M. A., Yahaya, J., Mansor, Z., & Hamdan, A. R. (2018). Determinants of Internet of Things Services Utilization in Health Information Exchange. *Journal of Engineering and Applied Sciences (Asian Research Publishing Network), 13*(24), 10490–10501.

Deloitte Centre for Health Solutions. (2018). *Medtech and the Internet of Medical Things How connected medical devices are transforming health care.* Deloitte.

Edquist, H., Goodridge, P., & Haskel, J. (2021). The Internet of Things and Economic Growth in a Panel of Countries. *Economics of Innovation and New Technology 30*(3), 262-283.

Emmanuel, N.O. & Dan-Muhammadu, I. (2017). *Acceptance and Rejection of Internet for Health Information Among Private Health Professionals in a Nigerian City.* New Media and Mass Communication.

Etukudoh, N. S., & Nelson, A. B. (2021). Health care delivery business and the role of Medical Laboratory Scientists. *IAR Journal of Medical Sciences*, 2(4), 76–80.

Etukudoh, N. S., & Obeta, M. U. (2021). Patients' (Clients) Satisfaction with Medical Laboratory Services Contributes to Health and Quality Improvement. Healthcare Access. IntechOpen, doi:10.5772/intechopen.99290

ITU (n.d.). Harnessing the Internet of Things for Global Development. *ITU/UNESCO Broadband Commission for Sustainable Development.* UNESCO.

Jia, C. (2015). Laboratory Management of the Internet based on the Technology of Internet of Things. *AASRI International Conference on Industrial Electronics and Applications.* Springer. 10.1007/978-981-16-0538-3_4

Kelly, J. T., Campbell, K. L., Gong, E., & Schuffham, P. (2020). The Internet of Things: Impact and Implications in Healthcare Delivery. *Journal of Medical Internet Research*, 22(11), e20135. doi:10.2196/20135 PMID:33170132

Khang, A. (2023). Enabling the Future of Manufacturing: Integration of Robotics and IoT to Smart Factory Infrastructure in Industry 4.0. AI-Based Technologies and Applications in the Era of the Metaverse. (1st Ed.). IGI Global Press. doi:10.4018/978-1-6684-8851-5.ch002

Khang, A., Abdullayev, V., Hrybiuk, O., & Shukla, A. K. (2024). *Computer Vision and AI-Integrated IoT Technologies in the Medical Ecosystem* (1st ed.). CRC Press. doi:10.1201/9781003429609

Khang, A., Hahanov, V., Abbas, G. L., & Hajimahmud, V. A. (2022). Cyber-Physical-Social System and İncident Management. AI-Centric Smart City Ecosystems: Technologies, Design and Implementation (1st Ed.). CRC Press. doi:10.1201/9781003252542-2

Khang, A., & Hajimahmud, V. A. (2024). *Advanced IoT Technologies and Applications in the Industry 4.0 Digital Economy* (1st ed.). CRC Press. doi:10.1201/9781003434269

Khang, A., & Muthmainnah, M. (2023). AI-Aided Teaching Model for the Education 5.0 Ecosystem" AI-Based Technologies and Applications in the Era of the Metaverse. (1st Ed.) IGI Global Press. doi:10.4018/978-1-6684-8851-5.ch004

Maheshwari, P., Kamble, S., Amine, A. P., Belhadi, A., Ndubisi, N. O., & Tiwari, S. (2021). Internet of things for perishable inventory management systems: An application and managerial insights for micro, small and medium enterprises. *Annals of Operations Research.* doi:10.1007/s10479-021-04277-9 PMID:34642526

Moloney, M. E., Dunfee, M., Rutledge, M., & Schoenberg, N. (2020). Evaluating the Feasibility and Acceptability of Internet-Based Cognitive Behavioral Therapy for Insomnia in Rural Women. *Women's Health Reports (New Rochelle, N.Y.)*, 1(1), 114–122. doi:10.1089/whr.2020.0053 PMID:32617531

Munir, T., Akbar, M. S., Ahmed, S., Sarfraz, A., Sarfraz, Z., Sarfraz, M., Felix, M., & Cherrez-Ojeda, I. (2022). A Systematic Review of Internet of Things in Clinical Laboratories: Opportunities, Advantages, and Challenges. *Sensors (Basel)*, *22*(20), 8051. doi:10.3390/s22208051 PMID:36298402

Obeta, M. U., Eze, E. M., Ofojekwu, M. N., Jwanse, R. I., & Maduka, M. K. (2019). Organogram for Medical Laboratory Services in Nigerian Public Health Institutions. *North American Academic Research*, *2*(6), 69–75. doi:10.5281/zenodo.3246909

Obeta, M. U., Maduka, K. M., Ofor, I. B., & Ofojekwu, N. M. (2019). Improving Quality and Cost Diminution in Modern Healthcare Delivery: The Role of the Medical Laboratory Scientists in Nigeria. [IJBMI]. *International Journal of Business and Management Invention*, *08*(03), 8–19.

Obeta, M. U., Nkereuwem, S. E., & Okoli, C. C. (2021). Nigerian Medical Laboratory Diagnosis of COVID-19; from Grass to Grace. Intelligent Computing Applications for COVID-19: Predictions, Diagnosis, and Prevention. CRC Press Tailor and Francis Group. doi:10.1201/9781003141105-5

Obeta, M. U., Umar, I. A., Ibanga, I. E., Okey-Orji, V. N., Ezeama, C. J., & Ejinaka, O. R. (2022). Acceptability of Internet of Medical Laboratory Things among Female Medical Laboratory Professionals in Jos-Nigeria. *Fifth International Conference for Women in Data Science (WiDS)*. Prince Sultan University. 10.1109/WiDS-PSU54548.2022.00026

Obeta, U. M., Ejinaka, O. R., & Etukudoh, N. S. (2022). Data Mining in Medical Laboratory Service Improves Disease Surveillance and Quality Healthcare. In T. Saba, (Eds.), Prognostic Models in Healthcare: AI and Statistical Approaches, Studies in Big Data 109. Springer. doi:10.1007/978-981-19-2057-8_17

Obeta, U. M., Njar, V. E., Etukudoh, N. S., & Obiora, O. R. (2023). Applications of Information Management Systems (IMSML) in Medical Laboratories. A. Khang (ed.) AI and IoT-Based Technologies for Precision Medicine. IGI Global. doi:10.4018/979-8-3693-0876-9.ch026

OECD Bridging the Digital Gender Divide Include. (2018). Upskill. *Innovate (North Miami Beach, Fla.)*.

Ozuruoke D.F.N. (2022). *History of Medical Laboratory Science: Nigerian Perspective*. Pundit Publishers Abuja.

Parteek. (2019). A Review Paper on IOT Advantages and Disadvantages. *International Journal of Research and Analytical Reviews, 6*(1)

Pradhan, B., Bharti, D., Chakravarty, S., Ray, S. S., Voinova, V. V., Bonartsev, A. P., & Kunal Pal, K. (2021). Internet of Things and Robotics in Transforming Current-Day Healthcare Services. *Journal of Healthcare Engineering*, *2021*, 1–15. doi:10.1155/2021/9999504 PMID:34104368

Pradhan, B., Bhattacharyya, S., & Pal, K. (2021). IoT-Based Applications in Healthcare Devices. *Journal of Healthcare Engineering*, *2021*, 1–18. doi:10.1155/2021/6632599 PMID:33791084

Rayan, R. A., Tsagkaris, C., & Iryna, R. B. (2021). The Internet of Things for Healthcare: Applications, Selected Cases and Challenges. G. Marques et al. (eds.), IoT in Healthcare and Ambient Assisted Living, Studies in Computational Intelligence. Springer. doi:10.1007/978-981-15-9897-5_1

Rehman, A., Haseeb, K., Saba, T., Lloret, J., & Tariq, U. (2021). Secured Big Data Analytics for Decision-Oriented Medical System Using Internet of Things. *Electronics (Basel)*, *10*(11), 1273. doi:10.3390/electronics10111273

Rehman, A., Saba, T., Haseeb, K., Marie-Sainte, S. L., & Lloret, J. (2021). Energy-Efficient IoT e-Health Using Artificial Intelligence Model with Homomorphic Secret Sharing. *Energies*, *14*(19), 6414. doi:10.3390/en14196414

Singh, H., & Sharma, A. (2019). Challenges of Internet of Things: Development and Application of Conceptual Framework. *International Journal of Recent Technology and Engineering*, *8*(3), 2277–3878. doi:10.35940/ijrte.C4719.098319

WHO. (2010). *Medical devices: managing the Mismatch An outcome of the Priority Medical Devices project*. WHO.

Zanella, A., Mason, F., Pluchino, P., & Cisotto, G. (2020). *Internet of Things for Elderly and Fragile People*. arXiv:2006.05709v1

Chapter 15
AI–Driven Content Developing and Designing for Teaching Materials of Digital Healthcare

M Muthmainnah
Universitas Al Asyariah Mandar, Indonesia

Ahmad Al Yakin
Universitas Al Asyariah Mandar, Indonesia

NurJannah
Universitas Islam Makassar, Indonesia

Muthmainnah Mursidin
🆔 https://orcid.org/0000-0002-9914-4447
Universitas Islam Makassar, Indonesia

Mohammed H. Al Aqad
Management and Science University, Malaysia

ABSTRACT

The aim of this research is to contribute knowledge on English language teaching materials with public health content based on AI-based design. The authors sought student input and information before starting to design modules for EFL based on AI-powered English classes. The subjects of this research were 51 public health students and two EFL lecturers to determine their needs. Based on these findings, all students strongly agree to provide teaching materials for AI-based English learning courses in higher education.

DOI: 10.4018/979-8-3693-3679-3.ch015

1. INTRODUCTION

AI migration has largely focused on integrating into conventional learning strategies, which often mirror or automate pre-existing educational beliefs and methods. Many AIED are also created (whether they realise it or not) to help teachers and learning become more effective because, here, undergraduate students are directed to understand using AI as a learning medium and technology, not as a substitute for teachers. Although this method can be applied in areas where the number of educators is limited, it clearly does not ignore the importance of the instructor's individual expertise and the importance of students' need for guidance and social learning (Khang, et al. 2023). On the other hand, AI has the potential to do more than just automate computer-assisted student teaching; it may pave the way for new approaches to education, pose new challenges to existing pedagogy, or even make educators more practical and efficient (Muthmainnah et al. 2023). Although AIED tools have hinted at some of these possibilities, we will hypothesise other new and challenging possibilities for implementation, including the involvement of AI as part of teaching materials and for collaborative learning, with the aim of helping us better understand learning and how to learn practical ones.

To improve education quality and adapt to the ever-changing digital world, higher education institutions have begun to embrace technology (Al Yakin et al. 2022). This shift in focus is a direct result of the impact that technological advancements have had on the education industry (Gill et al. 2024). International students from all over the world flock to the Asia Pasific for a variety of reasons, including its leadership in higher education technology adoption (Grájeda et al., 2024). However, concerns and opportunities regarding the benefits of technology are still considered when wanting to integrate technology in universities throughout Asia Pacific in line with existing global developments and global progress. The technology gap in Asia Pacific is a digital gap among lecturers, students, and staff, especially those in low economic categories. (Luo et al., 2024; Matahari et al., 2024). The proliferation of various digital applications, which are actually easy to access and relatively low cost, however, the significant gap in their use for students with low economic conditions, especially quota fees or free internet access, is still minimal (Nemorin et al., 2023) so this gap can reduce the efficiency of technology adaptation in Asian universities. . It is known that Vassilakopoulou and Hustad (2023) underlined that internet network constraints, including infrastructure, human resources, and very large costs, are supporting concerns about keeping up with developments in technological digitalization. (Alenezi et al., 2023).

Even though there are various obstacles, there are still various opportunities for higher education institutions to utilise this technology, such as increasing student involvement during the learning process, increasing collaboration and personalisation (Khang et al., 2023); Gupta et al. (2024); Ali et al. (2024); and metaverse interactive technologies (Al-Adwan et al., 2023; Rojas et al., 2023; Al Yakin et al., 2023). Designing metaverse-based learning in the era of generative AI is a challenge for universities, especially in Indonesia. The lack of adoption of virtual technology and the design of virtual learning activities still carry the stigma of inadequate technological literacy.

In fact, Indonesia has adapted to digital transformation with an independent curriculum that allows teachers to convert traditional classes to AI-based classes. So that undergraduate students have the potential of this metaverse technology, various efforts have been made to construct classes and mobilise AI into courses, focusing on 21st century skills, critical thinking, and preparing mentally to compete globally in the era of digital demands (Khang et al., 2023) and flexibility and maximum accessibility to advance with a very fast metaverse (Kaddoura and Al Husseiny, 2023).

Along with the obstacles and potential benefits of implementing technology in Indonesia higher education, the importance of laws and guidelines as a moderating factor becomes apparent. With the metaverse's potential influence on universities (Laine and Lee, 2023) and the speed with which technology is evolving, clear regulations and standards are needed to solve problems with accessibility and flexibility (Farmer, 2023). Bridging the digital divide among students, faculty, and staff can be achieved through fair access to necessary technology and software, which can be achieved through such regulations. These guidelines can also encourage professional development programmes for teachers so that they can become more adept at creating and leading metaverse-based experiential learning activities (Said, 2023; Huang et al., 2022; Onu et al., 2023). Therefore, the following objective is to be achieved through this investigation, namely, to examine how lecturers adopting AI digital innovations affects their ability to successfully implement metaverse initiatives in developing and designing AI-driven teaching materials for English courses in public health study program.

2. DESIGNING HEALTHCARE AI DRIVEN PEDAGOGY

The emergence of AI has sparked talk about the Fourth Industrial Revolution, which will focus on the extraction and exploitation of data, and many believe that artificial intelligence (AI), defined as "the theory and development of computer systems capable of performing tasks that typically require human intelligence" (Rajest et al., 2023) can provide solutions to critical problems in the field of technology, such as health, economy, housing, transportation, and including education. Its notable achievements in gaming and simulation have refocused attention on artificial intelligence (AI) in the classroom, with discussions on how best to use the AI ecosystem to further education around the world.

As a result, several AI-branded products are now competing for a place in the classroom. For example, according to UNESCO Mesmar and Badran (2022), intelligent assistants can handle tedious administrative tasks such as taking attendance and creating lessons and class activities, leaving teachers with more time to engage students (Aeni et al. 2023). Educators around the world are rushing to capitalise on educational technology opportunities that have increased demand for artificial intelligence (AI) in the classroom and its potential application in universities to facilitate more accessible distance learning. Although there is growing concern regarding the potential applications of AI in education (Muthmainnah et al., 2023), there appears to be a consensus among the media and online communities that AI will play an important role in the future in this field.

According to Fui-Hoon Nah et al. (2023) AI software that can mimic human conversational capabilities—such as chat rooms—in natural language via online platforms, messaging services, or mobile applications (apps) is known as artificial intelligence (AI). For instance, the well-known AI chatbot interface ChatGPT is available in AI Generative Pre-trained Transformer version 3 (GPT-3) by the AI research and implementation company OpenAI (Fayed et al. 2023) Robust models also have better understanding and response skills thanks to improved ML and natural language processing (NLP) capabilities, rather than being optimised for human-to-human communication interactions (Hohenstein et al. 2023).

Based on viewed from a public health perspective, AI-based applications have the potential to improve health promotion and education by providing solutions that are easily accessible, economically viable, and attractive (World Health Organization, 2023). Information on preventing chronic diseases such as diabetes, hypertension, and asthma can be self-managed with the help of AI (Alahi, et al. 2023), so that public health continues to improve.

The benefits and potential of AI for health services such as facilitating patient examinations, disease diagnosis, remote treatment or digital-based health consultations, monitoring, tracking health data, early symptoms, appropriate treatment, automation, and emotional support for mental illness Galetsi et al. (2023). Personalised health recommendations, check-up schedule reminders, healthy living behaviour, health promotion, disease prevention, rehabilitation, disease management, vaccination status, nutrition, and exercise are various pieces of information that can be managed by AI in the recommended health sector (Pedro et al., 2023); Karpov et al., 2023; and Vishwakarma et al., 2023; certainly have a positive impact on society (Beets et al., 2023; Aggarwal et al., (2023). data and information processing that can accelerate health information and appropriate decisions for their health.

However, data collection and information access can trigger social and ethical problems. Therefore, the use of AI still requires strict regulations and supervision. Although the emergence of AI is subject to various debates, its presence cannot be prevented in the academic and higher education communities (Asan et al., 2023). The presence of AI can improve the critical thinking skills of undergraduate students (Muthmainnah et al., 2022), and the computational skills of Muthmainnah et al. (2023) in the field of education can be achieved effectively and efficiently with the help of AI. On the other hand, they have claimed emphasised that AI needs to complement and support human instructors and researchers, not replace them.

Deiana et al. (2023) stated there is currently a lot of buzz in the scientific community about the application of artificial intelligence (AI) in academia. However, many concerns arise with these technological tools as well, namely more obvious problems such as plagiarism. In this preliminary study, we tested the hypothesis that the application of AI robot tutors and GPT-3 might be included as media and technology used to develop and design teaching materials, especially for public health study programmes could provide several benefits, such as more participation, easier collaboration, learning convenience, and easier accessibility. This research achieved several objectives: We began by evaluating EFL teaching materials, testing the efficacy of the English language tutor robot AI and GPT-3 features in terms of their potential to promote public health teaching materials. Second, to incorporate AI expertise into this field of study, we asked the AI model itself to write most of the textbook and serve as a co-author. Third, we study how to increase the production of AI teaching materials in the future and integrate AI tutor robots as a strategy to increase EFL learning motivation, engagement, self-confidence, and learning autonomy.

There are four primary ways in which artificial intelligence (AI) is influencing student learning: (1) task assignment according to individual competency, (2) human-machine discussions, (3) analysis of student work for feedback, and (4) increased flexibility and interaction in digital environments. Students have had their learning assignments tailored to their own strengths and interests through the usage of AI-powered learning environments Ifelebuegu, (2023) constructed an AI-integrated management system using AR, VR, and MR technologies to track students' progress in learning and assign adaptive tasks based on that data; Kouijzer, et al. (2023) used a virtual patient to train medical students; Monterubbianesi et al. (2023) designed and built an intelligent virtual lab to meet students' needs by giving them appropriately challenging lab work; and Hudson et al. (2023) employed an AI-enhanced pediatric to give medical students real-time feedback and adaptive tasks. One of the major obstacles to tailoring assignments to students' abilities, according to these studies, is an absence of helpful learning materials. Intelligence systems pre-made learning assignments weren't always up to snuff when it came to catering to students' unique requirements. These studies show that AI-powered personalised learning is still in its early stages of development and application, with the absence of suitable learning materials being the main obstacle.

Offering dialogues between machines and humans: Most of the research made use of AI chatbots and interactive books to facilitate student-machine dialogues over course material. Artificial intelligence methods use frameworks that store the expertise and knowledge of humans to simulate the way humans think. Language learners have found success with AI chatbots, and books developed using these methods by engaging in continuous interaction with the bots (Al-Obaydi et al., 2023). Using question-and-answer sessions, students engaged with AI agents. Most students thought this was a fun and effective way to get their questions answered. However, there are also certain difficulties with these conversations that these papers highlight, and they imply that there was a lack of research on the impact of these conversations on students' experiences. Chatbots have the potential to enhance learning and engage students, but it is yet uncertain whether and how to implement this strategy.

They have been to analyse student work and the learning process to provide timely feedback and advice (Montenegro et al., 2023). One study that employed an artificial intelligence notebook app to identify and learn kindergarteners' handwriting and examine its spatiotemporal properties (the form, order, and direction of the segments). Each writing session ended with the app providing students with feedback. By tracking the socially conscious emotions and actions of autistic students, Dergaa et al. (2023) were able to enhance their attention with the help of smart glasses powered by artificial intelligence. Unfortunately, these systems typically provided pre-written comments that did not address the requirements of individual students. Instead of receiving the same feedback repeatedly, both students and teachers would benefit from a system that is easier to use and gives better guidance.

The use of artificial intelligence (AI) has allowed for the collection of student learning data and the facilitation of interactions, leading to more adaptive digital environments that are both more interactive and more adaptable. Learning was made more flexible and interactive with the use of student profiles and personalities. Research on digital environments enhanced by artificial intelligence has focused on their design and implementation, but little is known about how these settings influence students' actual learning. The absence of a suitable evaluation strategy is the primary obstacle to the current state of exploratory research in this field. AI in the classroom function (1) providing adaptive teaching tactics; (2) enhancing instructors' abilities to teach; and (3) assisting teacher professional development are the three responsibilities that artificial intelligence (AI) has been ascribed in the field of education. Offering methods of personalised instruction: According to (Yang and Zhang, 2019) intelligent tutoring systems strive to suggest lesson plans and activities that are suitable for teaching purposes. For instance, in order to assist educators in determining the most effective ways to present material, conduct lessons, and communicate with students.

3. DEVELOPING TEACHING MATERIALS AI DRIVEN FOR PUBLIC HEALTH

Learning tools that are always developing include: a) learning materials; b) boundaries; c) methods; and d) evaluation techniques designed to achieve complex learning competency or sub-competency targets in an interesting, systematic, and principled manner. These are referred to as learning resources Deng and Wang (2023). Specifically, the purpose of this definition is to enlighten students about the studied theoretical principles, ideas, and results. According to Koraishi, (2023) the concept of applications, which function as learning resources, outline procedures for the teaching and learning process. Place emphasis on children learning by doing; this will help them develop their knowledge and abilities in a positive way.

In the broadest sense, "teaching materials" refer to all resources that educators use to convey knowledge to their students. The use of quality teaching materials can facilitate learning and boost student achievement. Students in a classroom come in all shapes and sizes, but they should all work towards the same learning goals; therefore, it is ideal if the lesson plan is tailored to the teacher's content (Yildiz, 2023). An alternative view (Wang and Zhang, 2023) argues that teaching materials are needed for teachers, supervisors, and students to carry out predetermined learning strategies by presenting information logically and sequentially. What resources do educators, or even students, utilise to enhance the learning process and this concept comes from Tomlinson (2023). Learning resources/learning activity resources that help each student's needs in the learning activity process. According to the author's analysis of the definitions provided, learning materials, or what helps students learn and carry out learning tasks, or what helps teachers understand teaching concepts, plans, and ideas more effectively, are all part of teaching.

When thinking about how to create virtual pedagogical tools, it is important to keep the following in mind: virtual pedagogies exist independently of each other; designers focus on ensuring that learning objects and their components are accessible to individuals and students; digital pedagogy (AI) tools that incorporate multimedia tools in real-time; digital pedagogical tools that represent things in their true form during the learning process; and finally, the visual form of digital pedagogical tools, such as two or three-dimensional images in analytical exposition materials, can make learning interesting and effective. The following are the stages of developing AI-driven teaching materials: (a) collecting and analysing students' learning material needs and required competencies; (b) preparation, where the teacher teaches students how to use AI and AI-driven teaching materials; and (c) maintenance, namely, the teacher carries out maintenance on the platform that accommodates AI-driven teaching materials. Various forms of electronic pedagogical resources, including but not limited to: YouTube, written materials, physical models, mind-mapping-based presentations, and interactive multimedia. Additionally, educational learning instructions, desired competencies, additional materials, activities, and assessments are the five pillars on which virtual pedagogy resources depend.

ASSURE following development steps: (1) pre-research, namely analysing student needs and collecting observations and field data to identify problems faced by both teachers and students during the learning process; (2) needs analysis, which involves understanding users to create products suitable for English language learners. The research investigation went through several phases, including literacy studies (which include expert opinions and related findings from previous research), comparative studies (which cover the how and why of product production), interviews, and observations. (3) There are three main schemes for preparing digital-based teaching materials: conceptual, procedural, and physical. (4) Expert assessments, small classes, and field group tests are used to validate, evaluate, and revise digital-based teaching materials. (5) Data collection and analysis are part of the research process involving the application of models. Conceptually, there is a plan for creating digital educational resources that combines the 3P model (user, process, and product) with design, conditions, and learning outcomes; procedurally, there is planning to use the ASSURE model.

This research seeks to increase the efficacy of pedagogical methodology in conventional classrooms by improving the learning design system process. This process serves as an important instrument for educators, facilitating the development of optimal learning environments designed to accommodate students with iGen characteristics. This research uses the ASSURE model, a comprehensive framework consisting of six interrelated components: analysing students, stating standards and goals, selecting strategies, technology, media, and materials, utilising technology, media, and Revise. In the context of this investigation, the foundational phase of ASSURE, referred to as learner analysis, takes precedence.

This initial stage has been carried out systematically to begin the development and formulation of pedagogical materials driven by artificial intelligence, with a special focus on improving learning strategies in the field of public health study programmes.

4. METHOD

Mix method used in this study adapts from Borg and Gall research and development design (R&D) (1986: 775-776) as a basic reference in developing and designing AI-driven public health teaching material products, which have never been done before. In this research, before researchers developed teaching material products, they investigated the needs of undergraduate students and conducted a survey regarding AI applications. The effectiveness of AI as an English tutor really helps undergraduate students understand the EFL language efficiently. The development principle begins with a survey to find out the opinions of students and lecturers regarding the products needed and developed based on the curriculum, as well as identify the challenges of learning English in public health study programmes that still use conventional methods. Based on this initial data, researchers needing AI-driven teaching materials then asked undergraduate students to provide their opinions through a survey questionnaire.

Figure 1. (a, b). Introducing AI driven for public health

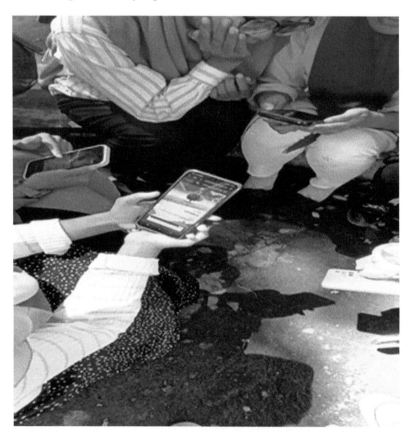

This research aims to create teaching materials in the public health study programme with artificial intelligence (AI)-driven teaching and learning at Al Asyariah Mandar University by surveying students and instructors. An online questionnaire with closed and open questions was used to conduct the survey. An analysis of undergraduate students' needs regarding AI in higher education formed the basis for creating the questionnaire as shown in Figure 1 (a, b).

Instrument

The research questionnaire covers the characteristics of undergraduate students' needs, readiness for transformation of AI-based teaching materials, success metrics, adoption intention factors, and learning activities, all of which originate from the hypothesis and scope of the research. The instrument consists of two segments, each aligned with a different investigative objective. The main part is conducting a comprehensive data survey, followed by tracing the syllabus and lesson plan, or performance readiness, as well as interviews. Using a 5-point Likert scale, respondents indicated their level of agreement, ranging from 1 to "strongly disagree" to 5 to "strongly agree." Further examination of the interactions between the identified factors was carried out.

5. DATA COLLECTION PROCEDURES

Research analysis unfolds through a two-level approach. Initially, field specialists examine questionnaire items to propose research hypotheses. This preliminary examination measures the observed variables, clarity of content, reliability, and validity of the scale. Further improvements to handle validity are filled in based on input. The second stage involved administering a formal questionnaire, which was distributed to 51 students in the public health studies programme at Universitas Al Asyariah Mandar and two English lecturers. By using a hybrid strategy that includes purposive sampling, this method ensures a comprehensive and representative sample.

To get a good idea of how people use and think about AI tools for English courses such as AI tutor Lily, Cici bot, Andy-AI, or generative ones such as ChatGPT, this survey has a variety of questions. Several questions probed participants' familiarity with forms of generative AI as well as their opinions on using these tools in classroom teaching. Survey data received from students and lecturers was analysed using descriptive statistics to learn more about how the development and design of teaching materials for EFL language courses in AI-driven integrated public health study programmes is used and perceived at universities. Statistical analysis is used to summarise and describe the main features of research samples and data; descriptive analysis is a good choice. When examining survey data, it can provide a good idea of the distribution of answers, central tendencies, and variability.

In addition to questionnaires, information was collected through in-depth interviews. In addition to numerical opinion polls, there were also open-ended questions designed to elicit responses that addressed the importance of incorporating AI-driven technology from respondents, and their unique viewpoints and experiences were carefully recorded. To find commonalities and trends in answers to free-form questions, researchers used a thematic analysis strategy. Rather than having planned themes, topics develop from the data because of using inductive techniques to examine replies.

6. DATA ANALYSIS

The analysis stage consists of four sequential steps that are adapted to the research objectives and the suitability of the measurement scale and statistical methods. Descriptive analysis and descriptive statistics using IBM SPSS 26. Initial exploratory analysis extracted respondent demographic information. A more complete picture of how and why AI-driven technologies are used and understood in universities as teaching materials is possible by combining quantitative and qualitative data. The results make it possible to identify possible needs, suggestions, and policy approaches for AI in higher education pedagogy. To ensure constructive and ethical use of this technology, understanding this is essential.

7. FINDINGS AND DISCUSSION

Over the language EFL course of 10 meeting from October 2023 to December 2023 questionnaires were sent out and 51 samples from respondents were collected. According to the gender breakdown in the descriptive analysis, men made up most respondents in terms of age, most respondents (95,9%) were female and (38%) in the 19-age bracket, 34% falling into the 17-18 age bracket, 28% were 20–25-year-old. Most respondents were instructors at the assistant professor level. Also, they were full-time teachers and almost were instructors low an information technology experience. The teachers surveyed had never used artificial intelligence before in teaching language EFL foreign language.

The data obtained in Figure 2 is known to depict the learning styles prevalent among the group of undergraduate students tested, presenting a portrait of their preferences and tendencies in the field of educational modalities that can be used as a basic reference for designing an EFL language learning syllabus. The survey results showed that students' inclination towards visual learning reached 24.5%, which shows a clear tendency to assimilate information through visual stimuli. This underlines the trend towards teaching materials that incorporate graphic representations, diagrams, pictures, and visual aids to enhance understanding.

At the same time, the kinaesthetic learning style, which accounts for 18.4% of the surveyed population, shows a great tendency towards tactile and hands-on experiences as the optimal channel for knowledge absorption. In contrast, the auditory learning style of 12.2% of respondents underlines the tendency towards auditory stimulation in the learning process. This group shows a tendency to assimilate information through auditory channels, such as lectures, discussions, and verbal articulations.

Remarkably, the prevalence of a combined auditory and visual learning style among students is very large; the data covers 44.9% of the total respondents. These data results indicate a preference for multimodal learning approaches that integrate auditory and visual elements, thereby accommodating a variety of sensory inputs to optimise the learning experience. This initial data on the known preferences of different learning styles serves as a basic framework for adapting teaching methodologies, allowing educators to skilfully design and implement pedagogical strategies that align with the diverse inherent preferences of the students under consideration, including AI-driven learning. The following questionnaire clearly shows the use of technology to improve English language teaching. The aim was to find out what students think and feel about an innovative teaching method that combines English language learning and artificial intelligence (AI). The thematic developments include a comprehensive 14-week curriculum, where AI integration is specifically designed to enhance understanding and appreciation of public health concepts. Delivered under the guidance of Tutor Lily, Cici bot and ChatGPT.

Figure 2. Students learning style

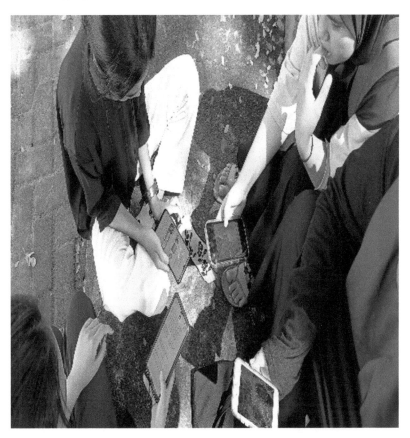

The questionnaire further explored subjective aspects of learning design, using refined academic discourse to find out how participants felt about the usefulness and impact of technology-based teaching materials. The responses are organized in a way that gives us a lot of different information about participants' feelings and opinions about this unique way of learning English and the use of AI to help teachers collaborate.

Based on descriptive statistics in Table 1 give us a lot of information about how the participants felt about using technology to improve their English language learning, especially when it came to integrating AI and making sure the lessons were relevant to teaching public health. Data collected from a sample size of 51 respondents showed consistently positive average scores across various dimensions, ranging from participants' desire to learn English with technology to their support for AI-based pedagogical interventions. Notably, the mean score for each item was consistently above 4 on a 5-point scale, indicating a high level of agreement and positive sentiment. Standard deviations, which reflect the degree of variability in responses, were generally moderate, thus indicating a degree of consensus among participants. What is interesting is the overarching theme that carefully designed teaching materials, enriched with AI elements, not only contribute significantly to participants' understanding of English and public health but also foster enthusiasm and confidence in the learning process. This empirical evidence underscores the potential efficacy of integrating AI into English education, particularly when contextualised within the domain of public health.

Table 1. The results of students need analysis on AI-Driven for public health materials

Descriptive Statistics	N	Minimum	Maximum	Mean	Std. Deviation
1. I need to learning English with technology	51	1.00	5.00	4.5490	.98618
2. I love learning English with AI	51	1.00	5.00	4.2941	.83172
3. I want English material based on public health	51	1.00	5.00	4.4314	.87761
4. Week 1: Introduction to Public Health and AI Integration	51	1.00	5.00	4.3529	.89047
5. Week 2: Epidemiological Foundations and AI Applications	51	1.00	5.00	4.3137	.92715
6. Weeks 3–4: Health Behavior and Promotion with AI Technology	51	1.00	5.00	4.3922	.87358
7. Weeks 5–6: Environmental Health Analysis and AI	51	2.00	5.00	4.3137	.86000
8. Weeks 7-8: AI Global Perspectives and Health in Global Health	51	2.00	5.00	4.3333	.73937
9. Weeks 9–10: Social Determinants of Health and AI Solutions	51	1.00	5.00	4.2941	.90098
10. Weeks 11–12: Public Health Policy, Advocacy, and AI Impact Assessment	51	3.00	5.00	4.3922	.75042
11. Weeks 13–14: Peaks and Future Directions in AI-Based Public Health	51	3.00	5.00	4.2941	.72922
12. The structural composition of teaching materials is inherently interesting.	51	3.00	5.00	4.3333	.73937
13. The design of teaching materials serves as a catalyst to grow my enthusiasm in mastering English.	51	1.00	5.00	4.2745	.87358
14. The teaching materials, designed with AI in mind, contributed significantly to my understanding of the nuances of AI driven English and basic public health concepts	51	3.00	5.00	4.4314	.70014
15. I believe that carefully designed teaching materials will increase the enjoyment of mastering English, especially because the teaching materials are aligned with my field of knowledge.	51	2.00	5.00	4.3922	.87358
16. The design of the teaching materials helped me understand English and public health.	51	2.00	5.00	4.3529	.82033
17. Carefully selected teaching materials really helped me understand EFL and healthcare	51	2.00	5.00	4.2941	.85543
18. This material will increase my confidence in mastering EFL	51	1.00	5.00	4.2353	.90749
19. Valid N (listwise)	51				

Table 2 presents descriptive statistics indicate a generally favourable outlook among participants, with the mean score well above the midpoint of the observed range. The narrow standard deviation suggests a degree of homogeneity in respondents' evaluations. Respondents generally showed a positive response based on a relatively high average score, which means they agreed that the EFL discussion material for the AI-driven public health study programme was useful and of high quality. The results of this statistical data provide valuable insight into the needs of undergraduate students and provide public health-specific teaching material content for the 1st semester EFL language course as an overall AI-driven.

Table 2. Descriptive Statistics

	N	Minimum	Maximum	Mean	Std. Deviation
EFL materials for public health AI driven	51	35.00	90.00	78.2745	12.49973
Valid N (listwise)	51				

Figure 3. The histogram of public health teaching materials

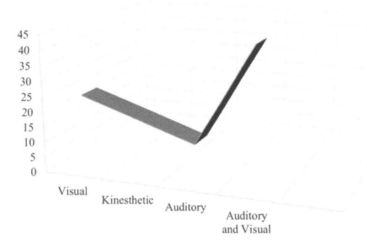

Based on the histogram and SPSS analysis results, it is known that the average value obtained is 78.2745, which is the answer from 51 respondents with a rating scale that is in the good category in Table 3 with a categorization framework starting from very low to very good. The results of this academic evaluation provide recommendations for the importance of developing and designing teaching materials according to student needs and more modern learning methods.

Table 3. Students' response toward the EFL-public health materials

Interval Score	Categories
90-100	Very Good
70-80	Good
60-70	Fairly
50-60	Low
<40	Very Low

After processing survey data regarding survey respondents regarding the development of AI-driven EFL language teaching materials for the public health study programme with excellent results and strong positive responses, semi-structured interviews were conducted. This interview selected six respondents from 51 total respondents and involved two EFL lecturers with teaching experience of between 5 and

10 years. This qualitative investigation was carried out outside the classroom and invited students to give their opinions on AI-driven teaching materials. In general, the six undergraduate students in the public health study programme who were interviewed had never had contact with AI technology while they were studying EFL, starting in junior high, senior high, and even at university. This novelty has an impact that raises their motivation to learn about EFL, which so far is still designed in the form of traditional and textual classes without any meaningful experience. The next question was about their opinion regarding the use of AI-driven learning in the classroom. Because AI-driven is something new, the researcher introduced AI-driven in class during two meetings.

The aim is for them to carefully understand the questions asked in the questionnaire. They showed their sentiments towards the use of AI-driven learning in the classroom. They both agreed that their EFL language learning content should focus on public health, for example, through readings or texts as well as artefact projects showing their knowledge of public health in EFL. Of course, they really appreciate this initiative because the material becomes easier to understand; for example, knowing the definition of tense and examples of its use in everyday life can be accommodated by the robot tutor, Lily. The implementation of this robot tutor maximises the personalisation of undergraduate students' learning. Of the six students interviewed, four respondents stated that it was very important to emphasise writing and reading practice independently and in groups.

Next, the respondents responded to the second question regarding whether they felt the benefits and effectiveness of AI-driven learning. They responded very well. Their answer was the same as the survey results; they added that the role of the EFL language tutor robot was very effective. Apart from that, ChatGPT also helps them find ideas, concepts, and criticism for public health. This AI-driven motivation motivates them to learn EFL, increases understanding, is interactive, fun, reduces anxiety and lack of self-confidence, and makes them feel like they are part of a language learning experience that actively involves them. Even though none of them mentioned negative impacts, quotas and internet access are really needed for this AI drive to be maximised.

The fourth question asked about public health content and activities, and they responded that they were very happy with the group and multimodal activities presented. The final question is regarding their suggestions and hopes. Their suggestion is to design EFL language teaching materials with very interesting AI-driven public health content that can be implemented next year, and they hope that lecturers in other courses can adopt this innovation. They hope that the aspirations and success of the dissemination of this teaching material will be sustainable, more advanced, interesting, oriented towards student-centred learning, and maintained. The results of this interview provide knowledge that overall students are very interested in the development and design of AI-driven teaching materials because they believe it can improve their EFL language skills and is very valuable for the progress of the EFL language learning model, which so far still adopts conventional methods.

Interviews with lecturers were conducted on December 17, 2023. Responses from lecturers who teach EFL in the public health study programme still use conventional methods and minimal media and technology. This is a new experience for them when they are introduced to AI, which is presented in the curriculum and lesson plans. The information obtained shows that so far, their teaching has emphasised textual and has not been based on a metaverse learning environment. Therefore, before conducting the interview, the researcher introduced several AIs that would be used in learning and instruction based on a student-centred learning approach and showed the results of data on the needs of undergraduate students and their responses, especially in applying learning in the context of incorporating AI robots.

The results of the interview responses obtained from the lecturers were that in the first question, the lecturers said that the integration of AI into EFL language learning would provide a pleasant atmosphere, and this would not only trigger the motivation of undergraduate students but also the lecturers who teach. They offered to be trained and guided in managing this AI-driven class. The second interview question asked about teaching materials or material content. They suggested that this content be presented in the study programme because they understand the scope of the material and its limitations of the material. Although researchers have evaluated the English language curriculum, they expressed the possibility that the development of teaching materials could be adapted to the core curriculum of study programmes and faculties of public health. The next question regarding their support for innovation in the development of teaching materials received a positive response; both lecturers strongly agreed.

The fourth question asked whether lecturers would be involved and support the development of this teaching material to make it more optimal and efficient. They responded with a commitment to participate and support optimally, and the use of these teaching materials will continue and be used forever. The last question expressed the lecturers' readiness to associate this AI-driven content with and prepare themselves to use applications that support EFL language learning with AI-driven public health content. In addition, overall, both lecturers and students agree with the development of AI-driven public health-based teaching materials.

8. DISCUSSION

The results of research based on statistical data and interviews revealed that 51 undergraduate students in the public health study program and two lecturers strongly agreed with the initiation of the development and design of EFL language teaching materials with AI-driven public health content. Involving AI in EFL language learning with the advantage of P, chatbots can be EFL language practice partners that are available 24/7 and can be implemented anytime and anywhere. Undergraduate students can practice their foreign language skills—their speaking and listening abilities—in a natural setting by engaging in dialogue with AI. AI can provide very practical feedback and help undergraduate students correct their mistakes so that their language skills can gradually improve. The AIEd tools that will be used in public health EFL classes are the Lily tutor robot, the Cici bot, and ChatGPT. Learning about public health starts with an introduction to public health, epidemiological foundations and AI apps, health behavior, environmental health analysis, global perspective and health in global health, determinants of health and AI solutions, public health policy, advocacy, and AI impact assessment, peaks, and future directions.

AI-based in public health is material content agreed upon by students according to the needs of learning EFL in the public health study program, which is welcomed by the public health faculty. Learning complex grammar with the help of AI robot tutors and other AIEd systems offers concrete explanations and grammatical examples with context-dependent sentences. The presence of AIEd really helps undergraduate students to increase vocabulary related to people's health, use new terms in a natural conversational atmosphere, and help them memorize the material and remember it very well.

Furthermore, AI-driven learning innovation motivates them to learn optimally (interview results). The capabilities of the robot tutor Lily, the Cici bot, and ChatGPT, which will be used during EFL language learning, have become very valuable and powerful tools for undergraduate students of public health study program Table 1. According to undergraduate students and lecturers in the public health study program, this AI-driven teaching material is very interesting and very useful for them, increasing EFL language productivity while still combining with other tools such as YouTube and Google sites.

Many of these processes can be automated with the use of AIEd tools, thereby increasing productivity and efficiency. Their ability to process natural language allows them to craft messages that are clear, professional, and contextually relevant; this makes it ideal for use in writing sentences, dialogue, and other types of communication similar with (Khang et al., 2023) investigation. While AI chatbots are great for many administrative jobs, humans are still needed for more complex tasks that involve judgement or decision-making, or for jobs where accuracy is a priority.

Development and design of public health teaching materials based on needs analysis in the public health study program with AI-based teaching material content described in Table 1. The data results show that respondents' comprehensive understanding and attitudes towards the use of AI technology are urgent, and the relevance of the material is in accordance with the study program on public health with AI pedagogical interventions. The empirical evidence shown in Table 1 is on a scale of 4–5 with high positive sentiment. The themes presented are carefully designed and enriched with AI elements that contribute significantly to public health English learning by fostering enthusiasm, motivation, self-confidence, and comfort in learning during the learning process. These findings contribute to a comprehensive understanding of the perceptions and responses of public health study program students towards the integration of AI-driven language acquisition.

This extensive review includes a perspective on AI-driven learning where participants, including students, lecturers, and faculty, support and identify the benefits that arise, such as feedback, personalization, increasing digital competence, learning innovation with virtual spaces that attract interest and motivation, and increasing EFL language proficiency, which results in Jayapal, J. (2024) conducted research that is comparable to this research.

The results of this research also explore the use of chatbots in education and their dual role as media, learning technology, and teaching materials, similar to the findings of several scholars such as Huseinović (2024) and Jiménez (2024) in efficiently improving the academic results of undergraduate students. This research exploration extends to metaverse adaptive environments so that universities can modernize their curricula by emphasizing teacher and student communication, predicting student performance, providing meaningful lessons and feedback, and creating an active and sustainable classroom atmosphere. This research also highlights the need for learning EFL in a public health context by integrating micro and macro language skills supported by AI driven. This research synthesis not only highlights the development of teaching materials but also the design of learning instructions that are varied, adaptive, and effective. Overall, the results of this comprehensive research support AI-driven contributions to public health, providing valuable insights into AI-driven applications in the metaverse era as well as the broader and deeper educational landscape.

9. CONCLUSION

The state of the art of this research is that constructing AI-driven teaching materials for public health is something new and an urgent need among university students. The development of this teaching material is strongly supported by instructors, faculties, and institutions. Based on the needs of undergraduate students, this AI-driven public health teaching material is interactive, efficient, effective, practical, interesting, motivating, authentic, easy to use, the instructions are clear, it involves 21st century skills, involves autonomy, self-direction, and self-determination in learning, can be applied in complex learning environments, is environmentally friendly, can be applied in formal, non-formal, and informal learning environments, can be evaluated online, and is affordable AI-driven technology.

EFL language learning activities are presented with interesting and contextual or real-life topics that present the concrete cultural background of undergraduate students and can be carried out at English level 1 semester 1, which emphasizes vocabulary construction, dialogue, grammar, and macro skills that can be used inside and outside the classroom, in independent study or group study, and have a global context. Instructors can use this teaching material and more varied instructions with collaborative learning that combines various IoT technologies, for example, YouTube and Google sites, and AI-driven learning is the main tool.

Here, the instructors do not only focus on EFL language skills themselves but also train 21st century skills, literacy skills, and leadership skills for their career development needs. Undergraduate students with iGen characteristics are more interested in learning by actively engaging them; they prefer to learn practically and increase their confidence to demonstrate their EFL language skills through AI-driven learning, which inspires them to learn more freely and creatively.

REFERENCES

Aeni, N., Khang, A., Al Yakin, A., Yunus, M., & Cardoso, L. (2024). Revolutionized Teaching by Incorporating Artificial Intelligence Chatbot for Higher Education Ecosystem. In *AI-Centric Modeling and Analytics* (pp. 43–76). CRC Press.

Aggarwal, A., Tam, C. C., Wu, D., Li, X., & Qiao, S. (2023). Artificial Intelligence–Based Chatbots for Promoting Health Behavioral Changes: Systematic Review. *Journal of Medical Internet Research*, *25*, e40789. doi:10.2196/40789 PMID:36826990

Al-Adwan, A. S., Li, N., Al-Adwan, A., Abbasi, G. A., Albelbisi, N. A., & Habibi, A. (2023). Extending the technology acceptance model (TAM) to Predict University Students' intentions to use metaverse-based learning platforms. *Education and Information Technologies*, 1–33. PMID:37361794

Al-Obaydi, L. H., Pikhart, M., & Klimova, B. (2023). ChatGPT and the General Concepts of Education: Can Artificial Intelligence-Driven Chatbots Support the Process of Language Learning? [iJET]. *International Journal of Emerging Technologies in Learning*, *18*(21), 39–50. doi:10.3991/ijet.v18i21.42593

Al Yakin, A., Muthmainnah, G., S., C., L., & Asrifan, A. (2023). Cybersocialization Through Smart Digital Classroom Management (SDCM) as a Pedagogical Innovation of "Merdeka Belajar Kampus Merdeka (MBKM)" Curriculum. In Digital Learning based Education: Transcending Physical Barriers (pp. 39-61). Singapore: Springer Nature Singapore.

Al Yakin, A., Obaid, A. J., Muthmainnah, R. S. A. M., Khalaf, H. A., & Al-Barzinji, S. M. (2022). Bringing technology into the classroom amid Covid 19, challenge and opportunity. *Journal of Positive School Psychology*, *6*(2), 1043–1052.

Alahi, M. E. E., Sukkuea, A., Tina, F. W., Nag, A., Kurdthongmee, W., Suwannarat, K., & Mukhopadhyay, S. C. (2023). Integration of IoT-Enabled Technologies and Artificial Intelligence (AI) for Smart City Scenario: Recent Advancements and Future Trends. *Sensors (Basel)*, *23*(11), 5206. doi:10.3390/s23115206 PMID:37299934

Alenezi, M., Wardat, S., & Akour, M. (2023). The Need of Integrating Digital Education in Higher Education: Challenges and Opportunities. *Sustainability (Basel)*, *15*(6), 4782. doi:10.3390/su15064782

Ali, O., Murray, P. A., Momin, M., Dwivedi, Y. K., & Malik, T. (2024). The effects of artificial intelligence applications in educational settings: Challenges and strategies. *Technological Forecasting and Social Change*, *199*, 123076. doi:10.1016/j.techfore.2023.123076

Asan, O., Choi, E., & Wang, X. (2023). Artificial Intelligence–Based Consumer Health Informatics Application: Scoping Review. *Journal of Medical Internet Research*, *25*, e47260. doi:10.2196/47260 PMID:37647122

Beets, B., Newman, T. P., Howell, E. L., Bao, L., & Yang, S. (2023). Surveying Public Perceptions of Artificial Intelligence in Health Care in the United States: Systematic Review. *Journal of Medical Internet Research*, *25*, e40337. doi:10.2196/40337 PMID:37014676

Borg, W. R., & Gall, M. D. (1986). Educational research: An introduction. *British Journal of Educational Studies*, *32*(3).

Deiana, G., Dettori, M., Arghittu, A., Azara, A., Gabutti, G., & Castiglia, P. (2023). Artificial intelligence and public health: Evaluating ChatGPT responses to vaccination myths and misconceptions. *Vaccines*, *11*(7), 1217. doi:10.3390/vaccines11071217 PMID:37515033

Deng, S., & Wang, X. (2023). Exploring locally developed ELT materials in the context of curriculum-based value education in China: Challenges and solutions. *Frontiers in Psychology*, *14*, 14. doi:10.3389/fpsyg.2023.1191420 PMID:37901095

Dergaa, I., Chamari, K., Zmijewski, P., & Saad, H. B. (2023). From human writing to artificial intelligence generated text: Examining the prospects and potential threats of ChatGPT in academic writing. *Biology of Sport*, *40*(2), 615–622. doi:10.5114/biolsport.2023.125623 PMID:37077800

Farmer, L. S. (2023). Technology use and its changing role in community education. In *Handbook of Research on Andragogical Leadership and Technology in a Modern World* (pp. 358–383). IGI Global. doi:10.4018/978-1-6684-7832-5.ch019

Fayed, A. M., Mansur, N. S. B., de Carvalho, K. A., Behrens, A., D'Hooghe, P., & de Cesar Netto, C. (2023). Artificial intelligence and ChatGPT in Orthopaedics and sports medicine. *Journal of Experimental Orthopaedics*, *10*(1), 74. doi:10.1186/s40634-023-00642-8 PMID:37493985

Fui-Hoon Nah, F., Zheng, R., Cai, J., Siau, K., & Chen, L. (2023). Generative AI and ChatGPT: Applications, challenges, and AI-human collaboration. *Journal of Information Technology Case and Application Research*, *25*(3), 277–304. doi:10.1080/15228053.2023.2233814

Galetsi, P., Katsaliaki, K., & Kumar, S. (2023). Exploring benefits and ethical challenges in the rise of mHealth (mobile healthcare) technology for the common good: An analysis of mobile applications for health specialists. *Technovation*, *121*, 102598. doi:10.1016/j.technovation.2022.102598

Gill, S. S., Xu, M., Patros, P., Wu, H., Kaur, R., Kaur, K., Fuller, S., Singh, M., Arora, P., Parlikad, A. K., Stankovski, V., Abraham, A., Ghosh, S. K., Lutfiyya, H., Kanhere, S. S., Bahsoon, R., Rana, O., Dustdar, S., Sakellariou, R., & Buyya, R. (2024). Transformative effects of ChatGPT on modern education: Emerging Era of AI Chatbots. *Internet of Things and Cyber-Physical Systems*, *4*, 19–23. doi:10.1016/j.iotcps.2023.06.002

Grájeda, A., Burgos, J., Córdova, P., & Sanjinés, A. (2024). Assessing student-perceived impact of using artificial intelligence tools: Construction of a synthetic index of application in higher education. *Cogent Education*, *11*(1), 2287917. doi:10.1080/2331186X.2023.2287917

Gupta, A. K., Aggarwal, V., Sharma, V., & Naved, M. (2024). Education 4.0 and Web 3.0 Technologies Application for Enhancement of Distance Learning Management Systems in the Post–COVID-19 Era. In The Role of Sustainability and Artificial Intelligence in Education Improvement (pp. 66-86). Chapman and Hall/CRC.

Hohenstein, J., Kizilcec, R. F., DiFranzo, D., Aghajari, Z., Mieczkowski, H., Levy, K., Naaman, M., Hancock, J., & Jung, M. F. (2023). Artificial intelligence in communication impacts language and social relationships. *Scientific Reports*, *13*(1), 5487. doi:10.1038/s41598-023-30938-9 PMID:37015964

Huang, Y., Zhao, Y., Zhu, L., Han, B., & Li, Z. (2022, December). Challenges and Reflections on Vocational Education in 6G Era. In *International Conference on 5G for Future Wireless Networks* (pp. 342-353). Cham: Springer Nature Switzerland.

Hudson, S., Nishat, F., Stinson, J., Litwin, S., Zeller, F., Wiles, B., Foster, M. E., & Ali, S. (2023). Perspectives of healthcare providers to inform the design of an AI-enhanced social robot in the pediatric emergency department. *Children (Basel, Switzerland)*, *10*(9), 1511. doi:10.3390/children10091511 PMID:37761472

Huseinović, L. (2024). The effects of gamification on student motivation and achievement in learning English as a foreign language in higher education. *MAP Education and Humanities*, *4*, 10–36.

Ifelebuegu, A. O., Kulume, P., & Cherukut, P. (2023). Chatbots and AI in Education (AIEd) tools: The good, the bad, and the ugly. *Journal of Applied Learning and Teaching*, *6*(2).

Jayapal, J. (2024). Artificial Intelligence in Education: A Critic on English Language Teaching. In Artificial Intelligence and Knowledge Processing (pp. 348-357). CRC Press.

Jiménez, W. C. (2024). El Assessing artificial intelligence and professors' calibration in English as a foreign language writing courses at a Costa Rican public university. *Actualidades Investigativas en Educación*, *24*(1), 1–25. doi:10.15517/aie.v24i1.55612

Kaddoura, S., & Al Husseiny, F. (2023). The rising trend of Metaverse in education: Challenges, opportunities, and ethical considerations. *PeerJ. Computer Science*, *9*, e1252. doi:10.7717/peerj-cs.1252 PMID:37346578

Karpov, O. E., Pitsik, E. N., Kurkin, S. A., Maksimenko, V. A., Gusev, A. V., Shusharina, N. N., & Hramov, A. E. (2023). Analysis of publication activity and research trends in the field of ai medical applications: Network approach. *International Journal of Environmental Research and Public Health*, *20*(7), 5335. doi:10.3390/ijerph20075335 PMID:37047950

Khang, A., Gupta, S. K., Rani, S., & Karras, D. A. (Eds.). (2023). *Smart Cities: IoT Technologies, Big Data Solutions, Cloud Platforms, and Cybersecurity Techniques*. CRC Press. doi:10.1201/9781003376064

Khang, A., Muthmainnah, M., Seraj, P. M. I., Al Yakin, A., & Obaid, A. J. (2023). AI-Aided teaching model in education 5.0. In *Handbook of Research on AI-Based Technologies and Applications in the Era of the Metaverse* (pp. 83–104). IGI Global. doi:10.4018/978-1-6684-8851-5.ch004

Khang, A., Shah, V., & Rani, S. (Eds.). (2023). *Handbook of Research on AI-Based Technologies and Applications in the Era of the Metaverse*. IGI Global. doi:10.4018/978-1-6684-8851-5

Koraishi, O. (2023). Teaching English in the age of AI: Embracing ChatGPT to optimize EFL materials and assessment. *Language Education and Technology, 3*(1).

Kouijzer, M. M., Kip, H., Bouman, Y. H., & Kelders, S. M. (2023). Implementation of virtual reality in healthcare: A scoping review on the implementation process of virtual reality in various healthcare settings. *Implementation Science Communications*, *4*(1), 1–29. doi:10.1186/s43058-023-00442-2 PMID:37328858

Laine, T. H., & Lee, W. (2023). Collaborative Virtual Reality in Higher Education: Students' Perceptions on Presence, Challenges, Affordances, and Potential. *IEEE Transactions on Learning Technologies*.

Luo, W., Yang, W., & Berson, I. R. (2024). Digital Transformations in Early Learning: From Touch Interactions to AI Conversations. *Early Education and Development*, *35*(1), 3–9. doi:10.1080/104092 89.2023.2280819

Mesmar, J., & Badran, A. (2022). The post-COVID classroom: Lessons from a pandemic. In *Higher Education in the Arab World: New Priorities in the Post COVID-19 Era* (pp. 11–41). Springer International Publishing. doi:10.1007/978-3-031-07539-1_2

Montenegro-Rueda, M., Fernández-Cerero, J., Fernández-Batanero, J. M., & López-Meneses, E. (2023). Impact of the implementation of ChatGPT in education: A systematic review. *Computers*, *12*(8), 153. doi:10.3390/computers12080153

Monterubbianesi, R., Tosco, V., Vitiello, F., Orilisi, G., Fraccastoro, F., Putignano, A., & Orsini, G. (2022). Augmented, virtual and mixed reality in dentistry: A narrative review on the existing platforms and future challenges. *Applied Sciences (Basel, Switzerland)*, *12*(2), 877. doi:10.3390/app12020877

Muthmainnah, O., A. J., Al Yakin, A., & Brayyich, M. (2023, June). Enhancing Computational Thinking Based on Virtual Robot of Artificial Intelligence Modeling in the English Language Classroom. In *International Conference on Data Analytics & Management* (pp. 1-11). Singapore: Springer Nature Singapore. 10.1007/978-981-99-6550-2_1

Nemorin, S., Vlachidis, A., Ayerakwa, H. M., & Andriotis, P. (2023). AI hyped? A horizon scan of discourse on artificial intelligence in education (AIED) and development. *Learning, Media and Technology*, *48*(1), 38–51. doi:10.1080/17439884.2022.2095568

Onu, P., Pradhan, A., & Mbohwa, C. (2023). Potential to use metaverse for future teaching and learning. *Education and Information Technologies*, 1–32. doi:10.1007/s10639-023-12167-9

Pedro, A. R., Dias, M. B., Laranjo, L., Cunha, A. S., & Cordeiro, J. V. (2023). Artificial intelligence in medicine: A comprehensive survey of medical doctor's perspectives in Portugal. *PLoS One*, *18*(9), e0290613. doi:10.1371/journal.pone.0290613 PMID:37676884

Rajest, S. S., Singh, B., Obaid, A. J., Regin, R., & Chinnusamy, K. (Eds.). (2023). *Advances in Artificial and Human Intelligence in the Modern Era*. IGI Global. doi:10.4018/979-8-3693-1301-5

Rojas, E., Hülsmann, X., Estriegana, R., Rückert, F., & Garcia-Esteban, S. (2023). Students' Perception of Metaverses for Online Learning in Higher Education: Hype or Hope? *Electronics (Basel)*, *12*(8), 1867. doi:10.3390/electronics12081867

Said, G. R. E. (2023). Metaverse-Based Learning Opportunities and Challenges: A Phenomenological Metaverse Human–Computer Interaction Study. *Electronics (Basel)*, *12*(6), 1379. doi:10.3390/electronics12061379

Sun, J., Wei, M., Feng, J., Yu, F., Li, Q., & Zou, R. (2024). Progressive knowledge tracing: Modeling learning process from abstract to concrete. *Expert Systems with Applications*, *238*, 122280. doi:10.1016/j.eswa.2023.122280

Tomlinson, B. (Ed.). (2023). *Developing materials for language teaching*. Bloomsbury Publishing.

Vassilakopoulou, P., & Hustad, E. (2023). Bridging digital divides: A literature review and research agenda for information systems research. *Information Systems Frontiers*, *25*(3), 955–969. doi:10.1007/s10796-020-10096-3 PMID:33424421

Vishwakarma, L. P., Singh, R. K., Mishra, R., & Kumari, A. (2023). Application of artificial intelligence for resilient and sustainable healthcare system: Systematic literature review and future research directions. *International Journal of Production Research*, 1–23. doi:10.1080/00207543.2023.2188101

Wang, Y., & Zhang, L. J. (2023). *The Routledge Handbook of Materials Development for Language Teaching*.

World Health Organization. (2023). *2023 emerging technologies and scientific innovations: a global public health perspective*. WHO.

Yang, J., & Zhang, B. (2019). Artificial intelligence in intelligent tutoring robots: A systematic review and design guidelines. *Applied Sciences (Basel, Switzerland)*, *9*(10), 2078. doi:10.3390/app9102078

Yildiz, A. (2023). *The Routledge Handbook of Materials Development for Language Teaching*. Routledge.

Chapter 16
An Integrated Approach to Next-Generation Telemedicine and Health Advice Systems Through AI Applications in Disease Diagnosis

Rita Komalasari
https://orcid.org/0000-0001-9963-2363
Universitas Yarsi, Indonesia

Alex Khang
https://orcid.org/0000-0001-8379-4659
Global Research Institute of Technology and Engineering, USA

ABSTRACT

This chapter explores the transformative potential of integrating knowledge engineering and artificial intelligence in healthcare, focusing on constructing a knowledge-based clinical decision support system (KBCDS). The primary objective is to design an AI-enabled health portal to enhance accessibility to medical advice globally. The study investigates the application of AI in diagnosing COVID-19 and pneumonia, aiming to improve diagnostic accuracy and speed, reducing the burden on healthcare systems, and saving lives. The research is based on extensive literature study, delving into the depths of knowledge engineering, AI applications in healthcare, and medical ontology. The findings underscore the transformative potential of the integrated approach, highlighting its impact on healthcare disparities globally. The AI-enabled health portal proves to be a reliable source of medical advice, demonstrating that the fusion of knowledge engineering and AI technologies empowers medical professionals and significantly enhances healthcare accessibility and diagnostic capabilities.

DOI: 10.4018/979-8-3693-3679-3.ch016

1. INTRODUCTION

In order to comprehend patients' illnesses, the cutting-edge healthcare support system (HSS) integrates technical hardware and software technologies (Shafiq et al., 2023). Diagnoses, treatments, monitoring, rehabilitation, clinical trials, epidemiology, and health education are just a few areas that have been transformed by the integration of AI in healthcare (Almotiri et al., 2023). Health telematics applications have profoundly affected all areas of medical care, including prevention, diagnosis, treatment, monitoring, rehabilitation, clinical trials, epidemiology, and health education (Zhao et al., 2023).

Research and development of artificial intelligence (AI) for healthcare has received active backing from the United States, the European Union, and the United Kingdom (Fatima et al., 2020). Intelligent systems that can make clinical decisions autonomously in healthcare are known as autonomous AI systems (Ghazal et al., 2021). To guarantee its advantages, autonomous AI must undergo a bioethical and responsible evaluation of its effects on patient outcomes, design, validation, data use, and responsibility (Festor et al., 2021).

Clinical decision support (CDS) systems provide healthcare providers, employees, and patients with important information and insights tailored to each individual's needs right at the point of treatment (Musen et al., 2021). These systems are vital parts of the healthcare support system. These systems improve the quality of treatment and decrease medical mistakes in various contexts, including reminders to maintain health, displays of pertinent information, screening for medication interactions, dosage modifications, order facilitators, workflow assistance, and more.

Knowledge engineering and AI, when combined, are causing a stir in the healthcare business at a time when unprecedented technical advancements are taking place. This research embarks on a visionary exploration, seeking to pioneer an integrated approach that seamlessly merges knowledge engineering and AI applications in healthcare. At the heart of this transformative endeavor lies the conceptualization and design of an Artificial Intelligence-enabled health portal—a Knowledge-Based Clinical Decision Support System (KBCDS) (Bashir et al., 2021). This innovative platform is meticulously designed to transcend geographical boundaries, offering enhanced accessibility to medical advice globally. The pressing need for a paradigm shift in healthcare delivery is the imperative driving this research. By focusing on developing an AI-driven health portal, we aim to address the challenges posed by the COVID-19 pandemic and pneumonia, specifically improving diagnostic accuracy and speed.

The overarching goal is to alleviate the strain on healthcare systems, thereby contributing to preserving precious human lives. Methodologically, this research stands on the solid foundation of an extensive literature study that delves into the intricate realms of knowledge engineering, AI applications in healthcare, and the nuanced domain of medical ontology. Rigorous analysis of existing studies and scholarly works has informed the conceptualization of our AI-enabled health portal and paved the way for a comprehensive understanding of the synergies between knowledge engineering and AI in healthcare (Khang & Hajimahmud et al., 2024).

The forthcoming chapters of this research unravel the intricacies of our integrated approach. We will navigate through the conceptual underpinnings of our Knowledge-Based Clinical Decision Support System, examining its potential to redefine healthcare accessibility and diagnostic capabilities. The research culminates in a profound exploration of the transformative impact of this integrated approach on healthcare disparities globally. As the reader embarks on this intellectual journey, our primary contention is that the fusion of knowledge engineering and AI technologies empowers medical professionals and catalyzes a paradigmatic shift in healthcare accessibility and diagnostic precision. This research, therefore, lays the groundwork for a future where healthcare transcends geographical constraints, bridging gaps and ensuring equitable access for diverse populations worldwide.

The following chapters illuminate the path towards this visionary future, marking a milestone in the evolution of healthcare. The new knowledge and information yielded by the research have the potential to impact and benefit various individuals, groups, and entities involved in the healthcare ecosystem. The primary stakeholders who can use this knowledge to change or improve the present situation include The Knowledge-Based Clinical Decision Support System and AI-enabled health portal, which may help doctors, nurses, and other medical staff make better decisions, have easier diagnostics, and better patients. This technology can be a valuable tool in supporting clinical decisions, particularly in complex cases. Hospitals, clinics, and healthcare systems can integrate the research findings into their existing infrastructure to optimize workflows, reduce diagnostic turnaround times, and manage patient loads efficiently.

The AI-driven health portal can potentially alleviate the burden on healthcare systems, especially during health crises like the COVID-19 pandemic. Public health authorities and policymakers can utilize the insights from the research to inform healthcare policies and strategies. Implementing AI technologies in healthcare delivery may lead to more effective and responsive public health interventions, contributing to better population health outcomes. Companies and innovators in the health technology sector can draw inspiration from the integrated approach proposed in the research.

The findings may guide the development of new AI applications, knowledge engineering systems, and health portals that prioritize accessibility, accuracy, and inclusivity. Patients and their caregivers stand to benefit from improved healthcare accessibility and diagnostic capabilities. The AI-enabled health portal can empower individuals by providing timely and reliable medical advice, facilitating proactive health management, and fostering a more collaborative relationship between patients and healthcare providers. The research contributes to the academic discourse on the intersection of knowledge engineering and AI in healthcare. Researchers can build upon these findings to explore further applications, refine methodologies, and contribute to the ongoing evolution of healthcare technologies.

International organizations, such as the World Health Organization (WHO), can consider the research findings in their initiatives to address global healthcare disparities. The integrated approach may offer insights into designing scalable solutions that can be implemented across diverse healthcare settings. Insurance companies and healthcare payers can assess the potential impact of the integrated approach on healthcare costs, efficiency, and outcomes.

The findings may inform decisions related to coverage, reimbursement models, and integrating advanced technologies into healthcare payment systems. By catering to diverse stakeholders, the research aims to contribute to a holistic healthcare transformation, fostering a more interconnected, efficient, and equitable healthcare ecosystem. This research can bring new ideas and technology to the healthcare industry, which might benefit patients and practitioners alike. Several important ways in which this study may advance the field are as follows: Diagnostic precision might be greatly improved using a Knowledge-Based Clinical Decision Support System (KBCDS) that combines knowledge engineering with artificial intelligence (Kannan, 2022).

Better and faster diagnoses are possible with AI-driven insights and decision assistance for medical practitioners. Improving access to medical advice internationally is the goal of developing an AI-enabled health portal, which aspires to transcend geographical restrictions. This has the potential to make a significant difference in areas where healthcare resources are scarce, allowing people to get prompt advice and assistance no matter where they are.

Medical practitioners may streamline their decision-making processes with the assistance of this study, which focuses on AI applications in healthcare. When every second counts, healthcare practitioners may use data analytics and cutting-edge algorithms to make quick, well-informed judgements. In times of public health emergency, such as the recent COVID-19 epidemic, the research highlights the burden on healthcare systems. Healthcare delivery may be made more efficient with the AI-driven health portal, which can manage patient loads, decrease waiting times, and optimize resource allocation.

Combining knowledge engineering with AI creates a powerful decision support system, which gives healthcare personnel more agency. In the long run, this benefits patients since it improves their diagnostic skills and encourages a team effort between humans and AI. Adding to what is already known about healthcare IT, this study lays the framework for an integrated strategy. New developments at the crossroads of knowledge engineering, artificial intelligence, and healthcare may be sparked by the insights obtained, which can provide the groundwork for such advancements.

The research adds to the academic and practical knowledge base in healthcare via its thorough literature review and analysis. Anyone interested in studying or working with cutting-edge healthcare technology may use the results as a reference. Promoting equitable healthcare is emphasized by the research's potential influence on healthcare inequities and its worldwide focus. Aiming to close gaps and guarantee a more equitable distribution of healthcare benefits across varied groups, the integrated approach provides accessible and accurate medical advice. Improvements in diagnostic skills and faster decision-making are two obvious practical uses of the research's findings. The study also has larger ramifications on the future path of healthcare innovation. The study's overarching goal is to influence healthcare providers and the industry as a whole for the better by using an integrated strategy.

2. BACKGROUND

Artificial intelligence (AI) is finding more and more applications in healthcare, with some initiatives aiming to enhance the effectiveness of treatments for critical conditions in fields including neurology, cardiology, and neurology (Bohr & Memarzadeh, 2020). Early detection and diagnosis, outcome prediction, prognosis appraisal, and prediction are areas where artificial intelligence is helping the healthcare business. Improved treatment results are possible using clinical data, which includes medical records, electronic recordings, pictures, data from clinical laboratories, and physical exams.

In order to conquer sickness and systemic obstacles, AI has also been created in several areas of medical practice, hospitals, and labs. Due to the large volume of X-rays, CT scans, MRIs, and other image data generated by the healthcare industry, machine learning (ML) has become an indispensable tool for image analysis (Khanna et al., 2022). Traditional image processing methods are upgraded to answer complicated issues and make them seem like someone solves them. Critical health issues are being resolved using publicly available picture datasets, standards, and ML image processing. Amidst the rapidly advancing healthcare landscape, a persistent and empirically supported problem emerges – the unequal distribution of healthcare resources and accessibility, particularly evident in the context of infectious disease diagnosis.

According to recent data from the World Health Organization (WHO) in 2022, there remains a significant global discrepancy in the timely diagnosis and management of infectious diseases, with vulnerable populations disproportionately affected (WHO, 2022). This empirical evidence underscores the urgent need for innovative solutions to address this healthcare disparity. Nearly 50% of the global population did not have access to primary healthcare in 2022, according to the World Health Organisation (WHO). This shocking inequity necessitates innovative approaches to expanding access to healthcare globally, according to the World Health Organisation (2022).

Global Burden of Disease Study data from 2017 shows that the prevalence of chronic diseases has been on the rise. Non-communicable diseases (NCDs) need advanced diagnosis and treatment methods, according to GBD 2019 Disease and Injury Incidence and Prevalence Collaborators (2022). These disorders account for a large share of the global disease burden. Since the COVID-19 pandemic was announced in March 2020 by the World Health Organization, pressure has been felt worldwide in healthcare systems. Due to the high demand for medical advice and diagnostic services, conventional healthcare delivery methods have proven inadequate, highlighting the need for innovative technology solutions (WHO, 2022). There has been a meteoric rise in the artificial intelligence (AI) healthcare business worldwide.

The growing awareness of AI's ability to revolutionize healthcare decision-making and delivery has predicted that the industry might reach $19.25 billion by 2026 (Chen et al., 2021). Infectious disorders, such as pneumonia and COVID-19, are known to be challenging to diagnose. Treatment and containment success depends on a prompt and precise diagnosis. There is hope that AI applications may improve the speed and accuracy of illness diagnostics (Mirbabaie et al., 2021).

The evolution of medical ontology has gained traction in recent years. Ontologies provide a structured framework for organizing medical knowledge, enabling more effective knowledge representation and sharing. Incorporating medical ontology in our study aligns with the growing trend of leveraging semantic technologies in healthcare informatics (Kaur et al., 2020). Machine learning algorithms, a subset of AI, are increasingly employed in predictive analytics for disease diagnosis.

The ability of these algorithms to analyze vast datasets and identify patterns contributes to more accurate predictions and personalized healthcare interventions (Mei et al., 2020). These statistics and trends collectively emphasize the timeliness and relevance of our research. The burgeoning global healthcare challenges and the increasing adoption of AI technologies position our integrated approach as a pioneering effort to address critical gaps in healthcare accessibility, diagnostic precision, and response to emerging health crises. The research aims to empirically investigate the transformative potential of an integrated approach, merging knowledge engineering and artificial intelligence, to contribute meaningfully to infectious disease diagnosis and bridge these gaps in healthcare accessibility (Anh & Vladimir et al., 2024).

3. METHOD

The foundation of this research rests upon an extensive literature study, exploring the depths of knowledge engineering, AI applications in healthcare, and the nuances of medical ontology. By comprehensively reviewing existing studies and scholarly works, the research draws upon a rich tapestry of insights to inform the conceptualization of the AI-enabled health portal. This method ensures that the proposed integrated approach aligns with established best practices and incorporates the latest advancements in the intersecting fields. Rigorous data analysis forms the backbone of our research, elucidating patterns, trends, and gaps in existing literature. By systematically synthesizing diverse sources, we derive actionable insights that guide the implementation of the Knowledge-Based Clinical Decision Support System. This analytical rigour ensures the robustness of our proposed solution, enhancing its potential impact on healthcare disparities, diagnostic capabilities, decision-making processes, professional empowerment, and the future landscape of healthcare innovation (Khang & Rana et al., 2023).

4. AN INTEGRATED APPROACH TO NEXT-GENERATION TELEMEDICINE

The incorporation of cutting-edge technology into the ever-changing world of healthcare has the potential to revolutionize medical practices and eliminate long-standing inequalities in access to medical treatment. The purpose of this study is to investigate how next-generation telemedicine, as part of an integrated strategy, may transform the way healthcare is provided. It is the hope of this research that by combining knowledge engineering with AI, we may improve diagnostic skills and close the current care gap.

As we explore this integrated approach further, we will keep an eye on how it can revolutionize healthcare inequities and bring about more efficient and fair telemedicine. Healthcare disparities represent a critical challenge in ensuring universal access to quality healthcare (Aranda et al., 2021). Rooted in socioeconomic factors, geographic constraints, and cultural nuances, these disparities have created substantial barriers to equitable healthcare. The ongoing COVID-19 pandemic has further accentuated these challenges, disproportionately affecting vulnerable populations. This section explores how integrating knowledge engineering and artificial intelligence (AI) can serve as a transformative solution to mitigate healthcare disparities. Socioeconomic factors, including income levels and education, often exacerbate healthcare disparities.

Individuals with lower socioeconomic status may need help accessing timely medical advice and services. This disparity is intended to be rectified using the knowledge engineering-based integrated AI-driven health site. Regardless of their financial situation, everyone may benefit from the system's intuitive design and tailored health recommendations. Healthcare accessibility is a common issue in rural and underserved urban regions because of the lack of infrastructure and resources. The integrated solution overcomes geographical limits by offering a centralized health site powered by AI. This site connects people in faraway places to professional medical advice as a virtual bridge.

The system's flexibility promotes accessibility and diversity by ensuring that healthcare resources are not limited to specific locations. Differences in healthcare access are primarily attributable to cultural factors. Healthcare providers and patients may need help communicating due to language obstacles, cultural norms, and divergent health ideas and practices. Using knowledge engineering concepts as a framework, the AI-powered health site considers cultural factors. Medical advice is accurate and meaningful to consumers since the system learns and adjusts to different cultural settings and language subtleties. This inclusivity enhances the overall effectiveness of healthcare interventions.

The COVID-19 pandemic has shown how vulnerable health emergencies hit communities the hardest (Mirbabaie, 2022). Access to timely and accurate information becomes critical in navigating these crises. The integrated AI-driven health portal emerges as a crucial tool during such times, providing real-time updates, personalized recommendations, and crisis-specific guidance. The method helps lessen the effect of health crises on different communities by tackling the specific problems experienced by disadvantaged groups. A technologically sophisticated, culturally sensitive, and internationally accessible system is needed to solve healthcare inequities via knowledge engineering and AI. This strategy showcases the commitment to achieving healthcare equity by ensuring that individuals from all backgrounds worldwide have access to reliable, personalized medical advice.

The realm of infectious diseases, exemplified by the challenges posed by the COVID-19 pandemic, underscores the critical importance of optimizing diagnostic capabilities (Aljedaani et al., 2023). Traditional diagnostic methods often struggle to meet the demand for rapid and accurate responses in the face of rapidly evolving infectious agents. This section explores the pivotal role that AI applications embedded within the proposed Knowledge-Based Clinical Decision Support System (KBCDS) play in revolutionizing diagnostic processes and alleviating the burden on healthcare systems. Knowledge-based AI (KBS) aims to use AI to supplement human decision-making by acquiring and converting expert knowledge (Hussain et al., 2021).

Knowledge-based systems, or KBS, typically include an inference engine and a knowledge base. In the healthcare industry, CDS is advancing its databases and SOA to enable ' mash-ups,' or the integration of large amounts of data, where CDS may provide cognitive support via the KBS. CDS's six facets are data, knowledge, inference, technology and architecture, integration and implementation, and users. Beginning at the base of the stack with data, further elements include knowledge, inference, architecture, technology, integration, implementation, and users.

Nevertheless, reprocessing CDS data is very difficult, and there currently needs to be universally accepted standards for integrating clinical data or interpreting clinical perceptions across various healthcare systems. Early CDS systems could not exchange information, the second component of the CDS dimension, knowledge. There has been a consistent progression in the application of AI in healthcare thanks to advancements in medical logic modules (MLMs), data mining, text processing, and computable biomedical knowledge (MCBK) (Manickam et al., 2022). Artificial intelligence (AI) has opened up a world of new possibilities in clinical decision support systems (CDS), including gene variant-clinical condition links, unique clinical correlations, and genome-specific medicine selection for personalized treatment (Khang & Medicine, 2023).

Due to the proliferation of application frameworks and technical environments, there has been a meteoric rise in the installation and incorporation of CDS into doctors' processes. Info buttons, order sets, documentation templates, data displays and flowsheets, alerts and reminders, and effective system connections have all performed remarkable services in the CDS. Unfortunately, despite the advancements in HIT, these features still need to be adequately integrated or implemented into more complex physician workflows (Azzi et al., 2020). A system gap has developed to prevent the CDS capabilities from progressing as expected, and users' lack of interest in technology relative to their jobs is a significant contributor.

The practical implementation of CDS interventions—AI, machine learning, and modern technology—in today's healthcare settings requires more participation from patients, therapists, nurses, and physicians. Many medical fields, including human biology, medical statistics, medical diagnostics, and HIT, have begun to use AI-assisted technologies. The shift from independent computer systems to client-server architectures in healthcare hardware and network technologies has coincided with the rise of architectural thinking and the creation of universal CDSs, such as OpenMRS and OpenEMR, which include AI, in today's healthcare systems (Shaikh et al., 2022).

A suitable integrated CDS across health facilities and care pathways is still in the works in this era of HIT, treatment complexity, the increasing ageing population, multimorbidity, therapeutic advancements, and sub-specialization of care. This area has been reluctant to adopt digital transformation from the top down due to its moderate growth and low level of continuous investment compared to other industries.

AI and KBS have worked together in healthcare for a while, thanks to years of experience and new information. Having sufficient resources for the system to function correctly is crucial for the latest advancements in AI. Artificial intelligence (AI) has a one-of-a-kind interaction with knowledge-based systems (KBS) since it augments human opinions with its knowledge by observing and learning internal patterns. With more and more healthcare data being publicly available and AI being used in various health analytic programs, the healthcare industry is shifting its focus to AI-supported technologies, where AI plays an essential role. Almost all healthcare clinicians have previously employed AI-assisted technologies when making decisions.

Regarding artificial intelligence (AI)-assisted technology, HIT relies on two main types: ML approaches and NLP techniques. Medical imaging, genetic, and EP data are examples of structured data that ML algorithms analyze (Menegotto et al., 2021). However, clinical notes and medical journals are examples of unstructured data in which NLP extracts information. With the advent of AI and ML, several new technological possibilities have opened up, such as the rapid expansion of telemedicine applications and the use of AI to aid in medical diagnosis, statistical analysis, human biology, and other fields. This is a significant area of study since it pertains to contemporary healthcare settings, where architectural thinking and the creation of a universal CDS with AI capabilities have arisen. An advancement on the traditional method of using neural networks, deep learning uses multi-layer neural networks to unearth intricate non-linear patterns in data.

Infectious diseases, marked by their contagious nature and swift transmission, necessitate diagnostic tools capable of providing rapid responses (Sharma et al., 2021). The KBCDS, enriched with AI applications, enables healthcare professionals to analyze clinical data and diagnostic information swiftly. In order to respond to new health risks in a timely and preventive manner, machine learning algorithms that have been trained on various datasets may help identify patterns linked to infectious illnesses. Various fields rely heavily on AI, including machine learning, data analysis, and image classification (Khang and Abuzarova et al., 2023). Researchers may make educated conclusions about the deployment of these models and possible advancements in AI technology by comprehending the circumstances and assessing their efficacy.

The healthcare sector has recognized the importance of AI as a technology that may enhance patient outcomes while simultaneously reducing expenses. Resampling techniques like cross-validation ensure that machine learning models function well on untrained data. To fit the model to the training data, one must first create K-groups from the provided data sample, use each group as a test data set or holdout, and then proceed with the fitting procedure. Next, the model is tested using the test data; the evaluation score is kept, and the model is then discarded.

AI has shown to be the most effective option for healthcare, offering a thorough grasp of the AI paradigm in HIT (Baker et al., 2022). Readers may acquire the necessary expertise to further their work in medical augmentation by examining pertinent portions of AI, ML, and Deep Learning. With the exceptional information and higher success rate it provides, this chapter is crucial for ongoing and future work in artificial intelligence (AI) in healthcare. Integrating AI applications into the KBCDS is the foundation of the suggested approach. These applications' range of machine learning methods allows them to handle and understand intricate medical data.

The technology improves diagnostic skills using these algorithms, providing doctors with data-driven insights and evidence-based suggestions to help them make quick, informed decisions. When combined, medical ontology and machine learning provide a solid basis for improving diagnostic skills. Machine learning algorithms are educated about the semantic context of medical data via medical ontology, which is organized information about medical things and their connections (Irfan et al., 2019). By allowing computers to pick up on subtleties and connections in the data, this semantic knowledge improves the accuracy of diagnostic predictions, leading to more accurate and trustworthy diagnoses (Khang & Hajimahmud et al., 2024).

The volume and complexity of medical data, particularly concerning infectious diseases, necessitate advanced analytical capabilities. Operating within the KBCDS framework, machine learning algorithms excel in analyzing vast datasets. This analytical skill enables the detection of trends, patterns, and anomalies that could otherwise go unnoticed by humans. A diagnostic instrument that learns from its mistakes and becomes better with time is the end outcome.

4.1 Knowledge Engineering and Artificial Intelligence Applications in Disease Diagnosis

The optimization of diagnostic capabilities through AI applications is not merely an enhancement in precision but a strategic move to reduce the burden on healthcare systems (Iqbal et al., 2021). By expediting the diagnostic process, the proposed system contributes to more efficient patient management, quicker initiation of treatment protocols, and improved resource allocation. This becomes especially pivotal during pandemics, where rapid and accurate diagnostics are instrumental in containment efforts.

Integrating AI applications, informed by medical ontology, within the KBCDS is a transformative approach to optimizing diagnostic capabilities. This tackles the problems caused by contagious illnesses and prepares medical personnel to react quickly and efficiently, which helps healthcare systems deal with health emergencies better. The need to simplify decision-making becomes critical in the complex healthcare system, where choices may have profound and even fatal effects.

The suggested Knowledge-Based Clinical Decision Support System (KBCDS) ushers in a new era by combining knowledge engineering with artificial intelligence (AI). This part will examine how this integration gives healthcare professionals the resources to make educated decisions quickly and efficiently. Numerous factors, including patient history, diagnostic data, therapy alternatives, and developing medical knowledge, have a role in healthcare choices. When every second counts, these judgements become much more complicated in life-or-death circumstances. As a remedy for the bewildering complexity, the simplified decision-making process offers a methodical way to sift through the mountain of medical data.

Knowledge engineering, which allows for establishing a structured knowledge base, is central to the suggested approach (Ahmad et al., 2021). This database organizes medical information, including recent studies, clinical recommendations, and case studies. Healthcare providers may create the framework for well-informed decision-making by organizing this knowledge into a comprehensive, standardized information source. Healthcare decision-making now includes real-time decision help thanks to AI solutions.

The KBCDS's built-in machine learning algorithms quickly assess patient data and contextual information. The ability to analyze data in real-time provides healthcare providers with valuable insights that can be used to evaluate various factors and possible consequences quickly. Healthcare providers seeking meaningful and current insights may find it challenging to sift through the vast amounts of medical information that are accessible. To overcome this obstacle, the integrated strategy uses AI tools to filter massive databases for relevant information. By organizing this data structure, knowledge engineering helps medical practitioners find the specific information they need to make informed decisions. Streamlining the decision-making process becomes crucial when time is of the essence in urgent healthcare circumstances.

Healthcare providers can make more prompt interventions with the help of the KBCDS, which combines knowledge engineering with AI. Healthcare delivery is made more efficient and thriving with the system's instant help, whether in an emergency or while making complicated treatment choices. To sum up, the KBCDS resolves the complexity of healthcare issues and transforms decision-making via integrating knowledge engineering and AI applications. In life-or-death circumstances, when every second counts, healthcare providers rely on this integrated approach's organized knowledge, real-time insights, and quick navigation of medical information.

Artificial intelligence (AI) applications and knowledge engineering are not meant to replace human expertise but to enhance it in the ever-changing healthcare sector (Ali et al., 2023). We will examine why this integration is critical to help healthcare practitioners have a solid decision support system. The health portal becomes a valued ally with the aid of AI, forging a link that benefits both parties and improves the competency of medical personnel. A significant change has occurred in knowledge engineering and AI, which aim to augment existing human knowledge rather than replace it.

Healthcare providers still have decision-making authority; the AI-powered site is only a tool to aid them in their work. Human intuition, empathy, and clinical judgement are priceless; when we work together, we can see this. With artificial intelligence, the health portal provides medical professionals with a wealth of data-driven insights, making it an effective decision-support tool. Fast analysis of massive volumes of medical data with evidence-based, patient-specific recommendations is the end objective of this system. Utilizing a blend of human expertise and AI capabilities gives healthcare practitioners a powerful decision-making tool.

AI technology has given healthcare professionals access to data-driven insights derived from large datasets. Among these discoveries are future-oriented analytics, trends, and relationships that could be difficult to see with the naked eye. This data may result in improved diagnosis, more efficient treatment plans, and awareness of emerging healthcare trends. Aligning with current medical research and well-established clinical guidelines, the AI-powered health site produces evidence-based suggestions. This ensures that doctors and nurses may draw on an accurate and current body of information when making choices. These suggestions are even more reliable and relevant now that knowledge engineering ideas are included.

The dynamic nature of medical science demands continuous learning and adaptation. The AI-enabled health portal is a conduit for healthcare professionals to stay abreast of the latest medical advancements. Through real-time updates, access to cutting-edge research, and insights from evolving healthcare data, professionals can maintain a proactive approach to their practice. The essence of the integration lies in fostering a symbiotic relationship between human expertise and AI technologies (Neethirajan, 2023).

While AI enhances analytical and data-processing capabilities, healthcare professionals contribute their nuanced understanding of patient histories, emotional nuances, and the broader socio-cultural context. This symbiosis optimally utilizes the strengths of both elements, creating a synergy that amplifies the overall proficiency of healthcare professionals. Integrating AI applications and knowledge engineering is an empowering force for healthcare professionals. Far from replacing human expertise, this integrated approach augments and enhances the capabilities of healthcare professionals, providing them with a sophisticated decision support system. The AI-enabled health portal becomes an indispensable ally, contributing to more informed, precise, and patient-centric healthcare practices.

This study lays the foundation for future advances in healthcare delivery via its pioneering combination of knowledge engineering, medical ontology, and artificial intelligence (AI). Insights from this study motivate healthcare researchers and developers to rethink healthcare delivery by revealing new options that may be explored and improved upon. Healthcare innovation is a dynamic story, and this study adds to it substantially with its integrated approach.

The research offers a comprehensive model that goes beyond traditional limits by combining knowledge engineering concepts with AI applications. This lays the groundwork for creative solutions to existing and future healthcare problems. Healthcare technology continues to progress thanks to the insights gained from this study. Researchers and developers may use the new information as a foundation to improve existing methods and look for new uses. The suggested integrated strategy is improved via this iterative process, promoting a never-ending healthcare innovation cycle. Researchers and developers are encouraged to explore new boundaries in healthcare technology by using the integrated approach. In order to pave the way for future endeavors, the study successfully integrates knowledge engineering, medical ontology and AI.

This motivation is crucial to encourage a culture of curiosity and experimentation among healthcare innovation professionals. Knowledge engineering, medical ontology, and artificial intelligence have provided a strong foundation for new developments. The medical ontology-enhanced structured knowledge base provides an ideal environment for using cutting-edge AI algorithms.

In addition to improving the planned AI-enabled health site, this synergy paves the way for new technology that can revolutionize healthcare delivery and flexibility. Healthcare delivery and flexibility may be redefined via knowledge engineering and AI, which tackle present difficulties and create the framework. Healthcare systems that are dynamic and sensitive to new information, technology, and patient demands may be possible thanks to advances that build on this integrated paradigm. Findings stress the significance of healthcare technology's ongoing innovation. This research establishes a standard for the ever-changing landscape of healthcare innovation with its comprehensive approach.

Knowledge engineering, medical ontology, and AI's revolutionary powers will likely shape the way technologies develop in the future so that they can meet new problems. Through laying the groundwork for future innovations in healthcare, this study goes beyond its immediate setting to become a catalyst for continuous progress. In addition to solving existing problems, the proposed integrated strategy may serve as a model for future work, opening up exciting new possibilities for healthcare innovation and reshaping its fundamental structure. With this review as a guide, researchers may improve their deep learning (DL) work and inspire others to do the same.

5. SOLUTIONS AND RECOMMENDATIONS

The study contributes significantly to the research landscape by showcasing the viability and effectiveness of an integrated approach. Researchers can build upon these insights to explore nuanced applications, refine methodologies, and delve deeper into the ethical considerations of deploying AI-driven health portals. The findings provide a solid foundation for future research endeavours to advance the intersection of knowledge engineering, AI, and healthcare. For healthcare practitioners, the implications are equally profound.

Integrating knowledge engineering and AI can revolutionize diagnostic accuracy, streamline decision-making processes, and empower professionals with a reliable decision-support system. The proposed AI-enabled health portal, informed by these findings, has the potential to become a cornerstone in everyday clinical practices, ensuring timely, data-driven, and patient-centric care. By embracing this integrated model, healthcare institutions can enhance efficiency, reduce healthcare disparities, and adapt to evolving medical landscapes. Patients stand to benefit from improved accessibility to accurate medical advice, timely diagnoses, and a healthcare system that is efficient and personalized to their needs.

6. FUTURE RESEARCH DIRECTIONS

Conducting longitudinal cohort studies can provide valuable insights into the sustained impact of integrated AI-driven health portals on healthcare disparities and patient outcomes over time. This design allows for the observation of trends, changes in diagnostic accuracy, and the long-term effectiveness of the proposed solution in diverse healthcare settings.

Randomized controlled trials may help determine how well the integrated strategy works compared to more conventional healthcare strategies. By randomly assigning participants to the AI-enabled health portal or standard care, researchers can systematically measure the impact on diagnostic capabilities, decision-making processes, and overall healthcare outcomes, ensuring a rigorous examination of causality.

Employing implementation science methodologies can help understand the factors influencing the successful integration of AI applications and knowledge engineering in real-world healthcare settings. Exploring barriers, facilitators, and variations in implementation outcomes will contribute to developing best practices for adopting and sustaining the proposed integrated model. Focusing on user experience research can provide insights into the acceptability and usability of the AI-enabled health portal among healthcare professionals and patients.

To gauge user happiness, spot problems, and fine-tune the portal for maximum engagement, researchers may utilize quantitative and qualitative approaches, including surveys, interviews, and usability testing. Ethnographic research is crucial to fully grasp the social and cultural aspects impacting the use of AI in healthcare. To further understand how the integrated model is implemented, researchers might visit healthcare facilities, observe interactions, and collect qualitative data to reveal subtleties that quantitative approaches might miss.

Big data analytics may improve the study's quality when applied to the massive datasets produced by the AI-powered health site. Using this method, we may find trends, correlations, and predictive insights showing how the system affects diagnostic precision, decision-making effectiveness, and patient outcomes in different groups. The integrated model's performance in different cultural settings may be better understood via cross-cultural comparative research (Khang & Ragimova et al., 2024).

A culturally customized deployment of the AI-enabled health portal may be achieved by comparing results across various locations and healthcare systems. This will allow researchers to uncover cultural elements that impact the efficacy and acceptability of the portal. In tackling healthcare inequalities, optimizing diagnostics, and educating healthcare workers, these different study methods jointly contribute to a thorough knowledge of the effect of the integrated strategy. In order to thoroughly investigate the observable results and the contextual elements impacting the suggested model's performance, a mix of quantitative and qualitative methodologies is used.

7. CONCLUSION

In summary, the integration of knowledge engineering and artificial intelligence, as showcased in this study, holds profound implications for research and practice in healthcare. The findings underscore the proposed AI-enabled health portal's transformative potential and pave the way for tangible improvements in patient care and healthcare delivery. The implications of this study extend beyond theoretical frameworks, offering tangible pathways for advancing research and practice in the healthcare field. Technology will be an essential tool in the quest for perfect patient care, and the suggested integrated strategy might revolutionize healthcare delivery, patient experience, and continuous improvement (Khang & Vladimir et al., 2024).

REFERENCES

Ahmad, Z., Rahim, S., Zubair, M., & Abdul-Ghafar, J. (2021). Artificial intelligence (AI) in medicine, current applications and future role with special emphasis on its potential and promise in pathology: Present and future impact, obstacles including costs and acceptance among pathologists, practical and philosophical considerations. A comprehensive review. *Diagnostic Pathology*, *16*(1), 1–16. doi:10.1186/s13000-021-01085-4 PMID:33731170

Ali Mohamad, T., Bastone, A., Bernhard, F., & Schiavone, F. (2023). How artificial intelligence impacts the competitive position of healthcare organizations. *Journal of Organizational Change Management*, *36*(8), 49–70. doi:10.1108/JOCM-03-2023-0057

Aljedaani, W., Krasniqi, R., Aljedaani, S., Mkaouer, M. W., Ludi, S., & Al-Raddah, K. (2023). If online learning works for you, what about deaf students? Emerging challenges of online learning for deaf and hearing-impaired students during COVID-19: A literature review. *Universal Access in the Information Society*, *22*(3), 1027–1046. doi:10.1007/s10209-022-00897-5 PMID:35910240

Almotiri, S. H., Nadeem, M., Al Ghamdi, M. A., & Khan, R. A. (2023). Analytic Review of Healthcare Software by Using Quantum Computing Security Techniques. *International Journal of Fuzzy Logic and Intelligent Systems*, *23*(3), 336–352. doi:10.5391/IJFIS.2023.23.3.336

Anh, P. T. N. (2024). *AI Models for Disease Diagnosis and Prediction of Heart Disease with Artificial Neural Networks. Computer Vision and AI-integrated IoT Technologies in Medical Ecosystem* (1st ed.). CRC Press. doi:10.1201/9781003429609-9

Aranda, M. P., Kremer, I. N., Hinton, L., Zissimopoulos, J., Whitmer, R. A., Hummel, C. H., Trejo, L., & Fabius, C. (2021). Impact of dementia: Health disparities, population trends, care interventions, and economic costs. *Journal of the American Geriatrics Society*, *69*(7), 1774–1783. doi:10.1111/jgs.17345 PMID:34245588

Azzi, S., Gagnon, S., Ramirez, A., & Richards, G. (2020). Healthcare applications of artificial intelligence and analytics: A review and proposed framework. *Applied Sciences (Basel, Switzerland)*, *10*(18), 6553. doi:10.3390/app10186553

Baker, R. E., Mahmud, A. S., Miller, I. F., Rajeev, M., Rasambainarivo, F., Rice, B. L., Takahashi, S., Tatem, A. J., Wagner, C. E., Wang, L.-F., Wesolowski, A., & Metcalf, C. J. E. (2022). Infectious disease in an era of global change. *Nature Reviews. Microbiology*, *20*(4), 193–205. doi:10.1038/s41579-021-00639-z PMID:34646006

Bashir, S., Almazroi, A. A., Ashfaq, S., Almazroi, A. A., & Khan, F. H. (2021). A knowledge-based clinical decision support system utilizing an intelligent ensemble voting scheme for improved cardiovascular disease prediction. *IEEE Access : Practical Innovations, Open Solutions*, *9*, 130805–130822. doi:10.1109/ACCESS.2021.3110604

Bohr, A., & Memarzadeh, K. (2020). The rise of artificial intelligence in healthcare applications. In *Artificial Intelligence in healthcare* (pp. 25–60). Academic Press. doi:10.1016/B978-0-12-818438-7.00002-2

Chen, J., Chen, C. B., Walther, J., & Sundar, S. S. (2021, May). Do you feel special when an AI doctor remembers you? Individuation effects of AI vs. human doctors on user experience. In *Extended Abstracts of the 2021 CHI Conference on Human Factors in Computing Systems* (pp. 1-7). ACM. 10.1145/3411763.3451735

Fatima, S., Desouza, K. C., & Dawson, G. S. (2020). National strategic artificial intelligence plans: A multi-dimensional analysis. *Economic Analysis and Policy*, *67*, 178–194. doi:10.1016/j.eap.2020.07.008

Festor, P., Habli, I., Jia, Y., Gordon, A., Faisal, A. A., & Komorowski, M. (2021). Levels of autonomy and safety assurance for AI-Based clinical decision systems. In Computer Safety, Reliability, and Security. SAFECOMP 2021 Workshops: DECSoS, MAPSOD, DepDevOps, USDAI, and WAISE, (pp. 291-296). Springer International Publishing. doi:10.1007/978-3-030-83906-2_24

GBD 2019 Ageing Collaborators. (2022). Global, regional, and national burden of diseases and injuries for adults 70 years and older: systematic analysis for the Global Burden of Disease 2019 Study. *BMJ*, 376.

Ghazal, T. M., Hasan, M. K., Alshurideh, M. T., Alzoubi, H. M., Ahmad, M., Akbar, S. S., Al Kurdi, B., & Akour, I. A. (2021). IoT for smart cities: Machine learning approaches in smart healthcare-A review. *Future Internet*, *13*(8), 218. doi:10.3390/fi13080218

Hussain, M., Satti, F. A., Ali, S. I., Hussain, J., Ali, T., Kim, H. S., Yoon, K.-H., Chung, T. C., & Lee, S. (2021). Intelligent knowledge consolidation: From data to wisdom. *Knowledge-Based Systems*, *234*, 107578. doi:10.1016/j.knosys.2021.107578

Iqbal, M. J., Javed, Z., Sadia, H., Qureshi, I. A., Irshad, A., Ahmed, R., Malik, K., Raza, S., Abbas, A., Pezzani, R., & Sharifi-Rad, J. (2021). Clinical applications of artificial intelligence and machine learning in cancer diagnosis: Looking into the future. *Cancer Cell International*, *21*(1), 1–11. doi:10.1186/s12935-021-01981-1 PMID:34020642

Irfan, R., Rehman, Z., Abro, A., Chira, C., & Anwar, W. (2019). Ontology learning in text mining for handling big data in healthcare systems. *Journal of Medical Imaging and Health Informatics*, *9*(4), 649–661. doi:10.1166/jmihi.2019.2681

Kannan, S. (2022). An automated clinical decision support system for predicting cardiovascular disease using ensemble learning approach. *Concurrency and Computation*, *34*(18), e7007. doi:10.1002/cpe.7007

Kaur, S., Singla, J., Nkenyereye, L., Jha, S., Prashar, D., Joshi, G. P., El-Sappagh, S., Islam, M. S., & Islam, S. R. (2020). Medical diagnostic systems using artificial intelligence (ai) algorithms: Principles and perspectives. *IEEE Access : Practical Innovations, Open Solutions*, 8, 228049–228069. doi:10.1109/ ACCESS.2020.3042273

Khang, A. (2023). *AI and IoT-Based Technologies for Precision Medicine* (1st ed.). IGI Global Press., doi:10.4018/979-8-3693-0876-9

Khang, A. (2024). *Using Big Data to Solve Problems in the Field of Medicine. Computer Vision and AI-integrated IoT Technologies in Medical Ecosystem* (1st ed.). CRC Press. doi:10.1201/9781003429609-21

Khang, A. (2024). *Medical and BioMedical Signal Processing and Prediction. Computer Vision and AI-integrated IoT Technologies in Medical Ecosystem* (1st ed.). CRC Press. doi:10.1201/9781003429609-7

Khang, A., Abdullayev, V., Hrybiuk, O., & Shukla, A. K. (2024). *Computer Vision and AI-Integrated IoT Technologies in the Medical Ecosystem* (1st ed.). CRC Press. doi:10.1201/9781003429609

Khang, A., & Abdullayev, V. A. (2023). *AI-Aided Data Analytics Tools and Applications for the Healthcare Sector. AI and IoT-Based Technologies for Precision Medicine* (1st ed.). IGI Global Press. doi:10.4018/979-8-3693-0876-9.ch018

Khang, A., & Hajimahmud, V. A. (2024). *Application of Computer Vision in the Healthcare Ecosystem. Computer Vision and AI-integrated IoT Technologies in Medical Ecosystem* (1st ed.). CRC Press. doi:10.1201/9781003429609-1

Khang, A., Rana, G., Tailor, R. K., & Hajimahmud, V. A. (2023). *Data-Centric AI Solutions and Emerging Technologies in the Healthcare Ecosystem* (1st ed.). CRC Press., doi:10.1201/9781003356189

Khanna, N. N., Maindarkar, M. A., Viswanathan, V., Fernandes, J. F. E., Paul, S., Bhagawati, M., & Suri, J. S. (2022, December). Economics of artificial intelligence in healthcare: diagnosis vs. treatment. In Healthcare (Vol. 10, No. 12, p. 2493). MDPI. doi:10.3390/healthcare10122493

Manickam, P., Mariappan, S. A., Murugesan, S. M., Hansda, S., Kaushik, A., Shinde, R., & Thipperudraswamy, S. P. (2022). Artificial intelligence (AI) and internet of medical things (IoMT) assisted biomedical systems for intelligent healthcare. *Biosensors (Basel)*, 12(8), 562. doi:10.3390/bios12080562 PMID:35892459

Mei, X., Lee, H. C., Diao, K. Y., Huang, M., Lin, B., Liu, C., Xie, Z., Ma, Y., Robson, P. M., Chung, M., Bernheim, A., Mani, V., Calcagno, C., Li, K., Li, S., Shan, H., Lv, J., Zhao, T., Xia, J., & Yang, Y. (2020). Artificial intelligence-enabled rapid diagnosis of patients with COVID-19. *Nature Medicine*, 26(8), 1224–1228. doi:10.1038/s41591-020-0931-3 PMID:32427924

Menegotto, A. B., Becker, C. D. L., & Cazella, S. C. (2021). Computer-aided diagnosis of hepatocellular carcinoma fusing imaging and structured health data. *Health Information Science and Systems*, 9(1), 20. doi:10.1007/s13755-021-00151-x PMID:33968399

Mhlanga, D. (2022). The role of artificial intelligence and machine learning amid the COVID-19 pandemic: What lessons are we learning on 4IR and the sustainable development goals. *International Journal of Environmental Research and Public Health*, 19(3), 1879. doi:10.3390/ijerph19031879 PMID:35162901

Mirbabaie, M., Stieglitz, S., & Frick, N. R. (2021). Artificial intelligence in disease diagnostics: A critical review and classification on the current state of research guiding future direction. *Health and Technology*, *11*(4), 693–731. doi:10.1007/s12553-021-00555-5

Musen, M. A., Middleton, B., & Greenes, R. A. (2021). Clinical decision-support systems. In *Biomedical informatics: computer applications in health care and biomedicine* (pp. 795–840). Springer International Publishing. doi:10.1007/978-3-030-58721-5_24

Neethirajan, S. (2023). Artificial Intelligence and Sensor Innovations: Enhancing Livestock Welfare with a Human-Centric Approach. *Human-Centric Intelligent Systems*, 1-16. Springer. doi:10.1007/s44230-023-00050-2

Shafiq, M., Du, C., Jamal, N., Abro, J. H., Kamal, T., Afsar, S., & Mia, M. S. (2023). Smart E-Health System for Heart Disease Detection Using Artificial Intelligence and Internet of Things Integrated Next-Generation Sensor Networks. *Journal of Sensors*, *2023*, 1–7. doi:10.1155/2023/6383099

Shaikh, M., Vayani, A. H., Akram, S., & Qamar, N. (2022). Open-source electronic health record systems: A systematic review of most recent advances. *Health Informatics Journal*, *28*(2), 14604582221099828. doi:10.1177/14604582221099828 PMID:35588400

Sharma, A., Mishra, R. K., Goud, K. Y., Mohamed, M. A., Kummari, S., Tiwari, S., Li, Z., Narayan, R., Stanciu, L. A., & Marty, J. L. (2021). Optical biosensors for diagnostics of infectious viral disease: A recent update. *Diagnostics (Basel)*, *11*(11), 2083. doi:10.3390/diagnostics11112083 PMID:34829430

World Health Organization. (2022). *Consolidated guidelines on HIV, viral hepatitis and STI prevention, diagnosis, treatment and care for key populations*. World Health Organization.

Zhao, Z., Li, X., Luan, B., Jiang, W., Gao, W., & Neelakandan, S. (2023). Secure internet of things (IoT) using a novel brooks Iyengar quantum byzantine agreement-centered blockchain networking (BIQBA-BCN) model in smart healthcare. *Information Sciences*, *629*, 440–455. doi:10.1016/j.ins.2023.01.020

KEY TERMS AND DEFINITIONS

AI Applications: AI applications are the practical use and implementation of artificial intelligence techniques, algorithms, and technologies to perform specific tasks, make decisions, or enhance processes across various domains. Diagnostic algorithms, decision support systems, and predictive analytics are some examples of AI applications in healthcare that aim to improve patient care.

Healthcare Disparities: When various demographic groups or populations have varied access to and experiences with healthcare, we say that healthcare disparities exist. Factors such as financial level, race/ethnicity, region, and cultural background may all shape these variations. Achieving universal healthcare access is a critical component in reducing healthcare inequities.

Knowledge Engineering: Knowledge engineers develop and execute strategies for gathering, organizing, and using information to address complex problems. The healthcare business relies on knowledge engineering to organize medical information, build decision support systems, and integrate knowledge-based technology like AI more easily into healthcare practices.

Medical Ontology: Medical ontology systematically represents medical concepts, entities, and relationships within a structured framework. It provides a standardized and formalized way to organize medical knowledge, enabling effective communication and sharing of information across different healthcare systems and applications. Medical ontology is integral to the development of semantic interoperability in

Transformative Healthcare: Bringing about significant and beneficial changes in healthcare delivery, accessibility, and outcomes is what we mean when we talk about transformative healthcare. All healthcare aspects, from treating individual patients to the whole system, may benefit from these innovative ideas and methods. Improved health outcomes, efficiency, and fairness in healthcare delivery are the goals of revolutionary healthcare.

Compilation of References

Abiodun, O. I., Jantan, A., Omolara, A. E., Dada, K. V., Umar, A. M., Linus, O. U., Arshad, H., Kazaure, A. A., Gana, U., & Kiru, M. U. (2019). Comprehensive review of artificial neural network applications to pattern recognition. *IEEE Access : Practical Innovations, Open Solutions, 7*, 158820–158846. doi:10.1109/ACCESS.2019.2945545

Abramson, N., Braverman, D. J., & Sebestyen, G. S. (2006). Pattern Recognition and Machine Learning. *Publications of the American Statistical Association, 103*(4), 886–887.

Abreu, P. H., Nunes, P., & Silva, M. J. (2022). Pervasive Health Care: Paving the Way to a Web of People Framework. *Procedia Technology, 5*, 454–461.

Achituv, D.B. & Haiman, L. (2016). Physicians' attitudes toward the use of IoT medical devices as part of their practice. *Online Journal of Applied Knowledge Management. 4*(2).

Aeni, N., Khang, A., Al Yakin, A., Yunus, M., & Cardoso, L. (2024). Revolutionized Teaching by Incorporating Artificial Intelligence Chatbot for Higher Education Ecosystem. In *AI-Centric Modeling and Analytics* (pp. 43–76). CRC Press.

Aggarwal, A., Tam, C. C., Wu, D., Li, X., & Qiao, S. (2023). Artificial Intelligence–Based Chatbots for Promoting Health Behavioral Changes: Systematic Review. *Journal of Medical Internet Research, 25*, e40789. doi:10.2196/40789 PMID:36826990

Aghaeeaval, M. (2021). Prediction of patient survival following postanoxic coma using EEG data and clinical features. In *2021 43rd Annual International Conference of the IEEE Engineering in Medicine & Biology Society (EMBC)*. IEEE. 10.1109/EMBC46164.2021.9629946

Ahamed, F., & Farid, F. (2018). Applying Internet of Things and Machine-Learning for Personalized Healthcare: Issues and Challenges. *2018 International Conference on Machine Learning and Data Engineering (iCMLDE)*. IEEE.

Ahishakiye, E., Wario, R., Mwangi, W., & Taremwa, D. (2020). Prediction of Cervical Cancer Basing on Risk Factors using Ensemble Learning. 2020 IST-Africa Conference (IST-Africa). IEEE.

Ahmadi, H. (2018). · Arji G, Shahmoradi L, Safdari R, Nilashi M, Alizadeh M. The application of internet of things in healthcare: A systematic literature review and classification. *Universal Access in the Information Society*. doi:10.1007/s10209-018-0618-4

Ahmad, Z., Rahim, S., Zubair, M., & Abdul-Ghafar, J. (2021). Artificial intelligence (AI) in medicine, current applications and future role with special emphasis on its potential and promise in pathology: Present and future impact, obstacles including costs and acceptance among pathologists, practical and philosophical considerations. A comprehensive review. *Diagnostic Pathology, 16*(1), 1–16. doi:10.1186/s13000-021-01085-4 PMID:33731170

Ahmeda, N., Ahammeda, R., Islama, M., & Uddina, A. (2021). Machine learning based diabetes prediction and development of smart web application. *International Journal of Cognitive Computing in Engineering, 2*, 229–241. doi:10.1016/j.ijcce.2021.12.001

Ahuja, S. P., Sindhu, M., & Jesus, Z. (2012). A Survey of the State of Cloud Computing in Healthcare. *Network CommunTechnol*, *1*(2), 12–19. doi:10.5539/nct.v1n2p12

Akobeng, A. K. (2007, May). Understanding diagnostic tests 3: Receiver operating characteristic curves. *Acta Paediatrica (Oslo, Norway)*, *96*(5), 644–647. doi:10.1111/j.1651-2227.2006.00178.x PMID:17376185

Al Rifai, Z., & Mulvey, D. (2016). Principles of total intravenous anaesthesia: Basic pharmacokinetics and model descriptions. *BJA Education*, *16*(3), 92–97. doi:10.1093/bjaceaccp/mkv021

Al Yakin, A., Muthmainnah, G., S., C., L., & Asrifan, A. (2023). Cybersocialization Through Smart Digital Classroom Management (SDCM) as a Pedagogical Innovation of "Merdeka Belajar Kampus Merdeka (MBKM)" Curriculum. In Digital Learning based Education: Transcending Physical Barriers (pp. 39-61). Singapore: Springer Nature Singapore.

Al Yakin, A., Obaid, A. J., Muthmainnah, R. S. A. M., Khalaf, H. A., & Al-Barzinji, S. M. (2022). Bringing technology into the classroom amid Covid 19, challenge and opportunity. *Journal of Positive School Psychology*, *6*(2), 1043–1052.

Alabdulkarim, A., Al-Rodhaan, M., & Al-Dhelaan, T. A. (2019). A Privacy-Preserving Algorithm for Clinical Decision Support Systems Using Random Forest. *Computers, Materials & Continua*, *58*(3), 585–601. doi:10.32604/cmc.2019.05637

Al-Adwan, A. S., Li, N., Al-Adwan, A., Abbasi, G. A., Albelbisi, N. A., & Habibi, A. (2023). Extending the technology acceptance model (TAM) to Predict University Students' intentions to use metaverse-based learning platforms. *Education and Information Technologies*, 1–33. PMID:37361794

Alahi, M. E. E., Sukkuea, A., Tina, F. W., Nag, A., Kurdthongmee, W., Suwannarat, K., & Mukhopadhyay, S. C. (2023). Integration of IoT-Enabled Technologies and Artificial Intelligence (AI) for Smart City Scenario: Recent Advancements and Future Trends. *Sensors (Basel)*, *23*(11), 5206. doi:10.3390/s23115206 PMID:37299934

Alaybeyi, S., & Lheureux, B. (2019). *Survey Analysis: Artificial Intelligence Establishes a Foothold in IoT Projects*. Gartner. https://www. gartner.com/en/documents/3968034/survey-analysisartificial-intelligence-establishes-a-fo

Alenezi, M., Wardat, S., & Akour, M. (2023). The Need of Integrating Digital Education in Higher Education: Challenges and Opportunities. *Sustainability (Basel)*, *15*(6), 4782. doi:10.3390/su15064782

Alghamdi, N. S., Hosni Mahmoud, H. A., Abraham, A., Alanazi, S. A., & Garcia-Hernandez, L. (2020). L. GarcíaHern´ andez, Predicting depression symptoms in an Arabic psychological forum. *IEEE Access : Practical Innovations, Open Solutions*, *8*, 57317–57334. https://ieeexplore.ieee.org/abstract/document/9040556/. doi:10.1109/ACCESS.2020.2981834

Alhanai, T., Ghassemi, M., & Glass, J. (2018). Detecting depression with audio/text sequence modeling of interviews. *Proc. Annu. Conf. Int. Speech Commun. Assoc. INTERSPEECH (September)* (pp. 1716–1720). IEEE.

Ali Mohamad, T., Bastone, A., Bernhard, F., & Schiavone, F. (2023). How artificial intelligence impacts the competitive position of healthcare organizations. *Journal of Organizational Change Management*, *36*(8), 49–70. doi:10.1108/JOCM-03-2023-0057

Ali, O., Murray, P. A., Momin, M., Dwivedi, Y. K., & Malik, T. (2024). The effects of artificial intelligence applications in educational settings: Challenges and strategies. *Technological Forecasting and Social Change*, *199*, 123076. doi:10.1016/j.techfore.2023.123076

Aljedaani, W., Krasniqi, R., Aljedaani, S., Mkaouer, M. W., Ludi, S., & Al-Raddah, K. (2023). If online learning works for you, what about deaf students? Emerging challenges of online learning for deaf and hearing-impaired students during COVID-19: A literature review. *Universal Access in the Information Society*, *22*(3), 1027–1046. doi:10.1007/s10209-022-00897-5 PMID:35910240

Alkhatib, H., Faraboschi, P., & Frachtenberg, E. (2014). *IEEE CS 2022 Report*. IEEE Computer Society.

Almeida, L. B. (2020). Multilayer perceptrons. In *Handbook of Neural Computation* (pp. C1–C2). CRC Press.

Almotiri, S. H., Nadeem, M., Al Ghamdi, M. A., & Khan, R. A. (2023). Analytic Review of Healthcare Software by Using Quantum Computing Security Techniques. *International Journal of Fuzzy Logic and Intelligent Systems*, 23(3), 336–352. doi:10.5391/IJFIS.2023.23.3.336

Al-Obaydi, L. H., Pikhart, M., & Klimova, B. (2023). ChatGPT and the General Concepts of Education: Can Artificial Intelligence-Driven Chatbots Support the Process of Language Learning? [iJET]. *International Journal of Emerging Technologies in Learning*, 18(21), 39–50. doi:10.3991/ijet.v18i21.42593

Alshammari, F., Almutairi, B., & Alonazi, B. (2019). A Review of Internet of Things Technologies for Ambient Assisted Living Environments. *Procedia Computer Science*, 65, 1040–1045.

Al-Shoukry, S., Rassem, T. H., & Makbol, N. M. (2020). Alzheimer's Diseases Detection by Using Deep Learning Algorithms: A Mini-Review. *IEEE Access : Practical Innovations, Open Solutions*, 8, 77131–77141. doi:10.1109/ACCESS.2020.2989396

Altinkaya, E., Polat, K., & Barakli, B. (2020). Detection of Alzheimer's disease and dementia states based on deep learning from MRI images: A comprehensive review. *Journal of the Institute of Electronics and Computer*, 1(1), 39–53.

Amadin, F. I., Egwuatu, J. O., Obienu, A. C., & Osazuwa, W. A. (2017). Internet of Things (IoT): Implications of a Wide Scale Use in Nigeria. *Computing, Information Systems, Development Informatics & Allied Research Journal*, 8(1), 95-102. www.cisdijournal.net

Ambarwari, A., Adrian, Q.J., & Herdiyeni, Y. (2020). Analysis of the Effect of Data Scaling on the Performance of the Machine Learning Algorithm for Plant Identification. *J. Resti (Rekayasa Sist. Dan Teknol. Inf.)*, 4, 117–122.

Amin, S. U., Hossain, M. S., Muhammad, G., Alhussein, M., & Rahman, M. A. (2019). Cognitive Smart Healthcare for Pathology Detection and Monitoring. *IEEE Access : Practical Innovations, Open Solutions*, 7, 10745–10753. doi:10.1109/ACCESS.2019.2891390

Anh, P. T. N. (2024). *AI Models for Disease Diagnosis and Prediction of Heart Disease with Artificial Neural Networks. Computer Vision and AI-integrated IoT Technologies in Medical Ecosystem* (1st ed.). CRC Press. doi:10.1201/9781003429609-9

Aqeel, K. H., Rahat, U. A., Mehmood, K. A., Tanveer, B. H., Saima, S., Wasim, A., Didier, S., & Faisal, S. (2022). The NMT Scalp EEG Dataset: An Open-Source Annotated Dataset of Healthy and Pathological EEG Recordings for Predictive Modeling. *Frontiers in Neuroscience*, 15, 755817. doi:10.3389/fnins.2021.755817 PMID:35069095

Aranda, M. P., Kremer, I. N., Hinton, L., Zissimopoulos, J., Whitmer, R. A., Hummel, C. H., Trejo, L., & Fabius, C. (2021). Impact of dementia: Health disparities, population trends, care interventions, and economic costs. *Journal of the American Geriatrics Society*, 69(7), 1774–1783. doi:10.1111/jgs.17345 PMID:34245588

Arora, D., Garg, M., & Gupta, M. (2020). Diving deep in Deep Convolutional Neural Network. In *2020 2nd International Conference on Advances in Computing, Communication Control and Networking (ICACCCN)* (pp. 749-751). IEEE. 10.1109/ICACCCN51052.2020.9362907

Arpita, N. (2023). Incorporating Artificial Intelligence (AI) for Precision Medicine: A Narrative Analysis. In AI and IoT-Based Technologies for Precision Medicine (1st ed.). IGI Global Press. doi:10.4018/979-8-3693-0876-9.ch002

Asan, O., Choi, E., & Wang, X. (2023). Artificial Intelligence–Based Consumer Health Informatics Application: Scoping Review. *Journal of Medical Internet Research*, 25, e47260. doi:10.2196/47260 PMID:37647122

Aslam, H., Ramashri, T., & Mohammed, I. (2013). A New Approach to Image Segmentation. *International Journal of Advanced Research in Computer and Communication Engineering*, 2(3), 1429-1436.

Avci, A., Bosch, S., & Marin-Perianu, M. (2010). *Activity Recognition Using Inertial Sensing for Healthcare, Wellbeing and Sports Applications: A Survey.* 23th International Conference on Architecture of Computing Systens 2010, Hannover, Germany.

Ayat, N. E., Cheriet, M., & Suen, C. Y. (2005). Automatic model selection for the optimization of SVM kernels. *Pattern Recognition, 38*(10), 1733–1745. doi:10.1016/j.patcog.2005.03.011

Azzi, S., Gagnon, S., Ramirez, A., & Richards, G. (2020). Healthcare applications of artificial intelligence and analytics: A review and proposed framework. *Applied Sciences (Basel, Switzerland), 10*(18), 6553. doi:10.3390/app10186553

Babu, G. C. N., Gupta, S., Bhambri, P., Leo, L. M., Rao, B. H., & Kumar, S. (2021). A Semantic Health Observation System Development Based on the IoT Sensors. *Turkish Journal of Physiotherapy and Rehabilitation, 32*(3), 1721–1729.

Babyak, M. A. (2004). What you see may not be what you get: A brief, nontechnical introduction to overfitting in regression-type models. *Psychosomatic Medicine, 66*, 411–421. PMID:15184705

Bag, D., Ghosh, A., & Saha, S. (2023). An Automatic Approach to Control Wheelchair Movement for Rehabilitation Using Electroencephalogram. In *Design and Control Advances in Robotics* (pp. 105–126). IGI Global.

Baker, R. E., Mahmud, A. S., Miller, I. F., Rajeev, M., Rasambainarivo, F., Rice, B. L., Takahashi, S., Tatem, A. J., Wagner, C. E., Wang, L.-F., Wesolowski, A., & Metcalf, C. J. E. (2022). Infectious disease in an era of global change. *Nature Reviews. Microbiology, 20*(4), 193–205. doi:10.1038/s41579-021-00639-z PMID:34646006

Bakshi, P., Bhambri, P., & Thapar, V. (2021). A Review Paper on Wireless Sensor Network Techniques in Internet of Things (IoT). *Wesleyan Journal of Research, 14*(7), 147–160.

Balabaeva, K., & Kovalchuk, S. (2019). Comparison of Temporal and Non-Temporal Features Effect on Machine Learning Models Quality and Interpretability for Chronic Heart Failure Patients. *Procedia Computer Science, 156*, 87–96. doi:10.1016/j.procs.2019.08.183

Bandyopadhyay, S. (2011). Detection of Brain Tumor – A Proposed Method. *Journal of Global Research in Computer Science, 2*(1), 55-63.

Bangui, H., Rakrak, S., Raghay, S., & Buhnova, B. (2018). Moving to the Edge-Cloud-of-Things: Recent Advances and Future Research Directions. *Electronics (Basel), 7*(11), 309. doi:10.3390/electronics7110309

Barbosa, M., & Chalmers, J. D. (2023). Bronchiectasis. *La Presse Medicale, 52*(3), 104174. doi:10.1016/j.lpm.2023.104174 PMID:37778637

Bashir, S., Almazroi, A. A., Ashfaq, S., Almazroi, A. A., & Khan, F. H. (2021). A knowledge-based clinical decision support system utilizing an intelligent ensemble voting scheme for improved cardiovascular disease prediction. *IEEE Access : Practical Innovations, Open Solutions, 9*, 130805–130822. doi:10.1109/ACCESS.2021.3110604

Beets, B., Newman, T. P., Howell, E. L., Bao, L., & Yang, S. (2023). Surveying Public Perceptions of Artificial Intelligence in Health Care in the United States: Systematic Review. *Journal of Medical Internet Research, 25*, e40337. doi:10.2196/40337 PMID:37014676

Bengtsson, E., & Malm, P. (2014). Screening for cervical cancer using automated analysis of PAP-smears. *Computational and Mathematical Methods in Medicine, 2014*, 1–12. doi:10.1155/2014/842037 PMID:24772188

Bentley, P., Ganesalingam, J., Carlton Jones, A. L., Mahady, K., Epton, S., Rinne, P., Sharma, P., Halse, O., Mehta, A., & Rueckert, D. (2014). Prediction of stroke thrombolysis outcome using CT brain machine learning. *NeuroImage. Clinical, 4*, 635–640. doi:10.1016/j.nicl.2014.02.003 PMID:24936414

Bera, S., & Shrivastava, V. K. (2020). Analysis of various optimizers on deep convolutional neural network model in the application of hyperspectral remote sensing image classification. *International Journal of Remote Sensing*, *41*(7), 2664–2683. doi:10.1080/01431161.2019.1694725

Bhambri, P. (2021). Electronic Evidence. In Textbook of Cyber Heal (pp. 86-120). AGAR Saliha Publication, Tamil Nadu. ISBN: 978-81-948141-7-7.

Bhambri, P., Singh, M., Dhanoa, I. S., & Kumar, M. (2022). Deployment of ROBOT for HVAC duct and Disaster Management. Oriental Journal of Computer Science and Technology, 15.

Bhambri, P., Kaur, H., Gupta, A., & Singh, J. (2020). Human Activity Recognition System. *Oriental Journal of Computer Science and Technology*, *13*(2-3), 91–96.

Bhambri, P., Singh, M., Jain, A., Dhanoa, I. S., Sinha, V. K., & Lal, S. (2021). Classification Of Gene Expression Data With The Aid Of Optimized Feature Selection. *Turkish Journal of Physiotherapy and Rehabilitation*, *32*, 3.

Bhambri, P., Singh, S., Sangwan, S., Devi, J., & Jain, S. (2023). Plants Recognition using Leaf Image Pattern Analysis. [Green Wave Publishing of Canada.]. *Journal of Survey in Fisheries Sciences*, *10*(2S), 3863–3871.

Bhardwaj, R., Nambiar, A. R., & Dutta, D. (2017). A Study of Machine Learning in Healthcare. *2017 IEEE 41st Annual Computer Software and Applications Conference (COMPSAC)*. IEEE.

Biswas, A., Mitra, A., Ghosh, A., Das, N., Ghosh, N., & Ghosh, A. (2022). A Deep Learning Approach to Classify the Causes of Depression from Reddit Posts. In *Machine Vision for Industry 4.0* (pp. 141–168). CRC Press. doi:10.1201/9781003122401-7

Bi, X., Li, S., Xiao, B., Li, Y., Wang, G., & Ma, X. (2020). Computer aided Alzheimer's disease diagnosis by an unsupervised deep learning technology. *Neurocomputing*, *392*, 296–304. doi:10.1016/j.neucom.2018.11.111

Bobdey, S., Sathwara, J., Jain, A., & Balasubramaniam, G. (2016). Burden of cervical cancer and role of screening in India. *Indian Journal of Medical and Paediatric Oncology : Official Journal of Indian Society of Medical & Paediatric Oncology*, *37*(4), 278–285. doi:10.4103/0971-5851.195751 PMID:28144096

Boden, M., & Hawkins, J. (2005, March). Improved access to sequential motifs: A note on the architectural bias of recurrent networks. *IEEE Transactions on Neural Networks*, *16*(2), 491–494. doi:10.1109/TNN.2005.844086 PMID:15787155

Bohr, A., & Memarzadeh, K. (2020). The rise of artificial intelligence in healthcare applications. In *Artificial Intelligence in healthcare* (pp. 25–60). Academic Press. doi:10.1016/B978-0-12-818438-7.00002-2

Bolhasani, H., Mohseni, M., & Rahmani, A. M. (2021). Deep learning applications for IoT in health care: A systematic review. *Informatics in Medicine Unlocked, 23*. doi:10.1016/j.imu.2021.100550

Bonato, P. (2010). Wearable sensors and systems. *IEEE Engineering in Medicine and Biology Magazine*, *29*(3), 25–36. doi:10.1109/MEMB.2010.936554 PMID:20659855

Borg, W. R., & Gall, M. D. (1986). Educational research: An introduction. *British Journal of Educational Studies*, *32*(3).

Bose, M. M., Yadav, D., Bhambri, P., & Shankar, R. (2021). Electronic Customer Relationship Management: Benefits and Pre-Implementation Considerations. [The Maharaja Sayajirao University of Baroda.]. *Journal of Maharaja Sayajirao University of Baroda*, *55*(01(VI)), 1343–1350.

Bosley M. (2018). *The Internet of Laboratory Equipment. Laboratory Products*. Labmate UK & Ireland.

BrainTumorInfo. (n.d.). *Info*. Brain Tumor Community.

Bray, F., Ferlay, J., Soerjomataram, I., Siegel, R. L., Torre, L. A., & Jemal, A. (2018). Global cancer statistics 2018: GLOBOCAN estimates of incidence and mortality worldwide for 36 cancers in 185 countries. *CA: a Cancer Journal for Clinicians*, *68*(6), 394–424. doi:10.3322/caac.21492 PMID:30207593

Breiman, L. (2001). Random forests. *Machine Learning*, *45*(1), 5–32. doi:10.1023/A:1010933404324

Brown, R., Cheng, Y., Haacke, M., Thompson, M., & Venkatesan, R. (2014). *Magnetic Resonance Imaging: Physical Principles and Sequence Design*. Wiley. doi:10.1002/9781118633953

Brown, A., & Jones, B. (2022). The Role of Wearable Devices in Patient Monitoring. *International Journal of Medical Informatics*, *98*, 1–8.

Cabrilo, I., Bijlenga, P., & Schaller, K. (2014, September). Augmented reality in the surgery of cerebral arteriovenous malformations: Technique assessment and considerations. *Acta Neurochirurgica*, *156*(9), 1769–1774. doi:10.1007/s00701-014-2183-9 PMID:25037466

Cafazzo, J. A., Barnsley, J., Masino, C., & Ross, H. J. (2012). Perceptions and experiences of heart failure patients and clinicians on the use of mobile phone-based telemonitoring. *Journal of Medical Internet Research*, *14*(1), e25. doi:10.2196/jmir.1912 PMID:22328237

Cai, L., Gao, J., & Zhao, D. (2020). A review of the application of deep Learning in medical image classification and segmentation. *Annals of Translational Medicine*, *8*(11), 713. doi:10.21037/atm.2020.02.44 PMID:32617333

Calvillo-Arbizu, J., Román-Martínez, I., & Reina-Tosina, J. (2021). Internet of things in health: Requirements, issues, and gaps. *Computer Methods and Programs in Biomedicine*, *208*, 106231. Advance online publication. doi:10.1016/j.cmpb.2021.106231 PMID:34186337

Cascone, S., Lamberti, G., Titomanlio, G., & Piazza, O. (2013). Pharmacokinetics of Remifentanil: A three-compartmental modeling approach. *Translational Medicine @ UniSa*, 18–22. PMID:24251247

Casson, A. J., & Rodriguez-Villegas, E. (2020). Machine learning and clinical analytics at the edge: Rethinking patient monitoring, telehealth and care delivery. *Sensors (Basel)*, *20*(21), 6272. PMID:33158047

Cavallaro, G., Riedel, M., Richerzhagen, M., Benediktsson, J. A., & Plaza, A. (2015). On understanding big data impacts in remotely sensed image classification using support vector machine methods. *IEEE Journal of Selected Topics in Applied Earth Observations and Remote Sensing*, *8*(10), 4634–4646. doi:10.1109/JSTARS.2015.2458855

Chakraborty, D., Ghosh, A., & Saha, S. (2020). A survey on Internet-of-Thing applications using electroencephalogram. In *Emergence of Pharmaceutical Industry Growth with Industrial IoT Approach* (pp. 21–47). Academic Press. doi:10.1016/B978-0-12-819593-2.00002-9

Chalak, L. F., Pavageau, L., Huet, B., & Hynan, L. (2020). Statistical rigor and kappa considerations: Which, when and clinical context matters. *Pediatric Research*, *88*(1), 5. doi:10.1038/s41390-020-0890-x PMID:32272485

Char, D. S., Shah, N. H., & Magnus, D. (2018, March 15). Implementing Machine Learning in Health Care - Addressing Ethical Challenges. *The New England Journal of Medicine*, *378*(11), 981–983. doi:10.1056/NEJMp1714229 PMID:29539284

Chartrand, G., Cheng, P. M., Vorontsov, E., Drozdzal, M., Turcotte, S., Pal, C. J., Kadoury, S., & Tang, A. (2017, November-December). Deep Learning: A Primer for Radiologists. *Radiographics*, *37*(7), 2113–2131. doi:10.1148/rg.2017170077 PMID:29131760

Chaudhuri, A. K., & Das, A. (2020). Variable Selection in Genetic Algorithm Model with Logistic Regression for Prediction of Progression to Diseases. *IEEE International Conference for Innovation in Technology (INOCON)*. IEEE. 10.1109/INOCON50539.2020.9298372

Chen, J., Chen, C. B., Walther, J., & Sundar, S. S. (2021, May). Do you feel special when an AI doctor remembers you? Individuation effects of AI vs. human doctors on user experience. In *Extended Abstracts of the 2021 CHI Conference on Human Factors in Computing Systems* (pp. 1-7). ACM. 10.1145/3411763.3451735

Chen, A. Y., Lu, T. Y., Ma, M. H., & Sun, W.-Z. (2016). Demand Forecast Using Data Analytics for the Preallocation of Ambulances. *IEEE Journal of Biomedical and Health Informatics*, *20*(4), 1178–1187. doi:10.1109/JBHI.2015.2443799 PMID:26087507

Chen, L., Wang, X., & Peng, T. (2022). Internet of Things in Healthcare: A Survey. *Journal of Medical Systems*, *41*(12), 199.

Chen, X., & Ishwaran, H. (2012). Random forests for genomic data analysis. *Genomics*, *99*(6), 323–329. doi:10.1016/j.ygeno.2012.04.003 PMID:22546560

Chen, Y., Jia, Z., Mercola, D., & Xie, X. (2013). A gradient boosting algorithm for survival analysis via direct optimization of concordance index. *Computational and Mathematical Methods in Medicine*, *2013*, 1–8. doi:10.1155/2013/873595 PMID:24348746

Cheung, C. Y., Ran, A. R., Wang, S., Chan, V. T. T., Sham, K., Hilal, S., Venketasubramanian, N., Cheng, C.-Y., Sabanayagam, C., Tham, Y. C., Schmetterer, L., McKay, G. J., Williams, M. A., Wong, A., Au, L. W. C., Lu, Z., Yam, J. C., Tham, C. C., Chen, J. J., & Wong, T. Y. (2022, November). A deep learning model for detection of Alzheimer's disease based on retinal photographs: A retrospective, multicentre case-control study. *The Lancet. Digital Health*, *4*(11), e806–e815. doi:10.1016/S2589-7500(22)00169-8 PMID:36192349

Cho, K., Van Merriënboer, B., Gülçehre, Ç., Bahdanau, D., Bougares, F., Schwenk, H., & Bengio, Y. (2014). Learning Phrase Representations using RNN Encoder-Decoder for Statistical Machine Translation. *arXiv (Cornell University)*. / arxiv.1406.1078 doi:10.3115/v1/D14-1179

Chong, & Ali, S. (2021). Schema Ontology Model to Support Semantic Interoperability in Healthcare Applications: Use Case of Depressive Disorder. In *2021 Twelfth International Conference on Ubiquitous and Future Networks (ICUFN)*, (pp. 409-412). IEEE. 10.1109/ICUFN49451.2021.9528708.s

Chowdhury, N. & Kashem, M. (2008). A comparative analysis of Feedforward neural network & Recurrent Neural network to detect intrusion. In *2008 International Conference on Electrical and Computer Engineering* (pp. 488-492). IEEE. . doi:10.1109/ICECE.2008.4769258

Cockshott, I. D., Douglas, E. J., & Prys-Roberts, C. (1987). Pharmacokinetics of propofol during and after intravenous infusion in man. *British Journal of Anaesthesia*, *59*, 941.

Coetzee, L., & Eksteen, J. (2011). The Internet of Things – Promise for the Future? An Introduction. *IST-Africa 2011 Conference Proceedings*. IIMC International Information Management Corporation.

Connelly, L. (2020). Logistic regression. *Medsurg Nursing*, *29*, 353–354.

Contreas, I., & Vehi, J. (2018). Artificial intelligence for diabetes management and decision support: Literature review. *Journal of Medical Internet Research*, *20*(5), e10775. doi:10.2196/10775 PMID:29848472

Cortes, C., & Vapnik, V. (1995). Support-vector networks. *Machine Learning*, *20*(3), 273–297. doi:10.1007/BF00994018

D'Elia, G., Caracchini, G., Cavalli, L., & Innocentia, P. (2009, September–December). Bone fragility and imaging techniques. *Clinical Cases in Mineral and Bone Metabolism*, *6*, 234–246. PMID:22461252

Darwish, A., & Hassanien, A. E. (2019). Wearable and implantable wireless sensor network solutions for healthcare monitoring. *Sensors (Basel)*, *19*(6), 5561–5595. doi:10.3390/s110605561 PMID:22163914

Das, S. & Bhattacharya, A. (2021). *ECG Assess Heartbeat rate. Classifying using BPNN while Watching Movie and send Movie Rating through Telegram.* Springer. . doi:10.1007/978-981-15-9774-9_43

Das, S., & Ghosh, L., & Saha, S. (2020). *Analyzing Gaming Effects on Cognitive Load Using Artificial Intelligent Tools.* IEEE. . doi:10.1109/CONECCT50063.2020.9198662

Das, S., Das, J., Modak, S., & Mazumdar, K. (2022). *Internet of Things with Machine Learning based smart Cardiovascular disease classifier for Healthcare in Secure platform.* Taylor & Francis.

Dash, S., Shakyawar, S. K., Sharma, M., & Kaushik, S. (2019). Big data in healthcare: Management, analysis and future prospects. *Journal of Big Data*, *6*(1), 54. doi:10.1186/s40537-019-0217-0

Dauwed, M. A., Yahaya, J., Mansor, Z., & Hamdan, A. R. (2018). Determinants of Internet of Things Services Utilization in Health Information Exchange. *Journal of Engineering and Applied Sciences (Asian Research Publishing Network)*, *13*(24), 10490–10501.

Deiana, G., Dettori, M., Arghittu, A., Azara, A., Gabutti, G., & Castiglia, P. (2023). Artificial intelligence and public health: Evaluating ChatGPT responses to vaccination myths and misconceptions. *Vaccines*, *11*(7), 1217. doi:10.3390/vaccines11071217 PMID:37515033

Deloitte Centre for Health Solutions. (2018). *Medtech and the Internet of Medical Things How connected medical devices are transforming health care.* Deloitte.

DeLong, E. R., DeLong, D. M., & Clarke-Pearson, D. L. (1988, September). Comparing the areas under two or more correlated receiver operating characteristic curves: A nonparametric approach. *Biometrics*, *44*(3), 837–845. doi:10.2307/2531595 PMID:3203132

Deng, S., & Wang, X. (2023). Exploring locally developed ELT materials in the context of curriculum-based value education in China: Challenges and solutions. *Frontiers in Psychology*, *14*, 14. doi:10.3389/fpsyg.2023.1191420 PMID:37901095

Dergaa, I., Chamari, K., Zmijewski, P., & Saad, H. B. (2023). From human writing to artificial intelligence generated text: Examining the prospects and potential threats of ChatGPT in academic writing. *Biology of Sport*, *40*(2), 615–622. doi:10.5114/biolsport.2023.125623 PMID:37077800

Desai, S. J., Shoaib, M., & Raychowdhury, A. (2015). An ultra-low power, "always-on" camera front-end for posture detection in body worn cameras using restricted boltzman machines. *IEEE Transactions on Multi-Scale Computing Systems*, *1*(4), 187–194. doi:10.1109/TMSCS.2015.2513741

Devadutta, K., Bhambri, P., Gountia, D., Mehta, V., Mangla, M., Patan, R., Kumar, A., Agarwal, P. K., Sharma, A., Singh, M., & Gadicha, A. B. (2020). *Method for Cyber Security in Email Communication among Networked Computing Devices* [Patent application number 202031002649].

Dhanalakshmi, P., & Kanimozhi, T. (2013). Automatic Segmentation of Brain Tumor using K-Means Clustering and its Area Calculation. *International Journal of Advanced Electrical and Electronics Engineering*, 130-134.

Diabetes.co. (n.d.). *Welcome!* Diabetes.co.uk. https://www.diabetes.co.uk/

Dimililer & Kamil. (2017). *IBFDS: Intelligent bone fracture detection system.* Elsevier.

Dinh-Le, C., Chuang, R., & Chokshi, S. (2020). Artificial Intelligence for Diabetes Management and Decision Support: Literature Review. *Journal of Medical Internet Research*, *21*(4), e12452.

Dodd, S., Berk, M., Kelin, K., Zhang, Q., Eriksson, E., Deberdt, W., & Nelson, J. C. (2014). Application of the Gradient Boosted method in randomised clinical trials: Participant variables that contribute to depression treatment efficacy of duloxetine, SSRIs or placebo. *Journal of Affective Disorders*, *168*, 284–293. doi:10.1016/j.jad.2014.05.014 PMID:25080392

Doi, K. (2007, June-July). Computer-aided diagnosis in medical imaging: Historical review, current status and future potential. *Computerized Medical Imaging and Graphics*, *31*(4-5), 198–211. doi:10.1016/j.compmedimag.2007.02.002 PMID:17349778

Du, W., Wang, Y., & Yu, Q. (2017). RPAN: An End-to-End Recurrent Pose-Attention Network for Action Recognition in Videos. *2017 IEEE International Conference on Computer Vision (ICCV)*. IEEE. 10.1109/ICCV.2017.402

Ebrahim, D., Ali-Eldin, A. M. T., Moustafa, H. E., & Arafat, H. (2020). Alzheimer Disease Early Detection Using Convolutional Neural Networks. In *2020 15th International Conference on Computer Engineering and Systems (ICCES)*. IEEE. 10.1109/ICCES51560.2020.9334594

Ebrahimighahnavieh, M. A., Luo, S., & Chiong, R. (2020). Deep learning to detect Alzheimer's disease from neuroimaging: A systematic literature review. *Computer Methods and Programs in Biomedicine*, *187*, 105242. doi:10.1016/j.cmpb.2019.105242 PMID:31837630

Edquist, H., Goodridge, P., & Haskel, J. (2021). The Internet of Things and Economic Growth in a Panel of Countries. *Economics of Innovation and New Technology 30*(3), 262-283.

Emanuel, E. J., & Wachter, R. M. (2019, June 18). Artificial Intelligence in Health Care: Will the Value Match the Hype? *Journal of the American Medical Association*, *321*(23), 2281–2282. doi:10.1001/jama.2019.4914 PMID:31107500

Emmanuel, N.O. & Dan-Muhammadu, I. (2017). *Acceptance and Rejection of Internet for Health Information Among Private Health Professionals in a Nigerian City*. New Media and Mass Communication.

Erickson, B. J., Korfiatis, P., Akkus, Z., & Kline, T. L. (2017, March-April). Machine Learning for Medical Imaging. *Radiographics*, *37*(2), 505–515. doi:10.1148/rg.2017160130 PMID:28212054

Esteva, A., Kuprel, B., Novoa, R. A., Ko, J., Swetter, S. M., Blau, H. M., & Thrun, S. (2018). Dermatologist-Level Classification of Skin Cancer with Deep Neural Networks. *Nature*, *542*(7639), 115–118. doi:10.1038/nature21056 PMID:28117445

Eswaran, U. (2023). Applying Machine Learning for Medical Image Processing. AI and IoT-Based Technologies for Precision Medicine (1st ed.). IGI Global Press. doi:10.4018/979-8-3693-0876-9.ch009

Etukudoh, N. S., & Obeta, M. U. (2021). Patients' (Clients) Satisfaction with Medical Laboratory Services Contributes to Health and Quality Improvement. Healthcare Access. IntechOpen, doi:10.5772/intechopen.99290

Etukudoh, N. S., & Nelson, A. B. (2021). Health care delivery business and the role of Medical Laboratory Scientists. *IAR Journal of Medical Sciences*, *2*(4), 76–80.

European Centre for Disease Prevention and Control. (2018). *Monitoring the use of whole-genome sequencing in infectious disease surveillance in Europe*. ECDC.

Falk, M., Andoralov, V., Silow, M., Toscano, M., & Shleev, S. (2013). Biofuel cells for biomedical applications: Colonizing the animal kingdom. *Analytical and Bioanalytical Chemistry*, *405*(11), 3791–3803. PMID:23241817

Fan, Z.-C., Chan, T.-S. T., Yang, Y.-H., & Jang, J.-S. R. (2020, July). Backpropagation With N -D Vector-Valued Neurons Using Arbitrary Bilinear Products. *IEEE Transactions on Neural Networks and Learning Systems*, *31*(7), 2638–2652. doi:10.1109/TNNLS.2019.2933882 PMID:31502991

Farmer, L. S. (2023). Technology use and its changing role in community education. In *Handbook of Research on Andragogical Leadership and Technology in a Modern World* (pp. 358–383). IGI Global. doi:10.4018/978-1-6684-7832-5.ch019

Fatima, S., Desouza, K. C., & Dawson, G. S. (2020). National strategic artificial intelligence plans: A multi-dimensional analysis. *Economic Analysis and Policy*, *67*, 178–194. doi:10.1016/j.eap.2020.07.008

Fayed, A. M., Mansur, N. S. B., de Carvalho, K. A., Behrens, A., D'Hooghe, P., & de Cesar Netto, C. (2023). Artificial intelligence and ChatGPT in Orthopaedics and sports medicine. *Journal of Experimental Orthopaedics*, *10*(1), 74. doi:10.1186/s40634-023-00642-8 PMID:37493985

Feng, C., Elazab, A., Yang, P., Wang, T., Zhou, F., Hu, H., Xiao, X., & Lei, B. (2019). Deep learning framework for Alzheimer's disease diagnosis via 3D-CNN and FSBi-LSTM. *IEEE Access : Practical Innovations, Open Solutions*, *7*, 63605–63618. doi:10.1109/ACCESS.2019.2913847

Feng, W., Halm-Lutterodt, N. V., Tang, H., Mecum, A., Mesregah, M. K., Ma, Y., Li, H., Zhang, F., Wu, Z., Yao, E., & Guo, X. (2020, June). Automated MRI-Based Deep Learning Model for Detection of Alzheimer's Disease Process. *International Journal of Neural Systems*, *30*(06), 2050032. doi:10.1142/S012906572050032X PMID:32498641

Ferdinand, A. S., Kelaher, M., Lane, C. R., da Silva, A. G., Sherry, N. L., Ballard, S. A., Andersson, P., Hoang, T., Denholm, J. T., Easton, M., Howden, B. P., & Williamson, D. A. (2021). An implementation science approach to evaluating pathogen whole genome sequencing in public health. *Genome Medicine*, *13*(1), 121. doi:10.1186/s13073-021-00934-7 PMID:34321076

Fernandes, K., Cardoso, J. S., & Fernandes, J. (June 2017). Transfer learning with partial observability applied to cervical cancer screening. In *Iberian conference on pattern recognition and image analysis* (pp. 243–250). Springer. doi:10.1007/978-3-319-58838-4_27

Fernández-Alemán, J. L., Señor, I. C., Lozoya, P. Á., & Toval, A. (2013, June). Security and privacy in electronic health records: A systematic literature review. *Journal of Biomedical Informatics*, *46*(3), 541–562. doi:10.1016/j.jbi.2012.12.003 PMID:23305810

Festor, P., Habli, I., Jia, Y., Gordon, A., Faisal, A. A., & Komorowski, M. (2021). Levels of autonomy and safety assurance for AI-Based clinical decision systems. In Computer Safety, Reliability, and Security. SAFECOMP 2021 Workshops: DECSoS, MAPSOD, DepDevOps, USDAI, and WAISE, (pp. 291-296). Springer International Publishing. doi:10.1007/978-3-030-83906-2_24

Flöck, A. N., & Walla, P. (2020). Think outside the box: small, enclosed spaces alter brain activity as measured with electroencephalography (EEG). In Information Systems and Neuroscience: NeuroIS Retreat 2020 (pp. 24-30). Springer International Publishing.

Franc, J. M., Ingrassia, P. L., Verde, M., Colombo, D., & Della Corte, F. (2015). A simple graphical method for quantification of disaster management surge capacity using computer simulation and process-control tools. *Prehospital and Disaster Medicine*, *30*(1), 9–15. doi:10.1017/S1049023X1400123X PMID:25407409

Friedman, J. H. (2001). Greedy function approximation: A gradient boosting machine. *Annals of Statistics*, *29*(5), 1189–1232. doi:10.1214/aos/1013203451

Fui-Hoon Nah, F., Zheng, R., Cai, J., Siau, K., & Chen, L. (2023). Generative AI and ChatGPT: Applications, challenges, and AI-human collaboration. *Journal of Information Technology Case and Application Research*, *25*(3), 277–304. doi:10.1080/15228053.2023.2233814

Galetsi, P., Katsaliaki, K., & Kumar, S. (2023). Exploring benefits and ethical challenges in the rise of mHealth (mobile healthcare) technology for the common good: An analysis of mobile applications for health specialists. *Technovation*, *121*, 102598. doi:10.1016/j.technovation.2022.102598

Galgano, M. T., Castle, P. E., Atkins, K. A., Brix, W. K., Nassau, S. R., & Stoler, M. H. (2010). Using biomarkers as objective standards in the diagnosis of cervical biopsies. *The American Journal of Surgical Pathology*, *34*(8), 1077–1087. doi:10.1097/PAS.0b013e3181e8b2c4 PMID:20661011

Gao, X., Wang, Y., Chen, X., & Gao, S. (2021). Interface, interaction, and intelligence in generalized brain–computer interfaces. *Trends in Cognitive Sciences*, *25*(8), 671–684. doi:10.1016/j.tics.2021.04.003 PMID:34116918

Gao, Z., Wang, X., Yang, Y., Li, Y., Ma, K., & Chen, G. (2021, December). A Channel-Fused Dense Convolutional Network for EEG-Based Emotion Recognition. *IEEE Transactions on Cognitive and Developmental Systems*, *13*(4), 945–954. doi:10.1109/TCDS.2020.2976112

Gayou, O., Das, S. K., Zhou, S. M., Marks, L. B., Parda, D. S., & Miften, M. (2008). A genetic algorithm for variable selection in logistic regression analysis of radiotherapy treatment outcomes. *Medical Physics*, *35*(12), 5426–5433. doi:10.1118/1.3005974 PMID:19175102

GBD 2019 Ageing Collaborators. (2022). Global, regional, and national burden of diseases and injuries for adults 70 years and older: systematic analysis for the Global Burden of Disease 2019 Study. *BMJ*, 376.

Gepts, E., Camu, F., Cockshott, I. D., & Douglas, E. J. (1987). Disposition of propofol administered as constant rate infusions in humans. *Anesthesia and Analgesia*, *66*(12), 1256–1263. doi:10.1213/00000539-198712000-00010 PMID:3500657

Ghazal, T. M. (2022). Alzheimer Disease Detection Empowered with Transfer Learning. *Computers, Materials & Continua*, *70*(3). https://www.researchgate.net/profile/Mohammad-Hasan-92/publication/355174632_Alzheimer_Disease_Detection_Empowered_with_Transfer_Learning/links/6165557aae47db4e57cbc3f2/Alzheimer-Disease-Detection-Empowered-with-Transfer-Learning.pdf

Ghazal, T. M., Hasan, M. K., Alshurideh, M. T., Alzoubi, H. M., Ahmad, M., Akbar, S. S., Al Kurdi, B., & Akour, I. A. (2021). IoT for smart cities: Machine learning approaches in smart healthcare-A review. *Future Internet*, *13*(8), 218. doi:10.3390/fi13080218

Ghosh, A., & Saha, S. (2021, August). Recurrent neural network based cognitive ability analysis in mental arithmetic task using electroencephalogram. In *2021 8th International Conference on Signal Processing and Integrated Networks (SPIN)* (pp. 1165-1170). IEEE. 10.1109/SPIN52536.2021.9566099

Ghosh, A., & Saha, S. (2022). Suppression of positive emotions during pandemic era: A deep learning framework for rehabilitation. *International Journal of Modelling Identification and Control*, *41*(1-2), 143–154. doi:10.1504/IJMIC.2022.127101

Gillies, R. J., Kinahan, P. E., & Hricak, H. (2016, February). Radiomics: Images Are More than Pictures, They Are Data. *Radiology*, *278*(2), 563–577. doi:10.1148/radiol.2015151169 PMID:26579733

Gill, S. S., Xu, M., Patros, P., Wu, H., Kaur, R., Kaur, K., Fuller, S., Singh, M., Arora, P., Parlikad, A. K., Stankovski, V., Abraham, A., Ghosh, S. K., Lutfiyya, H., Kanhere, S. S., Bahsoon, R., Rana, O., Dustdar, S., Sakellariou, R., & Buyya, R. (2024). Transformative effects of ChatGPT on modern education: Emerging Era of AI Chatbots. *Internet of Things and Cyber-Physical Systems*, *4*, 19–23. doi:10.1016/j.iotcps.2023.06.002

Glas, A. S., Lijmer, J. G., Prins, M. H., Bonsel, G. J., & Bossuyt, P. M. (2003, November). The diagnostic odds ratio: A single indicator of test performance. *Journal of Clinical Epidemiology*, *56*(11), 1129–1135. doi:10.1016/S0895-4356(03)00177-X PMID:14615004

Gondy, L. A., Thomas, C., & Bayes, N. (1993). Programs for machine learning. *Advances in Neural Information Processing Systems*, *79*(2), 937–944.

Gong, Y., & Poellabauer, C. (2017). "Topic modeling based multi-modaldepression detection. Proceedings of the 7th Annual Workshopon Audio/Visual Emotion Challenge. ACM.

Gong, M., Liu, J., Qin, A. K., Zhao, K., & Tan, K. C. (2021, January). Evolving Deep Neural Networks via Cooperative Coevolution With Backpropagation. *IEEE Transactions on Neural Networks and Learning Systems*, *32*(1), 420–434. doi:10.1109/TNNLS.2020.2978857 PMID:32217489

Goodfellow, I. J., Pouget-Abadie, J., Mirza, M., Xu, B., Warde-Farley, D., Ozair, S., Courville, A., & Bengio, Y. (2014). Generative adversarial networks. *arXiv (Cornell University)*. https://doi.org//arxiv.1406.2661 doi:10.48550

Goodfellow, I., Bengio, Y., & Courville, A. (2016). *Deep learning*. MIT Press.

Goularas, D., & Kamis, S. (2019). Evaluation of Deep Learning Techniques in Sentiment Analysis from Twitter Data. In *2019 International Conference on Deep Learning and Machine Learning in Emerging Applications (Deep-ML)* (pp. 12-17). IEEE. 10.1109/Deep-ML.2019.00011

Grájeda, A., Burgos, J., Córdova, P., & Sanjinés, A. (2024). Assessing student-perceived impact of using artificial intelligence tools: Construction of a synthetic index of application in higher education. *Cogent Education*, *11*(1), 2287917. doi:10.1080/2331186X.2023.2287917

Green, M., Bjrk, J., & Forberg, J. (2006). Comparison between neural networks and multiple logistic regression to predict acute coronary syndrome in the emergency room. *Artificial Intelligence in Medicine*, *38*(3), 305–318. doi:10.1016/j.artmed.2006.07.006 PMID:16962295

Gubbi, J., Buyya, R., Marusic, S., & Palaniswami, M. (2013). Internet of Things (IoT): A Vision, Architectural Elements, and Future Directions. *Future Generation Computer Systems*, *29*(7), 1645–1660. doi:10.1016/j.future.2013.01.010

Gulshan, V., Peng, L., Coram, M., Stumpe, M. C., Wu, D., Narayanaswamy, A., Venugopalan, S., Widner, K., Madams, T., Cuadros, J., Kim, R., Raman, R., Nelson, P. C., Mega, J. L., & Webster, D. R. (2016, December 13). Development and Validation of a Deep Learning Algorithm for Detection of Diabetic Retinopathy in Retinal Fundus Photographs. *Journal of the American Medical Association*, *316*(22), 2402–2410. doi:10.1001/jama.2016.17216 PMID:27898976

Gupta, A. K., Aggarwal, V., Sharma, V., & Naved, M. (2024). Education 4.0 and Web 3.0 Technologies Application for Enhancement of Distance Learning Management Systems in the Post–COVID-19 Era. In The Role of Sustainability and Artificial Intelligence in Education Improvement (pp. 66-86). Chapman and Hall/CRC.

Gupta, R., & Jain, P. (2019). Applications of Artificial Intelligence in Monitoring Chronic Diseases. *Journal of Healthcare Informatics Research*, *10*(3), 213–229.

Guvenc, G., Akyuz, A., & Açikel, C. H. (2011). Health belief model scale for cervical cancer and Pap smear test: Psychometric testing. *Journal of Advanced Nursing*, *67*(2), 428–437. doi:10.1111/j.1365-2648.2010.05450.x PMID:20946564

Haider, F. (2014). Cellular architecture and key technologies for 5G wireless communication networks. *J Chongqing Univ Posts Telecommun*, *52*(2), 122–130.

Hamburg, M. A., & Collins, F. S. (2010, July 22). The path to personalized medicine. *The New England Journal of Medicine*, *363*(4), 301–304. doi:10.1056/NEJMp1006304 PMID:20551152

Harris, M.L., Oldmeadow, C., Hure, A., Luu, J., Loxton, D., & Attia, J. (2017). Stress increases the risk of type 2 diabetes onset in women: A 12-year longitudinal study using causal modelling. *PLoS One, 12*(2), e0172126. doi:.pone.0172126 doi:10.1371/journal

Helaly, H. A., Badawy, M., & Haikal, A. Y. (2022, September). Deep Learning Approach for Early Detection of Alzheimer's Disease. *Cognitive Computation*, *14*(5), 1711–1727. doi:10.1007/s12559-021-09946-2 PMID:34745371

Higgins, L. (2019). The evolution of smart biosensor technology. *Chemical Society Reviews*, *48*(9), 2327–2338.

Hingmire, M., Bagjilewale, M., & Dakhole, M. (2017). What is Cloud Computing. *Springer VerlagNy*, *17*(1), 3–20.

Hiraku, Y., Kawanishi, S., & Ohshima, H. (Eds.). (2014). *Cancer and inflammation mechanisms: chemical, biological, and clinical aspects*. John Wiley & Sons. doi:10.1002/9781118826621

Hohenstein, J., Kizilcec, R. F., DiFranzo, D., Aghajari, Z., Mieczkowski, H., Levy, K., Naaman, M., Hancock, J., & Jung, M. F. (2023). Artificial intelligence in communication impacts language and social relationships. *Scientific Reports*, *13*(1), 5487. doi:10.1038/s41598-023-30938-9 PMID:37015964

Holmes, D. R., & Oetgen, W. J. (2021). Health Care 2020: Reengineering Health Care Delivery to Combat Chronic Disease. *The American Journal of Medicine*, *128*(4), 337–343. PMID:25460529

Hopkins Medicine. (n.d.). *Fractures*. Hopkins Medicine. https://www.hopkinsmedicine.org/health/conditions-anddiseases/fractures

Hosny, A., Parmar, C., Quackenbush, J., Schwartz, L. H., & Aerts, H. J. W. L. (2018, August). Artificial intelligence in radiology. *Nature Reviews. Cancer*, *18*(8), 500–510. doi:10.1038/s41568-018-0016-5 PMID:29777175

Huang, Y., Zhao, Y., Zhu, L., Han, B., & Li, Z. (2022, December). Challenges and Reflections on Vocational Education in 6G Era. In *International Conference on 5G for Future Wireless Networks* (pp. 342-353). Cham: Springer Nature Switzerland.

Huang, H. K., Aberle, D. R., Lufkin, R., Grant, E. G., Hanafee, W. N., & Kangarloo, H. (1990, February 1). Advances in medical imaging. *Annals of Internal Medicine*, *112*(3), 203–220. doi:10.7326/0003-4819-112-3-203 PMID:2404446

Huang, J., Saleh, S., & Liu, Y. (2021). A review on Artificial intelligence in education. *Academic Journal of Interdisciplinary Studies*, *10*(3), 206. doi:10.36941/ajis-2021-0077

Hua, X., Aldrich, M. C., & Chen, Q. (2015). Validating drug repurposing signals using electronic health records: A case study of metformin associated with reduced cancer mortality. *Journal of the American Medical Informatics Association : JAMIA*, (1), 179–191. PMID:25053577

Hudson, S., Nishat, F., Stinson, J., Litwin, S., Zeller, F., Wiles, B., Foster, M. E., & Ali, S. (2023). Perspectives of healthcare providers to inform the design of an AI-enhanced social robot in the pediatric emergency department. *Children (Basel, Switzerland)*, *10*(9), 1511. doi:10.3390/children10091511 PMID:37761472

Hung, P., Zhang, Y., & Zhang, H. (2023). Healthcare Data Gateways: Found Healthcare Intelligence on Blockchain with Novel Privacy Risk Control. *Journal of Medical Systems*, *40*(10), 218. PMID:27565509

Huseinović, L. (2024). The effects of gamification on student motivation and achievement in learning English as a foreign language in higher education. *MAP Education and Humanities*, *4*, 10–36.

Hussain, M., Satti, F. A., Ali, S. I., Hussain, J., Ali, T., Kim, H. S., Yoon, K.-H., Chung, T. C., & Lee, S. (2021). Intelligent knowledge consolidation: From data to wisdom. *Knowledge-Based Systems*, *234*, 107578. doi:10.1016/j.knosys.2021.107578

Ifelebuegu, A. O., Kulume, P., & Cherukut, P. (2023). Chatbots and AI in Education (AIEd) tools: The good, the bad, and the ugly. *Journal of Applied Learning and Teaching*, *6*(2).

Ijjina, E. P., & Mohan, C. K. (2016). Hybrid deep neural network model for human action recognition. *Applied Soft Computing*, *46*, 936–952. doi:10.1016/j.asoc.2015.08.025

Iqbal, M. J., Javed, Z., Sadia, H., Qureshi, I. A., Irshad, A., Ahmed, R., Malik, K., Raza, S., Abbas, A., Pezzani, R., & Sharifi-Rad, J. (2021). Clinical applications of artificial intelligence and machine learning in cancer diagnosis: Looking into the future. *Cancer Cell International*, *21*(1), 1–11. doi:10.1186/s12935-021-01981-1 PMID:34020642

Irfan, R., Rehman, Z., Abro, A., Chira, C., & Anwar, W. (2019). Ontology learning in text mining for handling big data in healthcare systems. *Journal of Medical Imaging and Health Informatics*, *9*(4), 649–661. doi:10.1166/jmihi.2019.2681

Isard, A. B. A. M. (1998). *Active Contours*. Springer Verlag.

Ishikawa, T., Takahashi, J., Takemura, H., Mizoguchi, H., & Kuwata, T. (2014). Gastric lymph node cancer detection using multiple features support vector machine for pathology diagnosis support system. *The 15th International Conference on Biomedical Engineering*, Cham: Springer. 10.1007/978-3-319-02913-9_31

Islam, J., & Zhang, Y. (2017). A Novel Deep Learning Based Multi-class Classification Method for Alzheimer's Disease Detection Using Brain MRI Data. In Y. Zeng, Y. He, J. H. Kotaleski, M. Martone, B. Xu, H. Peng, & Q. Luo (Eds.), *Lecture Notes in Computer Science* (Vol. 10654, pp. 213–222). Springer International Publishing. doi:10.1007/978-3-319-70772-3_20

Islam, M., Hossain, M., & Haque, I. (2021). Mathematical Comparison of Defuzzification of Fuzzy Logic Controller for Intelligence Air Conditioning System. *Int. J. Sci. Res. Math. Stat. Sci.*, *8*, 29–37.

Islam, S. R., Kwak, D., Kabir, M. H., Hossain, M., & Kwak, K. S. (2015). The internet of things for health care: A comprehensive survey. *IEEE Access : Practical Innovations, Open Solutions*, *3*, 678–708. doi:10.1109/ACCESS.2015.2437951

Istepanian, R. S., Zitouni, K., & Harry, D. (2022). Evaluation of a Mobile Phone Telemonitoring System for Glycaemic Control in Patients with Diabetes. *Journal of Telemedicine and Telecare*, *17*(7), 340–343. PMID:19364893

ITU (n.d.). Harnessing the Internet of Things for Global Development. *ITU/UNESCO Broadband Commission for Sustainable Development*. UNESCO.

Jabbar, M. A., & Samreen, S. (2016). Heart disease prediction system based on hidden naïve bayes classifier. *International Conference on Circuits, Controls, Communications and Computing (I4C)*. IEEE. 10.1109/CIMCA.2016.8053261

Jabeen, A., Pallathadka, H., Pallathadka, L. K., & Bhambri, P. (2021). E-CRM Successful Factors for Business Enterprises CASE STUDIES. [The Maharaja Sayajirao University of Baroda.]. *Journal of Maharaja Sayajirao University of Baroda*, *55*(01(VI)), 1332–1342.

Jacob, N. E., & Wyawahare, M. (2013, June). Survey of bone fracture detection techniques. *Int. J. Comput. Appl.*, *71*(17), 31–34.

Javeed Hussain, S., Satya Savitr, T., & Sree Devi, P. (2012). Segmentation of Tissues in Brain MRI Images using Dynamic Neuro – Fuzzy Technique. *International Journal of Soft Computing and Engineering*.

Jayapal, J. (2024). Artificial Intelligence in Education: A Critic on English Language Teaching. In Artificial Intelligence and Knowledge Processing (pp. 348-357). CRC Press.

Jemal, A., Center, M. M., DeSantis, C., & Ward, E. M. (2010). Global patterns of cancer incidence and mortality rates and trends. *Cancer Epidemiology, Biomarkers & Prevention*, *19*(8), 1893–1907. doi:10.1158/1055-9965.EPI-10-0437 PMID:20647400

Jia, C. (2015). Laboratory Management of the Internet based on the Technology of Internet of Things. *AASRI International Conference on Industrial Electronics and Applications*. Springer. 10.1007/978-981-16-0538-3_4

Jiang, Z., & Shen, G. (2019). Prediction of House Price Based on The Back Propagation Neural Network in The Keras Deep Learning Framework. In *2019 6th International Conference on Systems and Informatics (ICSAI)*. IEEE. 10.1109/ICSAI48974.2019.9010071

Jiang, P., & Zhao, K. (2017). Real-time biomedical signal transmission of IoT-based wearable sensor network for mobile healthcare. *IEEE Access : Practical Innovations, Open Solutions, 6*, 18236–18242.

Jiménez, W. C. (2024). El Assessing artificial intelligence and professors' calibration in English as a foreign language writing courses at a Costa Rican public university. *Actualidades Investigativas en Educación, 24*(1), 1–25. doi:10.15517/aie.v24i1.55612

Ji, Y., Yu, S., & Zhang, Y. (2011). A novel naive bayes model: Packaged hidden naive bayes. *6th IEEE Joint International Information Technology and Artificial Intelligence Conference*. IEEE. 10.1109/ITAIC.2011.6030379

Johnson, A., Pollard, T., Shen, L., Lehman, L. H., Feng, M., Ghassemi, M., Moody, B., Szolovits, P., Anthony Celi, L., & Mark, R. G. (2023). MIMIC-III, a Freely Accessible Critical Care Database. *Scientific Data, 3*(1), 160035. doi:10.1038/sdata.2016.35 PMID:27219127

Jo, T., Nho, K., & Saykin, A. J. (2019). Deep learning in Alzheimer's disease: Diagnostic classification and prognostic prediction using neuroimaging data. *Frontiers in Aging Neuroscience, 11*, 220. doi:10.3389/fnagi.2019.00220 PMID:31481890

Joyia, G. J., Liaqat, R. M., & Farooq, A. (2017). Internet of medical things (IOMT): Applications, benefits and future challenges in healthcare domain. *Journal of Communication, 12*(4), 240–247.

Judith, E., & James, M. (2001). Artificial neural networks. *Cancer, 91*(S8), 1615–1635. doi:10.1002/1097-0142(20010415)91:8+<1615::AID-CNCR1175>3.0.CO;2-L PMID:11309760

Kaddoura, S., & Al Husseiny, F. (2023). The rising trend of Metaverse in education: Challenges, opportunities, and ethical considerations. *PeerJ. Computer Science, 9*, e1252. doi:10.7717/peerj-cs.1252 PMID:37346578

Kahn, C. E. Jr, Langlotz, C. P., Channin, D. S., & Rubin, D. L. (2011, January-February). Informatics in radiology: An information model of the DICOM standard. *Radiographics, 31*(1), 295–304. doi:10.1148/rg.311105085 PMID:20980665

Kamalov, F., Pourghebleh, B., Gheisari, M., Liu, Y., & Moussa, S. (2023). Internet of Medical Things Privacy and Security: Challenges, Solutions, and Future Trends from a New Perspective. *Sustainability (Basel), 15*(4), 3317. doi:10.3390/su15043317

Kamil, N., & Kamil, S. (2015). Global cancer incidences, causes and future predictions for subcontinent region. *Systematic Reviews in Pharmacy, 6*, 13.

Kamruzzaman, J., & Begg, R. K. (2006). Support vector machines and other pattern recognition approaches to the diagnosis of cerebral palsy gait. *IEEE Transactions on Biomedical Engineering, 53*(12), 2479–2490. doi:10.1109/TBME.2006.883697 PMID:17153205

Kannan, S. (2022). An automated clinical decision support system for predicting cardiovascular disease using ensemble learning approach. *Concurrency and Computation, 34*(18), e7007. doi:10.1002/cpe.7007

Karpov, O. E., Pitsik, E. N., Kurkin, S. A., Maksimenko, V. A., Gusev, A. V., Shusharina, N. N., & Hramov, A. E. (2023). Analysis of publication activity and research trends in the field of ai medical applications: Network approach. *International Journal of Environmental Research and Public Health, 20*(7), 5335. doi:10.3390/ijerph20075335 PMID:37047950

Kartono, A., Anggraini, D., Wahyudi, S. T., Setiawan, A. A., & Irmansyah. (2021). Study of Parameters Estimation of The Three-Compartment Pharmacokinetic Model using Particle Swarm Optimization Algorithm. *Journal of Physics: Conference Series, 1805*(1), 012032. doi:10.1088/1742-6596/1805/1/012032

Kaur, H., & Kumari, V. (2018). Predictive Modelling and analytics for diabetes using a machine learning approach. *Applied Computing and Informatics*, *12*(1/2), 90–100. doi:10.1016/j.aci.2018.12.004

Kaur, J., & Bhambri, P. (2020). *Hybrid Classification Model for the Reverse Code Generation in Software Engineering. Jalandhar*. I.K. Gujral Punjab Technical University.

Kaur, S., Singla, J., Nkenyereye, L., Jha, S., Prashar, D., Joshi, G. P., El-Sappagh, S., Islam, M. S., & Islam, S. R. (2020). Medical diagnostic systems using artificial intelligence (ai) algorithms: Principles and perspectives. *IEEE Access : Practical Innovations, Open Solutions*, *8*, 228049–228069. doi:10.1109/ACCESS.2020.3042273

Kawala-Sterniuk, A., Podpora, M., Pelc, M., Blaszczyszyn, M., Gorzelanczyk, E. J., Martinek, R., & Ozana, S. (2020). Comparison of smoothing filters in analysis of EEG data for the medical diagnostics purposes. *Sensors (Basel)*, *20*(3), 807. doi:10.3390/s20030807 PMID:32024267

Keerthika, K., Kannan, M., & Khang, A. (2023). Medical Data Analytics: Roles, Challenges, and Analytical Tools. In AI and IoT-Based Technologies for Precision Medicine (1st ed.). IGI Global Press. doi:10.4018/979-8-3693-0876-9.ch001

Kelly, J. T., Campbell, K. L., Gong, E., & Schuffham, P. (2020). The Internet of Things: Impact and Implications in Healthcare Delivery. *Journal of Medical Internet Research*, *22*(11), e20135. doi:10.2196/20135 PMID:33170132

Kerkar, R. A., & Kulkarni, Y. V. (2006). Screening for cervical cancer: An overview. *Journal of Obstetrics and Gynecology of India*, *56*, 115–122.

Khang, A. (2023b). Enabling the Future of Manufacturing: Integration of Robotics and IoT to Smart Factory Infrastructure in Industry 4.0. In AI-Based Technologies and Applications in the Era of the Metaverse. (1st Ed.). IGI Global Press. doi:10.4018/978-1-6684-8851-5.ch002

Khang, A. (2024b). The Era of Digital Healthcare System and Its Impact on Human Psychology. In *AI and IoT Technology and Applications for Smart Healthcare Systems*. Taylor and Francis. doi:10.1201/9781032686745-1

Khang, A., & Hajimahmud, V. A. (2024). Cloud Platform and Data Storage Systems in Healthcare Ecosystem. Medical Robotics and AI-Assisted Diagnostics for a High-Tech Healthcare Industry (1st ed.). IGI Global Press. doi:10.4018/979-8-3693-2105-8.ch022

Khang, A., & Muthmainnah, M. (2023). AI-Aided Teaching Model for the Education 5.0 Ecosystem. AI-Based Technologies and Applications in the Era of the Metaverse. (1st Ed.) IGI Global Press. doi:10.4018/978-1-6684-8851-5.ch004

Khang, A., Hahanov, V., Abbas, G. L., & Hajimahmud, V. A. (2022). Cyber-Physical-Social System and İncident Management. AI-Centric Smart City Ecosystems: Technologies, Design and Implementation (1st Ed.). CRC Press. doi:10.1201/9781003252542-2

Khang, A., Rath, K. C., Anh, P. T. N., Rath, S. K., & Bhattacharya, S. (2024). Quantum-Based Robotics in High-Tech Healthcare Industry: Innovations and Applications. Medical Robotics and AI-Assisted Diagnostics for a High-Tech Healthcare Industry (1st ed.). IGI Global Press. doi:10.4018/979-8-3693-2105-8.ch001

Khang, A. (2023). *AI and IoT-Based Technologies for Precision Medicine* (1st ed.). IGI Global Press., doi:10.4018/979-8-3693-0876-9

Khang, A. (2024). *Medical and BioMedical Signal Processing and Prediction. Computer Vision and AI-integrated IoT Technologies in Medical Ecosystem* (1st ed.). CRC Press. doi:10.1201/9781003429609-7

Khang, A. (2024). *Medical Robotics and AI-Assisted Diagnostics for a High-Tech Healthcare Industry* (1st ed.). IGI Global Press. doi:10.4018/979-8-3693-2105-8

Khang, A. (2024). *Using Big Data to Solve Problems in the Field of Medicine. Computer Vision and AI-integrated IoT Technologies in Medical Ecosystem* (1st ed.). CRC Press. doi:10.1201/9781003429609-21

Khang, A. (Ed.). (2024a). *AI and IoT Technology and Applications for Smart Healthcare Systems* (1st ed.). Auerbach Publications. doi:10.1201/9781032686745

Khang, A., & Abdullayev, V. A. (2023). *AI-Aided Data Analytics Tools and Applications for the Healthcare Sector, "AI and IoT-Based Technologies for Precision Medicine* (1st ed.). IGI Global Press. doi:10.4018/979-8-3693-0876-9.ch018

Khang, A., Abdullayev, V., Hrybiuk, O., & Shukla, A. K. (2024). *Computer Vision and AI-Integrated IoT Technologies in the Medical Ecosystem* (1st ed.). CRC Press. doi:10.1201/9781003429609

Khang, A., Gupta, S. K., Rani, S., & Karras, D. A. (Eds.). (2023). *Smart Cities: IoT Technologies, Big Data Solutions, Cloud Platforms, and Cybersecurity Techniques.* CRC Press. doi:10.1201/9781003376064

Khang, A., & Hajimahmud, V. A. (2024). *Advanced IoT Technologies and Applications in the Industry 4.0 Digital Economy* (1st ed.). CRC Press. doi:10.1201/9781003434269

Khang, A., & Hajimahmud, V. A. (2024). *Application of Computer Vision in the Healthcare Ecosystem. Computer Vision and AI-integrated IoT Technologies in Medical Ecosystem* (1st ed.). CRC Press. doi:10.1201/9781003429609-1

Khang, A., Rana, G., Tailor, R. K., & Hajimahmud, V. A. (2023). *Data-Centric AI Solutions and Emerging Technologies in the Healthcare Ecosystem* (1st ed.). CRC Press. doi:10.1201/9781003356189

Khang, A., Shah, V., & Rani, S. (2023). *AI-Based Technologies and Applications in the Era of the Metaverse* (1st ed.). IGI Global Press. doi:10.4018/978-1-6684-8851-5

Khanna, N. N., Maindarkar, M. A., Viswanathan, V., Fernandes, J. F. E., Paul, S., Bhagawati, M., & Suri, J. S. (2022, December). Economics of artificial intelligence in healthcare: diagnosis vs. treatment. In Healthcare (Vol. 10, No. 12, p. 2493). MDPI. doi:10.3390/healthcare10122493

Kim, D. H., & MacKinnon, T. (2018, May). Artificial intelligence in fracture detection: Transfer learning from deep convolutional neural networks. *Clinical Radiology*, *73*(5), 439–445. doi:10.1016/j.crad.2017.11.015 PMID:29269036

Kim, D., Oh, G., Seo, Y., & Kim, Y. (2017). Reinforcement Learning-Based optimal flat spin recovery for unmanned aerial vehicle. *Journal of Guidance, Control, and Dynamics*, *40*(4), 1076–1084. doi:10.2514/1.G001739

Kim, S., & Kim, H. (2023). Wearable Biosensors for Healthcare Monitoring. *RSC Advances*, *8*(52), 29844–29855.

Kirkpatrick, T., Cockshott, I. D., Douglas, E. J., & Nimmo, W. S. (1988). Pharmacokinetics of propofol (Diprivan) in elderly patients. *British Journal of Anaesthesia*, *6O*, i46–i150. PMID:3257879

Kjær, A., Loft, A., Law, I., Berthelsen, A. K., Borgwardt, L., Löfgren, J., Johnbeck, C. B., Hansen, A. E., Keller, S., Holm, S., & Højgaard, L. (2013, February). PET/MRI in cancer patients: First experiences and vision from Copenhagen. *Magma (New York, N.Y.)*, *26*(1), 37–47. doi:10.1007/s10334-012-0357-0 PMID:23266511

Kjellberg, L., Hallmans, G., Åhren, A. M., Johansson, R., Bergman, F., Wadell, G., & Dillner, J. (2000). Smoking, diet, pregnancy and oral contraceptive use as risk factors for cervical intra-epithelial neoplasia in relation to human papillomavirus infection. *British Journal of Cancer*, *82*(7), 1332–1338. doi:10.1054/bjoc.1999.1100 PMID:10755410

Kohli, M., Prevedello, L. M., Filice, R. W., & Geis, J. R. (2017, April). Implementing Machine Learning in Radiology Practice and Research. *AJR. American Journal of Roentgenology*, *208*(4), 754–760. doi:10.2214/AJR.16.17224 PMID:28125274

Koraishi, O. (2023). Teaching English in the age of AI: Embracing ChatGPT to optimize EFL materials and assessment. *Language Education and Technology, 3*(1).

Kosmatos, E. A., Tselikas, N. D., & Boucouvalas, A. C. (2011). Integrating RFIDs and Smart Objects into a UnifiedIn-ternet of Things Architecture. *Adv Internet Things, 1*(1), 5–12. doi:10.4236/ait.2011.11002

Kouijzer, M. M., Kip, H., Bouman, Y. H., & Kelders, S. M. (2023). Implementation of virtual reality in healthcare: A scoping review on the implementation process of virtual reality in various healthcare settings. *Implementation Science Communications, 4*(1), 1–29. doi:10.1186/s43058-023-00442-2 PMID:37328858

Kourou, K., Exarchos, T. P., Exarchos, K. P., Karamouzis, M. V., & Fotiadis, D. I. (2021). Machine Learning Applica-tions in Cancer Prognosis and Prediction. *Computational and Structural Biotechnology Journal, 13*, 8–17. doi:10.1016/j.csbj.2014.11.005 PMID:25750696

Krallinger, M., Leitner, F., Vazquez, M., & Valencia, A. (2014). Text Mining. *Compr Biomed Phys, 6*(10, Supplement), 51–66. doi:10.1016/B978-0-444-53632-7.01107-2 PMID:15998455

Kufrin, R. (1997). Decision trees on parallel processors. *Machine Intelligence Pattern Recognition, 20*, 279–306.

Kulkarni, M., & Kalaskar, A. (2021). The Internet of Things in Healthcare: An Overview." *Advances in Human Factors and Ergonomics*, 484-495.

Kuzhaloli, S., Devaneyan, P., Sitaraman, N., Periyathanbi, P., Gurusamy, M., & Bhambri, P. (2020). *IoT based Smart Kitchen Application for Gas Leakage Monitoring* [Patent application number 202041049866A].

Lai, H., Huang, H., Keshavjee, K., Guergachi, A., & Gao, X. (2019). Predictive models for diabetes mellitus using machine learning techniques. *BMC Endocrine Disorders, 19*(1), 1–9. doi:10.1186/s12902-019-0436-6 PMID:31615566

Laine, T. H., & Lee, W. (2023). Collaborative Virtual Reality in Higher Education: Students' Perceptions on Presence, Challenges, Affordances, and Potential. *IEEE Transactions on Learning Technologies*.

LeCun, Y., Bengio, Y., & Hinton, G. (2015, May 28). Deep learning. *Nature, 521*(7553), 436–444. doi:10.1038/nature14539 PMID:26017442

Lee, J. M., Hwang, Y., & Kang, Y. (2023). A Survey of Healthcare Applications and the Supporting Platforms in the Internet of Things. *Journal of Medical Systems, 40*(12), 286.

Le, H.-N., & Boyd, R. C. (2022). Prevention of Major Depression. *Early Detection and Early Intervention in the General Population, 2006*, 23.

Leung, K. Y. (2021, July 6). Applications of Advanced Ultrasound Technology in Obstetrics. *Diagnostics (Basel), 11*(7), 1217. doi:10.3390/diagnostics11071217 PMID:34359300

Liaw, A., & Wiener, M. (2002). Classification and regression by randomForest. *R News, 2*, 18–22.

Lin, L., Chen, X., Shen, Y. L., & Zhang, L. (2020). Zhang, towards automatic depression detection: A bilstm/1d cnn-based model. *Applied Sciences (Basel, Switzerland), 10*(23), 1–20. doi:10.3390/app10238701

Litjens, G., Kooi, T., Bejnordi, B. E., Setio, A. A. A., Ciompi, F., Ghafoorian, M., van der Laak, J. A. W. M., van Gin-neken, B., & Sánchez, C. I. (2017, December). A survey on deep learning in medical image analysis. *Medical Image Analysis, 42*, 60–88. doi:10.1016/j.media.2017.07.005 PMID:28778026

Liu, F., Xu, F., & Yang, S. (2017). A Flood Forecasting Model Based on Deep Learning Algorithm via Integrating Stacked Autoencoders with BP Neural Network. In *2017 IEEE Third International Conference on Multimedia Big Data (BigMM)* (pp. 58-61). IEEE. 10.1109/BigMM.2017.29

Liu, X., Faes, L., Kale, A. U., Wagner, S. K., Fu, D. J., Bruynseels, A., Mahendiran, T., Moraes, G., Shamdas, M., Kern, C., Ledsam, J. R., Schmid, M. K., Balaskas, K., Topol, E. J., Bachmann, L. M., Keane, P. A., & Denniston, A. K. (2019, October). A comparison of deep learning performance against health-care professionals in detecting diseases from medical imaging: A systematic review and meta-analysis. *The Lancet. Digital Health*, *1*(6), e271–e297. doi:10.1016/S2589-7500(19)30123-2 PMID:33323251

Liu, X., & Yang, X. D. (2018). *Multi-stream with deep convolutional neural networks for human action recognition in videos.Neural Information Processing*. Springer International Publishing.

Li, X., Chen, Q., Hao, J.-H., Chen, X., & He, K.-L. (2019). Heat current method for analysis and optimization of a refrigeration system for aircraft environmental control system. *International Journal of Refrigeration*, *106*, 163–180. doi:10.1016/j.ijrefrig.2019.06.004

Logswari, T., & Karnan, M. (2010). An improved implementation of brain tumor detection using segmentation based on soft computing. *Journal of Cancer Research and Experimental Oncology, 2*(1), 6-14.

Loh, W. Y. (2011). Classification and regression trees. *Wiley Interdisciplinary Reviews. Data Mining and Knowledge Discovery*, *1*(1), 14–23. doi:10.1002/widm.8

Luhn, P., Walker, J., Schiffman, M., Zuna, R. E., Dunn, S. T., Gold, M. A., & Wentzensen, N. (2013). The role of co-factors in the progression from human papillomavirus infection to cervical cancer. *Gynecologic Oncology*, *128*(2), 265–270. doi:10.1016/j.ygyno.2012.11.003 PMID:23146688

Lu, J., Song, E., Ghoneim, A., & Alrashoud, M. (2020). Machine learning for assisting cervical cancer diagnosis: An ensemble approach. *Future Generation Computer Systems*, *106*, 199–205. doi:10.1016/j.future.2019.12.033

Lundervold, A. S., & Lundervold, A. (2019, May). An overview of deep learning in medical imaging focusing on MRI. *Zeitschrift für Medizinische Physik*, *29*(2), 102–127. doi:10.1016/j.zemedi.2018.11.002 PMID:30553609

Luo, W., Yang, W., & Berson, I. R. (2024). Digital Transformations in Early Learning: From Touch Interactions to AI Conversations. *Early Education and Development*, *35*(1), 3–9. doi:10.1080/10409289.2023.2280819

Lydia, A., & Francis, F. S. (2019). Convolutional Neural Network with an Optimized Backpropagation Technique. In *2019 IEEE International Conference on System, Computation, Automation and Networking (ICSCAN)* (pp. 1-5). IEEE. 10.1109/ICSCAN.2019.8878719

Ma, X., Yang, H., Chen, Q., Huang, D., & Wang, Y. (2016). DepAudioNet: an efficient deep model for audio based depression classification. AVEC 2016 - Proc. 6th Int. Work. Audio/Visual Emot. Challenge, Co-located with ACM Multimed. ACM. doi:10.1145/2988257.2988267

Ma, X., Yang, H., Chen, Q., Huang, D., & Wang, Y. (2016). Depaudionet:An efficient deep model for audio based depression classifica-tion, *Proceedings of the 6th International Workshop on Au-dio/Visual Emotion Challenge*. ACM.

Madakam, S., Ramaswamy, R., & Tripathi, S. (2015). Internet of Things (IoT): A Literature Review. *J Comp Commun*, *3*(3), 164–173. doi:10.4236/jcc.2015.35021

Mahabub, A. (2019). A robust voting approach for diabetes prediction using traditional machine learning techniques. *SN Applied Sciences*, *1*(12), 1667. doi:10.1007/s42452-019-1759-7

Maheshwari, P., Kamble, S., Amine, A. P., Belhadi, A., Ndubisi, N. O., & Tiwari, S. (2021). Internet of things for perishable inventory management systems: An application and managerial insights for micro, small and medium enterprises. *Annals of Operations Research*. doi:10.1007/s10479-021-04277-9 PMID:34642526

Maier, O., Wilms, M., von der Gablentz, J., Krämer, U. M., Münte, T. F., & Handels, H. (2015). Extra tree forests for sub-acute ischemic stroke lesion segmentation in MR sequences. *Journal of Neuroscience Methods*, *240*, 89–100. doi:10.1016/j.jneumeth.2014.11.011 PMID:25448384

Majumder, S., Mondal, T., & Deen, M. J. (2017). Wearable sensors for remote health monitoring. *Sensors (Basel)*, *17*(1), 130. doi:10.3390/s17010130 PMID:28085085

Maldonado, S., López, J., Jimenez-Molina, A., & Lira, H. (2020). *Simultaneous feature selection and heterogeneity control for SVM classification: An application to mental workload assessment* (Vol. 143). Expert Syst. Appl.

Manickam, P., Mariappan, S. A., Murugesan, S. M., Hansda, S., Kaushik, A., Shinde, R., & Thipperudraswamy, S. P. (2022). Artificial intelligence (AI) and internet of medical things (IoMT) assisted biomedical systems for intelligent healthcare. *Biosensors (Basel)*, *12*(8), 562. doi:10.3390/bios12080562 PMID:35892459

Marjani, M., Nasaruddin, F., & Gani, A. (2017). Big IoT Data Analytics: Architecture, Opportunities, and Open Research Challenges. *IEEE Access : Practical Innovations, Open Solutions*, *5*(99), 5247–5261.

Martinez-Millana, A., Fernandez-Llatas, C., & Traver, V. (2023). Internet of Things for Adaptive and Personalized Health Monitoring. *Studies in Health Technology and Informatics*, *236*, 123–135.

Martin, R., Rose, D., Yu, K., & Barros, S. (2006). Toxicogenomics Strategies for Predicting Drug Toxicity. *Pharmacogenomics*, *7*(7), 1003–1016. doi:10.2217/14622416.7.7.1003 PMID:17054411

Masood, A. (2013). Fuzzy C Mean Thresholding based Level Set for Automated Segmentation of Skin Lesions. *Journal of Signal and Information Processing*, *4*, 66-71. https://www.scirp.org/journal/jsip doi:10.4236/jsip.2013.43B012

McCrackin, L. (2018). Early Detection of Alzheimer's Disease Using Deep Learning. In E. Bagheri & J. C. K. Cheung (Eds.), *Lecture Notes in Computer Science* (Vol. 10832, pp. 355–359). Springer International Publishing. doi:10.1007/978-3-319-89656-4_40

McKinney, S. M., Sieniek, M., Godbole, V., Godwin, J., Antropova, N., Ashrafian, H., Back, T., Chesus, M., Corrado, G. S., Darzi, A., Etemadi, M., Garcia-Vicente, F., Gilbert, F. J., Halling-Brown, M., Hassabis, D., Jansen, S., Karthikesalingam, A., Kelly, C. J., King, D., & Shetty, S. (2020, January). International evaluation of an AI system for breast cancer screening. *Nature*, *577*(7788), 89–94. doi:10.1038/s41586-019-1799-6 PMID:31894144

Mei, X., Lee, H. C., Diao, K. Y., Huang, M., Lin, B., Liu, C., Xie, Z., Ma, Y., Robson, P. M., Chung, M., Bernheim, A., Mani, V., Calcagno, C., Li, K., Li, S., Shan, H., Lv, J., Zhao, T., Xia, J., & Yang, Y. (2020). Artificial intelligence-enabled rapid diagnosis of patients with COVID-19. *Nature Medicine*, *26*(8), 1224–1228. doi:10.1038/s41591-020-0931-3 PMID:32427924

Menegotto, A. B., Becker, C. D. L., & Cazella, S. C. (2021). Computer-aided diagnosis of hepatocellular carcinoma fusing imaging and structured health data. *Health Information Science and Systems*, *9*(1), 20. doi:10.1007/s13755-021-00151-x PMID:33968399

Meng, H., Huang, D., Wang, H., Yang, H., Ai Shuraifi, M., & Wang, Y. (2013). Depression recognition based on dynamic facial and vocal expression features using partial least square regression. *Proceedings of the 3rd ACM international workshop on Audio/visual emotion challenge*. ACM. 10.1145/2512530.2512532

Mesmar, J., & Badran, A. (2022). The post-COVID classroom: Lessons from a pandemic. In *Higher Education in the Arab World: New Priorities in the Post COVID-19 Era* (pp. 11–41). Springer International Publishing. doi:10.1007/978-3-031-07539-1_2

Mhlanga, D. (2022). The role of artificial intelligence and machine learning amid the COVID-19 pandemic: What lessons are we learning on 4IR and the sustainable development goals. *International Journal of Environmental Research and Public Health, 19*(3), 1879. doi:10.3390/ijerph19031879 PMID:35162901

Miotto, R., Wang, F., Wang, S., Jiang, X., & Dudley, J. T. (2023). Deep Learning for Healthcare: Review, Opportunities, and Challenges. *Briefings in Bioinformatics, 19*(6), 1236–1246. doi:10.1093/bib/bbx044 PMID:28481991

Mirbabaie, M., Stieglitz, S., & Frick, N. R. (2021). Artificial intelligence in disease diagnostics: A critical review and classification on the current state of research guiding future direction. *Health and Technology, 11*(4), 693–731. doi:10.1007/s12553-021-00555-5

Mishra, G. A., Pimple, S. A., & Shastri, S. S. (2011). An overview of prevention and early detection of cervical cancers. *Indian Journal of Medical and Paediatric Oncology : Official Journal of Indian Society of Medical & Paediatric Oncology, 32*(3), 125–132. doi:10.4103/0971-5851.92808 PMID:22557777

Mitra, A., Biswas, A., Chakraborty, K., Ghosh, A., Das, N., Ghosh, N., & Ghosh, A. (2022). A Machine Learning Approach to Identify Personality Traits from Social Media. In *Machine Learning and Deep Learning in Efficacy Improvement of Healthcare Systems* (pp. 31–60). CRC Press. doi:10.1201/9781003189053-2

Moloney, M. E., Dunfee, M., Rutledge, M., & Schoenberg, N. (2020). Evaluating the Feasibility and Acceptability of Internet-Based Cognitive Behavioral Therapy for Insomnia in Rural Women. *Women's Health Reports (New Rochelle, N.Y.), 1*(1), 114–122. doi:10.1089/whr.2020.0053 PMID:32617531

Montenegro-Rueda, M., Fernández-Cerero, J., Fernández-Batanero, J. M., & López-Meneses, E. (2023). Impact of the implementation of ChatGPT in education: A systematic review. *Computers, 12*(8), 153. doi:10.3390/computers12080153

Monterubbianesi, R., Tosco, V., Vitiello, F., Orilisi, G., Fraccastoro, F., Putignano, A., & Orsini, G. (2022). Augmented, virtual and mixed reality in dentistry: A narrative review on the existing platforms and future challenges. *Applied Sciences (Basel, Switzerland), 12*(2), 877. doi:10.3390/app12020877

Moreno, V., Bosch, F. X., Muñoz, N., Meijer, C. J., Shah, K. V., Walboomers, J. M., Herrero, R., & Franceschi, S.International Agency for Research on Cancer (IARC) Multicentric Cervical Cancer Study Group. (2002). Effect of oral contraceptives on risk of cervical cancer in women with human papillomavirus infection: The IARC multicentric case-control study. *Lancet, 359*(9312), 1085–1092. doi:10.1016/S0140-6736(02)08150-3 PMID:11943255

Muhammad, G., Alshehri, F., Karray, F., El Saddik, A., Alsulaiman, M., & Falk, T. H. (2021). A comprehensive survey on multimodal medical signals fusion for smart healthcare systems. *Information Fusion, 76*, 355–375. doi:10.1016/j.inffus.2021.06.007

Munir, T., Akbar, M. S., Ahmed, S., Sarfraz, A., Sarfraz, Z., Sarfraz, M., Felix, M., & Cherrez-Ojeda, I. (2022). A Systematic Review of Internet of Things in Clinical Laboratories: Opportunities, Advantages, and Challenges. *Sensors (Basel), 22*(20), 8051. doi:10.3390/s22208051 PMID:36298402

Musen, M. A., Middleton, B., & Greenes, R. A. (2021). Clinical decision-support systems. In *Biomedical informatics: computer applications in health care and biomedicine* (pp. 795–840). Springer International Publishing. doi:10.1007/978-3-030-58721-5_24

Muthmainnah, O., A. J., Al Yakin, A., & Brayyich, M. (2023, June). Enhancing Computational Thinking Based on Virtual Robot of Artificial Intelligence Modeling in the English Language Classroom. In *International Conference on Data Analytics & Management* (pp. 1-11). Singapore: Springer Nature Singapore. 10.1007/978-981-99-6550-2_1

Nagalkar, V.J. & Asole, S.S. (2012). Brain tumor detection using digital image processing based on soft computing. *Journal of Signal and Image Processing, 3*(3).

Nahmias, D. O., Civillico, E. F., & Kontson, K. L. (2020). Deep learning and feature based medication classifications from EEG in a large clinical data set. *Scientific Reports*, *10*(1), 14206. doi:10.1038/s41598-020-70569-y PMID:32848165

Najdi, S., Gharbali, A. A., & Fonseca, J. M. (2017). Feature transformation based on stacked sparse autoencoders for sleep stage classification. In *Doctoral Conference on Computing, Electrical and Industrial Systems* (pp. 191-200). Springer. 10.1007/978-3-319-56077-9_18

Namita, P. (2023). Application of Machine Learning for Image Processing in the Healthcare Sector. AI and IoT-Based Technologies for Precision Medicine (1st ed.). IGI Global Press. doi:10.4018/979-8-3693-0876-9.ch004

Narendra Kumar Rao, B., Ranjana, R., Panini Challa, N., & Sreenivasa Chakravarthi, S. (2023). *Convolutional Neural Network Model for Traffic Sign Recognition*. 2023 3rd International Conference on Advance Computing and Innovative Technologies in Engineering (ICACITE), Greater Noida, India. 10.1109/ICACITE57410.2023.10182966

Narendra Kumar Rao, B. (2023). Factors influencing Mental Health due to Climate Change & Role of Artificial Intelligence. *Factors influencing Mental Health due to Climate Change & Role of Artificial Intelligence, CRC Press Taylor & Francis (T&F)*. doi:10.4018/978-1-0034-2960-9

Narendra Kumar Rao, B., Partheeban, P., Naseeba, B., & Raju, H. P. (2022). ML Approaches to Detect Email Spam Anamoly. *2022 International Conference on Data Science, Agents & Artificial Intelligenc (ICDSAAI)*, Chennai, India. 10.1109/ICDSAAI55433.2022.10028911

Nasution, M. Z. F., Sitompul, O. S., & Ramli, M. (2018). PCA based feature reduction to improve the accuracy of decision tree c4.5 classification. *Journal of Physics: Conference Series*, *978*, 012058. doi:10.1088/1742-6596/978/1/012058

Natarajan, P., Krishnan, N., Kenkre, N. S., Nancy, S., & Singh, B. P. (2012). Tumor detection using threshold operation in MRI brain images. *Computational Intelligence & Computing Research (ICCIC)*. IEEE. 10.1109/ICCIC.2012.6510299

Neethirajan, S. (2023). Artificial Intelligence and Sensor Innovations: Enhancing Livestock Welfare with a Human-Centric Approach. *Human-Centric Intelligent Systems*, 1-16. Springer. doi:10.1007/s44230-023-00050-2

Nemorin, S., Vlachidis, A., Ayerakwa, H. M., & Andriotis, P. (2023). AI hyped? A horizon scan of discourse on artificial intelligence in education (AIED) and development. *Learning, Media and Technology*, *48*(1), 38–51. doi:10.1080/17439884.2022.2095568

Newell, M. E., Adhikari, S., & Halden, R. U. (2022). Systematic and state-of the science review of the role of environmental factors in Amyotrophic Lateral Sclerosis (ALS) or Lou Gehrig's Disease. *The Science of the Total Environment*, *817*, 152504. doi:10.1016/j.scitotenv.2021.152504 PMID:34971691

Newson, J. J., & Thiagarajan, T. C. (2019). EEG frequency bands in psychiatric disorders: A review of resting state studies. *Frontiers in Human Neuroscience*, *12*, 521. doi:10.3389/fnhum.2018.00521 PMID:30687041

Nguyen, K., Fookes, C., & Sridharan, S. (2015). Improving deep convolutional neural networks with unsupervised feature learning. *2015 IEEE International Conference on Image Processing (ICIP)*, (pp. 2270-2274). IEEE. 10.1109/ICIP.2015.7351206

Nguyen, M., Sun, N., Alexander, D. C., Feng, J., & Yeo, B. T. (2018). Modeling Alzheimer's disease progression using deep recurrent neural networks. In *2018 International Workshop on Pattern Recognition in Neuroimaging (PRNI)* (pp. 1-4). IEEE. 10.1109/PRNI.2018.8423955

Ng, Y. H., Hausknecht, M., & Vijayanarasimhan, S. (2015). Beyond short snippets: Deep networks for video classification. *2015 IEEE Conference on Computer Vision and Pattern Recognition (CVPR)*. IEEE.

Niewiadomski, R., & Anderson, D. (2017). The rise of artificial intelligence. In Advances in computational intelligence and robotics book series (pp. 29–49). IGI Global. doi:10.4018/978-1-5225-1656-9.ch003

Obermeyer, Z., & Emanuel, E. J. (2016, September 29). Predicting the Future - Big Data, Machine Learning, and Clinical Medicine. *The New England Journal of Medicine*, *375*(13), 1216–1219. doi:10.1056/NEJMp1606181 PMID:27682033

Obermeyer, Z., Powers, B., Vogeli, C., & Mullainathan, S. (2019, October 25). Dissecting racial bias in an algorithm used to manage the health of populations. *Science*, *366*(6464), 447–453. doi:10.1126/science.aax2342 PMID:31649194

Obeta, M. U., Nkereuwem, S. E., & Okoli, C. C. (2021). Nigerian Medical Laboratory Diagnosis of COVID-19; from Grass to Grace. Intelligent Computing Applications for COVID-19: Predictions, Diagnosis, and Prevention. CRC Press Tailor and Francis Group. doi:10.1201/9781003141105-5

Obeta, U. M., Ejinaka, O. R., & Etukudoh, N. S. (2022). Data Mining in Medical Laboratory Service Improves Disease Surveillance and Quality Healthcare. In T. Saba, (Eds.), Prognostic Models in Healthcare: AI and Statistical Approaches, Studies in Big Data 109. Springer. doi:10.1007/978-981-19-2057-8_17

Obeta, U. M., Njar, V. E., Etukudoh, N. S., & Obiora, O. R. (2023). Applications of Information Management Systems (IMSML) in Medical Laboratories. A. Khang (ed.) AI and IoT-Based Technologies for Precision Medicine. IGI Global. doi:10.4018/979-8-3693-0876-9.ch026

Obeta, M. U., Eze, E. M., Ofojekwu, M. N., Jwanse, R. I., & Maduka, M. K. (2019). Organogram for Medical Laboratory Services in Nigerian Public Health Institutions. *North American Academic Research*, *2*(6), 69–75. doi:10.5281/zenodo.3246909

Obeta, M. U., Maduka, K. M., Ofor, I. B., & Ofojekwu, N. M. (2019). Improving Quality and Cost Diminution in Modern Healthcare Delivery: The Role of the Medical Laboratory Scientists in Nigeria. [IJBMI]. *International Journal of Business and Management Invention*, *08*(03), 8–19.

Obeta, M. U., Umar, I. A., Ibanga, I. E., Okey-Orji, V. N., Ezeama, C. J., & Ejinaka, O. R. (2022). Acceptability of Internet of Medical Laboratory Things among Female Medical Laboratory Professionals in Jos-Nigeria. *Fifth International Conference for Women in Data Science (WiDS)*. Prince Sultan University. 10.1109/WiDS-PSU54548.2022.00026

OECD Bridging the Digital Gender Divide Include. (2018). Upskill. *Innovate (North Miami Beach, Fla.)*.

Olichney, J., Xia, J., Church, K. J., & Moebius, H. J. (2022). Predictive power of cognitive biomarkers in neurodegenerative disease drug development: Utility of the P300 event-related potential. *Neural Plasticity*, *2022*, 2022. doi:10.1155/2022/2104880 PMID:36398135

Onu, P., Pradhan, A., & Mbohwa, C. (2023). Potential to use metaverse for future teaching and learning. *Education and Information Technologies*, 1–32. doi:10.1007/s10639-023-12167-9

Ozuruoke D.F.N. (2022). *History of Medical Laboratory Science: Nigerian Perspective*. Pundit Publishers Abuja.

Panchbhai, A. S. (2015). Wilhelm Conrad Röntgen and the discovery of X-rays: Revisited after centennial. *Journal of Indian Academy of Oral Medicine and Radiology, 27*(1), 90-95. doi:10.4103/0972-1363.167119

Park, S. U., Park, J. H., Al-Masni, M. A., Al-Antari, M. A., Uddin, M. Z., & Kim, T. S. (2016). A depth camera-based human activity recognition via deep learning recurrent neural network for health and social care services. *Procedia Computer Science*, *100*, 78–84. doi:10.1016/j.procs.2016.09.126

Parteek. (2019). A Review Paper on IOT Advantages and Disadvantages. *International Journal of Research and Analytical Reviews, 6*(1)

Patil, P., & Shah, L. (2019). Assessment of risk of type 2 diabetes mellitus with stress as a risk factor using classification algorithms. *International Journal of Recent Technology and Engineering, 8*(4), 11273–11277. doi:10.35940/ijrte.D9509.118419

Pedro, A. R., Dias, M. B., Laranjo, L., Cunha, A. S., & Cordeiro, J. V. (2023). Artificial intelligence in medicine: A comprehensive survey of medical doctor's perspectives in Portugal. *PLoS One, 18*(9), e0290613. doi:10.1371/journal.pone.0290613 PMID:37676884

Pesapane, F., Volonté, C., Codari, M., & Sardanelli, F. (2018, October). Artificial intelligence as a medical device in radiology: Ethical and regulatory issues in Europe and the United States. *Insights Into Imaging, 9*(5), 745–753. doi:10.1007/s13244-018-0645-y PMID:30112675

Petersen, R. C., Aisen, P. S., Beckett, L. A., Donohue, M. C., Gamst, A. C., Harvey, D. J., Jack, C. R. Jr, Jagust, W. J., Shaw, L. M., Toga, A. W., Trojanowski, J. Q., & Weiner, M. W. (2010, January). Alzheimer's Disease Neuroimaging Initiative (ADNI): Clinical characterization. *Neurology, 74*(3), 201–209. doi:10.1212/WNL.0b013e3181cb3e25 PMID:20042704

Petry, K. U. (2014). HPV and cervical cancer. *Scandinavian Journal of Clinical and Laboratory Investigation, 74*(sup244), 59–62. doi:10.3109/00365513.2014.936683 PMID:25083895

Pima Indians Diabetes dataset. (n.d.). UC Irving. http://archive.ics.uci.edu/ml/machine learning-databases/pima-indiansdiabetes/pima-indians-diabetes

Plissiti, M. E., & Nikou, C. (2013). A review of automated techniques for cervical cell image analysis and classification. In U. Andreaus & D. Iacoviello (Eds.), *Biomedical Imaging and Computational Modeling in Biomechanics* (pp. 1–18). Springer. doi:10.1007/978-94-007-4270-3_1

Plummer, M., Herrero, R., Franceschi, S., Meijer, C. J., Snijders, P., Bosch, F. X., & Muñoz, N. (2003). Smoking and cervical cancer: Pooled analysis of the IARC multi-centric case–control study. *Cancer Causes & Control, 14*(9), 805–814. doi:10.1023/B:CACO.0000003811.98261.3e PMID:14682438

Pradhan, B., Bharti, D., Chakravarty, S., Ray, S. S., Voinova, V. V., Bonartsev, A. P., & Kunal Pal, K. (2021). Internet of Things and Robotics in Transforming Current-Day Healthcare Services. *Journal of Healthcare Engineering, 2021*, 1–15. doi:10.1155/2021/9999504 PMID:34104368

Pradhan, B., Bhattacharyya, S., & Pal, K. (2021). IoT-Based Applications in Healthcare Devices. *Journal of Healthcare Engineering, 2021*, 1–18. doi:10.1155/2021/6632599 PMID:33791084

Pradhan, S. R., Mahata, S., Ghosh, D., Sahoo, P. K., Sarkar, S., Pal, R., & Nasare, V. D. (2020). Human Papillomavirus Infections in Pregnant Women and Its Impact on Pregnancy Outcomes: Possible Mechanism of Self-Clearance. In R. Rajkumar (Ed.), *Human Papillomavirus* (pp. 1–27). IntechOpen. doi:10.5772/intechopen.90197

Preskill, J. (2018, August 6). Quantum Computing in the NISQ era and beyond. *Quantum : the Open Journal for Quantum Science, 2*, 79. doi:10.22331/q-2018-08-06-79

Priyanka, B. (2013). A Review on Brain Tumor Detection using segmentation. *International Journal of Computer Science and Mobile Computing, 2*(7).

Priya, S., & Karthikeyan, N. K. (2020). A Heuristic and ANN based Classification Model for Early Screening of Cervical Cancer. *Int. J. Comput. Intell. Syst., 13*(1), 1092–1100. doi:10.2991/ijcis.d.200730.003

Puente-Castro, A., Fernandez-Blanco, E., Pazos, A., & Munteanu, C. R. (2020). Automatic assessment of Alzheimer's disease diagnosis based on deep learning techniques. *Computers in Biology and Medicine, 120*, 103764. doi:10.1016/j.compbiomed.2020.103764 PMID:32421658

Qiu, T., Yang, Y., Qiu, J., Huang, Y., Xu, T., Xiao, H., Wu, D., Zhang, Q., Zhou, C., Zhang, X., Tang, K., Xu, J., & Cao, Z. (2018). CE-BLAST makes it possible to compute antigenic similarity for newly emerging pathogens. *Nature Communications*, *9*(1), 1772. doi:10.1038/s41467-018-04171-2 PMID:29720583

Qi, Y., Zhao, J., Shi, Y., Zuo, G., Zhang, H., Long, Y., Wang, F., & Wang, W. (2020). Ground Truth Annotated Femoral X-Ray Image Dataset and Object Detection Based Method for Fracture Types Classification. *IEEE Access : Practical Innovations, Open Solutions*, *8*, 189436–189444. doi:10.1109/ACCESS.2020.3029039

Quan, X.X., Yang, J. F., & Luo, Z. (2021). Models in digital business and economic forecasting based on big data IoT data visualization technology. *PersUbiquitComput, Current Medical Science, 41*(6), 1149 2021. doi:10.1007/s00779-021-01603-7

Rachna, B. P., & Chhabra, Y. (2022). Deployment of Distributed Clustering Approach in WSNs and IoTs. In Cloud and Fog Computing Platforms for Internet of Things (pp. 85-98). Chapman and Hall/CRC.

Rachna, C. Y., & Bhambri, P. (2021). Various Approaches and Algorithms for Monitoring Energy Efficiency of Wireless Sensor Networks. In Lecture Notes in Civil Engineering (Vol. 113, pp. 761-770). Springer, Singapore.

Račić, L., & Popović, T. S. (2021). Pneumonia Detection Using Deep Learning Based on Convolutional Neural Network. *2021 25th International Conference on Information Technology (IT)*, (pp. 1-4). IEEE. 10.1109/IT51528.2021.9390137

Raees, P. M., & Thomas, V. (2021). Automated detection of Alzheimer's Disease using Deep Learning in MRI. Journal of Physics: Conference Series. https://iopscience.iop.org/article/10.1088/1742-6596/1921/1/012024/meta

Rajest, S. S., Singh, B., Obaid, A. J., Regin, R., & Chinnusamy, K. (Eds.). (2023). *Advances in Artificial and Human Intelligence in the Modern Era*. IGI Global. doi:10.4018/979-8-3693-1301-5

Rajkomar, A., Dean, J., & Kohane, I. (2020). Machine Learning in Medicine. *The New England Journal of Medicine*, *380*(14), 1347–1358. doi:10.1056/NEJMra1814259 PMID:30943338

Ramaraju, H., Nagaveni, Y., & Khazi, A. (2017). Use of Schiller's test versus Pap smear to increase the detection rate of cervical dysplasias. *International Journal of Reproduction, Contraception, Obstetrics and Gynecology*, *5*, 1446–1450.

Rana, R., Chabbra, Y., & Bhambri, P. (2020). Comparison of Clustering Approaches for Enhancing Sustainability Performance in WSNs: A Study. In *Proceedings of the International Congress on Sustainable Development through Engineering Innovations* (pp. 62-71). Springer.

Rasamoelina, A. D., Adjailia, F., & Sinčák, P. (2020). A review of activation function for artificial neural network. In *2020 IEEE 18th World Symposium on Applied Machine Intelligence and Informatics (SAMI)* (pp. 281-286). IEEE. 10.1109/SAMI48414.2020.9108717

Rash, B. (2010). The Brain MR Image Segmentation Techniques And Use Of Diagnostic Packages. *Proceedings Of The Academic Radiology*, *17*(May).

Ray, A., & Chaudhuri, A. K. (2021). *Smart healthcare disease diagnosis and patient management: Innovation, improvement and skill development* (Vol. 3). Machine Learning with Applications.

Rayan, R. A., Tsagkaris, C., & Iryna, R. B. (2021). The Internet of Things for Healthcare: Applications, Selected Cases and Challenges. G. Marques et al. (eds.), IoT in Healthcare and Ambient Assisted Living, Studies in Computational Intelligence. Springer. doi:10.1007/978-981-15-9897-5_1

Razali, N., Mostafa, S. A., Mustapha, A., Abd Wahab, M. H., & Ibrahim, N. A. (2020, April). Risk Factors of Cervical Cancer using Classification in Data Mining. *Journal of Physics: Conference Series*, *1529*(2), 022102. doi:10.1088/1742-6596/1529/2/022102

Rehman, A., Haseeb, K., Saba, T., Lloret, J., & Tariq, U. (2021). Secured Big Data Analytics for Decision-Oriented Medical System Using Internet of Things. *Electronics (Basel)*, *10*(11), 1273. doi:10.3390/electronics10111273

Rehman, A., Saba, T., Haseeb, K., Marie-Sainte, S. L., & Lloret, J. (2021). Energy-Efficient IoT e-Health Using Artificial Intelligence Model with Homomorphic Secret Sharing. *Energies*, *14*(19), 6414. doi:10.3390/en14196414

Ren, F., & Bao, Y. (2020). A review on human-computer interaction and intelligent robots. *International Journal of Information Technology & Decision Making*, *19*(01), 5–47. doi:10.1142/S0219622019300052

Ren, Z. H., Xu, H. Y., & Feng, S. L. (2017). Sequence labeling Chinese word segmentation method based on LSTM networks. *ComputAppl Res*, *34*(5), 1321–1324.

Riccio, A., Simione, L., Schettini, F., Pizzimenti, A., Inghilleri, M., Belardinelli, M. O., Mattia, D., & Cincotti, F. (2013). Attention and P300-based BCI performance in people with amyotrophic lateral sclerosis. *Frontiers in Human Neuroscience*, *7*, 732. doi:10.3389/fnhum.2013.00732 PMID:24282396

Ritu, & Bhambri, P. (2022). *A CAD System for Software Effort Estimation. Paper presented at the International Conference on Technological Advancements in Computational Sciences*, 140-146. IEEE.. doi:10.1109/ICTACS56270.2022.9988123

Rodríguez, A. C., Schiffman, M., Herrero, R., Hildesheim, A., Bratti, C., Sherman, M. E., & Burk, R. D. (2010). Longitudinal study of human papillomavirus persistence and cervical intraepithelial neoplasia grade 2/3: Critical role of duration of infection. *Journal of the National Cancer Institute*, *102*(5), 315–324. doi:10.1093/jnci/djq001 PMID:20157096

Rodríguez-Ruiz, A., Krupinski, E., Mordang, J. J., Schilling, K., Heywang-Köbrunner, S. H., Sechopoulos, I., & Mann, R. M. (2019, February). Detection of Breast Cancer with Mammography: Effect of an Artificial Intelligence Support System. *Radiology*, *290*(2), 305–314. doi:10.1148/radiol.2018181371 PMID:30457482

Rohit, S. (2013). Segmentation of Brain Tumor and Its Area Calculation in Brain MR Images using K – Mean Clustering and Fuzzy C – Mean Algorithm. *International Journal of Computer Science & Engineering Technology, 4*(5).

Rojas, E., Hülsmann, X., Estriegana, R., Rückert, F., & Garcia-Esteban, S. (2023). Students' Perception of Metaverses for Online Learning in Higher Education: Hype or Hope? *Electronics (Basel)*, *12*(8), 1867. doi:10.3390/electronics12081867

Ronco, G., Dillner, J., Elfström, K. M., Tunesi, S., Snijders, P. J., Arbyn, M., Kitchener, H., Segnan, N., Gilham, C., Giorgi-Rossi, P., Berkhof, J., Peto, J., & Meijer, C. J. L. M.International HPV Screening Working Group. (2014). Efficacy of HPV-based screening for prevention of invasive cervical cancer: Follow-up of four European randomised controlled trials. *Lancet*, *383*(9916), 524–532. doi:10.1016/S0140-6736(13)62218-7 PMID:24192252

Rowe, S. P., & Pomper, M. G. (2022, July). Molecular imaging in oncology: Current impact and future directions. *CA: a Cancer Journal for Clinicians*, *72*(4), 333–352. doi:10.3322/caac.21713 PMID:34902160

Rudin, C. (2019). Stop explaining black box machine learning models for high stakes decisions and use interpretable models instead. *Nature Machine Intelligence*, *1*(5), 206–215. doi:10.1038/s42256-019-0048-x PMID:35603010

Ryeu, J. K., Tak, H. Y., Heo, N. W., & Chung, H. S. (1993). Recognition of Korean spoken digit using single layer recurrent neural networks. *Proceedings of 1993 International Conference on Neural Networks (IJCNN-93-Nagoya, Japan)*. IEEE. 10.1109/IJCNN.1993.713908

Said, G. R. E. (2023). Metaverse-Based Learning Opportunities and Challenges: A Phenomenological Metaverse Human–Computer Interaction Study. *Electronics (Basel)*, *12*(6), 1379. doi:10.3390/electronics12061379

Salani, M., Roy, S., & Fissell, W. H. IV. (2018, November). Innovations in Wearable and Implantable Artificial Kidneys. *American Journal of Kidney Diseases*, *72*(5), 745–751. doi:10.1053/j.ajkd.2018.06.005 PMID:30146422

Sampath, B. (2023). AI-Integrated Technology for a Secure and Ethical Healthcare Ecosystem. AI and IoT-Based Technologies for Precision Medicine (1st ed.). IGI Global Press. doi:10.4018/979-8-3693-0876-9.ch003

Santos, K. C., Fernandes, C. A., & Costa, J. R. (2022). Feasibility of Bone Fracture Detection Using Microwave Imaging. *IEEE Open Journal of Antennas and Propagation*, 3, 836–847. doi:10.1109/OJAP.2022.3194217

Sarwar, M. U., Hanif, M. K., Talib, R., Mobeen, A., & Aslam, M. (2017). A survey of big data analytics in healthcare. *International Journal of Advanced Computer Science and Applications*, 8, 355–359.

Schiffman, M., Castle, P. E., Jeronimo, J., Rodriguez, A. C., & Wacholder, S. (2007). Human papillomavirus and cervical cancer. *Lancet*, 370(9590), 890–907. doi:10.1016/S0140-6736(07)61416-0 PMID:17826171

Schölkopf, B., Smola, A. J., Williamson, R. C., & Bartlett, P. L. (2000). New support vector algorithms. *Neural Computation*, 12(5), 1207–1245. doi:10.1162/089976600300015565 PMID:10905814

Sellors, J. W., & Sankaranarayanan, R. (2003). *Colposcopy and treatment of cervical intraepithelial neoplasia: a beginner's manual*. International Agency for Research on Cancer.

Shafer, A., Doze, V. A., Shafer, S. L., & White, P. F. (1988). Pharmacokinetics and pharmacodynamics of propofol infusions during general anesthesia. *Anesthesiology*, 69(3), 348–356. doi:10.1097/00000542-198809000-00011 PMID:3261954

Shafiq, M., Du, C., Jamal, N., Abro, J. H., Kamal, T., Afsar, S., & Mia, M. S. (2023). Smart E-Health System for Heart Disease Detection Using Artificial Intelligence and Internet of Things Integrated Next-Generation Sensor Networks. *Journal of Sensors*, 2023, 1–7. doi:10.1155/2023/6383099

Shahriyari, L. (2019). Effect of normalization methods on the performance of supervised learning algorithms applied to HTSeq-FPKM-UQ data sets: 7SK RNA expression as a predictor of survival in patients with colon adenocarcinoma. *Briefings in Bioinformatics*, 20(3), 985–994. doi:10.1093/bib/bbx153 PMID:29112707

Shah, V., Turkbey, B., Mani, H., Pang, Y., Pohida, T., Merino, M. J., & Bernardo, M. (2012). Decision support system for localizing prostate cancer based on multiparametric magnetic resonance imaging. *Medical Physics*, 39(7Part1), 4093–4103. doi:10.1118/1.4722753 PMID:22830742

Shaikhina, T., Lowe, D., Daga, S., Briggs, D., Higgins, R., & Khovanova, N. (2019). Decision tree and random forest models for outcome prediction in antibody incompatible kidney transplantation. *Biomedical Signal Processing and Control*, 52, 456–462. doi:10.1016/j.bspc.2017.01.012

Shaikh, M., Vayani, A. H., Akram, S., & Qamar, N. (2022). Open-source electronic health record systems: A systematic review of most recent advances. *Health Informatics Journal*, 28(2), 14604582221099828. doi:10.1177/14604582221099828 PMID:35588400

Shao, H. (2008, September). Delay-Dependent Stability for Recurrent Neural Networks With Time-Varying Delays. *IEEE Transactions on Neural Networks*, 19(9), 1647–1651. doi:10.1109/TNN.2008.2001265 PMID:18779095

Sharma, G., & Joshi, A. M. (2021). Novel EEG based Schizophrenia Detection with IoMT Framework for Smart Healthcare. *arXiv preprint arXiv:2111.11298*.

Sharma, A. (2016). Univariate short term forecasting of solar irradiance using modified online backpropagation through time. *2016 International Computer Science and Engineering Conference (ICSEC)*, (pp. 1-6). IEEE. 10.1109/ICSEC.2016.7859922

Sharma, A., Mishra, R. K., Goud, K. Y., Mohamed, M. A., Kummari, S., Tiwari, S., Li, Z., Narayan, R., Stanciu, L. A., & Marty, J. L. (2021). Optical biosensors for diagnostics of infectious viral disease: A recent update. *Diagnostics (Basel)*, 11(11), 2083. doi:10.3390/diagnostics11112083 PMID:34829430

Sharma, R., & Bhambri, P. (2020). *Energy Aware Bio Inspired Routing Technique for Mobile Adhoc Networks. Jalandhar.* I.K. Gujral Punjab Technical University.

Sharma, S., Kelly, T. K., & Jones, P. A. (2010, January). Epigenetics in cancer. *Carcinogenesis, 31*(1), 27–36. doi:10.1093/carcin/bgp220 PMID:19752007

Sheikh, A., & Bates, D. W. (2016). Assessing the Impact of Health Information Technology on Quality of Care: What Can Be Learned from the NHS? *BMJ (Clinical Research Ed.), 331*(7522), 982–986.

Shen, Y., & Wang, J. (2008, March). An Improved Algebraic Criterion for Global Exponential Stability of Recurrent Neural Networks With Time-Varying Delays. *IEEE Transactions on Neural Networks, 19*(3), 528–531. doi:10.1109/TNN.2007.911751 PMID:18334371

Shickel, B., Tighe, P. J., Bihorac, A., & Rashidi, P. (2020). Deep EHR: A Survey of Recent Advances in Deep Learning Techniques for Electronic Health Record (EHR) Analysis. *IEEE Journal of Biomedical and Health Informatics, 22*(5), 1589–1604. doi:10.1109/JBHI.2017.2767063 PMID:29989977

Shin, H., Roth, H. R., Gao, M., Lü, L., Xu, Z., Nogues, I., Yao, J., Mollura, D. J., & Summers, R. M. (2016). Deep Convolutional Neural Networks for Computer-Aided Detection: CNN architectures, dataset characteristics and transfer learning. *IEEE Transactions on Medical Imaging, 35*(5), 1285–1298. doi:10.1109/TMI.2016.2528162 PMID:26886976

Shi, Y., & Liu, Z. (2023). Evolution from Medical Imaging to Visualized Medicine. *Advances in Experimental Medicine and Biology, 1199*, 1–13. doi:10.1007/978-981-32-9902-3_1 PMID:37460724

Shouman, M., Turner, T., & Stocker, R. (2012). Applying k-nearest neighbour in diagnosing heart disease patients. *International Journal of Information and Education Technology (IJIET), 2*, 220–223. doi:10.7763/IJIET.2012.V2.114

Siegel, R. L., Miller, K. D., & Jemal, A. (2016). Cancer statistics, 2016. *CA: a Cancer Journal for Clinicians, 66*(1), 7–30. doi:10.3322/caac.21332 PMID:26742998

Singh, G., Singh, M., & Bhambri, P. (2020). Artificial Intelligence based Flying Car. In *Proceedings of the International Congress on Sustainable Development through Engineering Innovations* (pp. 216-227). Springer. ISBN 978-93-89947-14-4.

Singh, H. D. (2018). *Diagnosis of Cervical Cancer using Hybrid Machine Learning Models.* [Doctoral dissertation, Dublin, National College of Ireland].

Singh, P., & Bhadauria, H. S. (2014). Automatic brain MRI image segmentation using FCM and LSM", Reliability, Infocom Technologies and Optimization. *2014 3rd International Conference on.* IEEE.

Singh, H., & Sharma, A. (2019). Challenges of Internet of Things: Development and Application of Conceptual Framework. *International Journal of Recent Technology and Engineering, 8*(3), 2277–3878. doi:10.35940/ijrte.C4719.098319

Singh, M., Bhambri, P., Lal, S., Singh, Y., Kaur, M., & Singh, J. (2021). Design of the Effective Technique to Improve Memory and Time Constraints for Sequence Alignment. [Roman Science Publications and Distributions.]. *International Journal of Applied Engineering Research (Netherlands), 6*(02), 127–142.

Sisodia, D., & Sisodia, D. (2018). Prediction of diabetes using classification algorithms. *Procedia Computer Science, 132*, 1578–1585. doi:10.1016/j.procs.2018.05.122

Smith, J., & Johnson, A. (2020). Artificial Intelligence in Healthcare: A Comprehensive Review. *Journal of Digital Medicine, 7*(2), 123–145.

Sneha, N., & Gangil, T. (2019). Analysis of diabetes mellitus for early prediction using optimal features selection. *Journal of Big Data, 6*(1), 13. doi:10.1186/s40537-019-0175-6

Sokolova, M., & Lapalme, G. (2009). A systematic analysis of performance measures for classification tasks. *Information Processing & Management*, *45*(4), 427–437. doi:10.1016/j.ipm.2009.03.002

Son, Y. J., Kim, H. G., Kim, E. H., Choi, S., & Lee, S. K. (2010). Application of support vector machine for prediction of medication adherence in heart failure patients. *Healthcare Informatics Research*, *16*(4), 253–259. doi:10.4258/hir.2010.16.4.253 PMID:21818444

Soualmi, A., Alti, A., & Laouamer, L. (2020). *Medical Data Protection Using BlindWatermarking Technique*. Enabl AI Appl Data Sci.

Srinivas, K., Rani, B. K., & Govrdhan, A. (2010). Applications of data mining techniques in healthcare and prediction of heart attacks. *International Journal on Computer Science and Engineering*, *2*, 250–255.

Steyerberg, E. W. (2019). *Clinical prediction models*. Springer International Publishing. doi:10.1007/978-3-030-16399-0

Subramanian, S., Sankaranarayanan, R., Esmy, P. O., Thulaseedharan, J. V., Swaminathan, R., & Thomas, S. (2016). Clinical trial to implementation: Cost and effectiveness considerations for scaling up cervical cancer screening in low- and middle-income countries. *Journal of Cancer Policy*, *7*, 4–11. doi:10.1016/j.jcpo.2015.12.006

Suchita, G. (2013). Brain Tumor Detection using Unsupervised Learning based Neural Network. In *International conference on communication system and networking technologies*. IEEE.

Suganthan, P. N., & Katuwal, R. (2021). On the origins of randomization-based feedforward neural networks. *Applied Soft Computing*, *105*, 107239. doi:10.1016/j.asoc.2021.107239

Sultan, N. (2014). Making use of cloud computing for healthcare provision: Opportunities and challenges. *International Journal of Information Management*, *34*(2), 177–184. doi:10.1016/j.ijinfomgt.2013.12.011

Sumathi, N., Thirumagal, J., Jagannathan, S., Bhambri, P., & Ahamed, I. N. (2021). A Comprehensive Review on Bionanotechnology for the 21st Century. *Journal of the Maharaja Sayajirao University of Baroda*, *55*(1), 114–131.

Sun, B., Zhang, Y., He, J., Yu, L., Xu, Q., Li, D., & Wang, Z. (2017). A random forest regression method with selected text feature for de-pression assessment. Proceedings of the 7th Annual Workshop on Audio/Visual Emotion Challenge. ACM.

Sung, H., Ferlay, J., Siegel, R. L., Laversanne, M., Soerjomataram, I., Jemal, A., & Bray, F. (2021). Global cancer statistics 2020: GLOBOCAN estimates of incidence and mortality worldwide for 36 cancers in 185 countries. *CA: a Cancer Journal for Clinicians*, *71*(3), 209–249. doi:10.3322/caac.21660 PMID:33538338

Sun, J., Wei, M., Feng, J., Yu, F., Li, Q., & Zou, R. (2024). Progressive knowledge tracing: Modeling learning process from abstract to concrete. *Expert Systems with Applications*, *238*, 122280. doi:10.1016/j.eswa.2023.122280

Szilagyi, L. (2003). *MR brain image segmentation using an enhanced fuzzy c-means algorithm*. Engineering in Medicine and Biology Society. doi:10.1109/IEMBS.2003.1279866

Tackley, R. M., Lewis, G. T. R., Prys-Roberts, C., Boaden, R. W., Dixon, J., & Harvey, J. T. (1989). Computer-controlled infusion of propofol. *British Journal of Anaesthesia*, *62*(1), 46–53. doi:10.1093/bja/62.1.46 PMID:2783854

Takase, H., Gouhara, K., & Uchikawa, Y. (1993). Time sequential pattern transformation and attractors of recurrent neural networks. *Proceedings of 1993 International Conference on Neural Networks (IJCNN-93-Nagoya, Japan)* (pp. 2319-2322). IEEE. 10.1109/IJCNN.1993.714189

Tama, B. A., & Lim, S. (2020). A Comparative Performance Evaluation of Classification Algorithms for Clinical Decision Support Systems. *Mathematics*, *8*(8), 1814. doi:10.3390/math8101814

Tang, Y., & Zhou, J. (2015). The performance of PSO-SVM in inflation forecasting. *12th International Conference on Service Systems and Service Management (ICSSSM)*. IEEE.

Thangarajan, R., Harichandran, K. N., & Srinivas, K. (2022). AI Enabled Healthcare: A Review. *Materials Today: Proceedings, 29*, 270–274.

Tharwat, A. (2021). Independent component analysis: An introduction. *Applied Computing and Informatics, 17*(2), 222–249. doi:10.1016/j.aci.2018.08.006

Toltzis, P., Soto-Campos, G., & Shelton, C. (2015). Evidence Based Pediatric Outcome Predictors to Guide the Allocation of Critical Care Resources in a Mass Casualty Event. *Pediatric Critical Care Medicine, 16*(7), e207–e216. doi:10.1097/PCC.0000000000000481 PMID:26121100

Tomlinson, B. (Ed.). (2023). *Developing materials for language teaching*. Bloomsbury Publishing.

Topol, E. J. (2021). High-Performance Medicine: The Convergence of Human and Artificial Intelligence. *Nature Medicine, 25*(1), 44–56. doi:10.1038/s41591-018-0300-7 PMID:30617339

Trambaiolli, L. R., Lorena, A. C., Fraga, F. J., Kanda, P. A. M., Anghinah, R., & Nitrini, R. (2011, July). Improving Alzheimer's Disease Diagnosis with Machine Learning Techniques. *Clinical EEG and Neuroscience, 42*(3), 160–165. doi:10.1177/155005941104200304 PMID:21870467

Tsien, C. L., Fraser, H. S., & Long, W. J. (1998). Using classification tree and logistic regression methods to diagnose myocardial infarction. *Studies in Health Technology and Informatics, 52*(1), 493–497. PMID:10384505

Tubishat, M., Idris, N., Shuib, L., Abushariah, M. A., & Mirjalili, S. (2020). *Improved Salp Swarm Algorithm based on opposition based learning and novel local search algorithm for feature selection* (Vol. 145). Expert Syst. Appl.

Tuli, S., Tuli, S., Wander, G., Wander, P., Gill, S. S., Dustdar, S., Sakellariou, R., & Rana, O. (2020). Next Generation Technologies for Smart Healthcare: Challenges, Vision, Model, Trends and Future Directions. *Internet Technology Letters, 3*(2), e145. doi:10.1002/itl2.145

Tuya Inc, & the Gartner Group. (2020). *2021 Global AIoT Developers Ecosystem White Paper*. Tech Show Developers Conference, Hangzhou, China

Tzeng, E., Devin, C., Hoffman, J., Finn, C., Abbeel, P., Levine, S., & Darrell, T. (December 2016). Adapting deep visuomotor representations with weak pairwise constraints. In *Algorithmic Foundations of Robotics XII* (pp. 688–703). Springer.

Uçkun, F. A., Özer, H., Nurbaş, E., & Onat, E. (2020). Direction Finding Using Convolutional Neural Networks and Convolutional Recurrent Neural Networks. *2020 28th Signal Processing and Communications Applications Conference (SIU)*, 1-4. 10.1109/SIU49456.2020.9302448

Van der Schaar, M., & Choi, E. (2021). Predicting Healthcare Trajectories from Medical Records: A Deep Learning Approach. *Journal of the American Medical Informatics Association : JAMIA, 26*(4), 339–346.

Vandewiele, G., Dehaene, I., Kovács, G., Sterckx, L., Janssens, O., Ongenae, F., & Demeester, T. (2021). *Overly optimistic prediction results on imbalanced data: a case study of flaws and benefits when applying over-sampling* (Vol. 111). Artif. Intell. Med.

Vassilakopoulou, P., & Hustad, E. (2023). Bridging digital divides: A literature review and research agenda for information systems research. *Information Systems Frontiers, 25*(3), 955–969. doi:10.1007/s10796-020-10096-3 PMID:33424421

Vayena, E., Blasimme, A., & Cohen, I. G. (2018, November 6). Machine learning in medicine: Addressing ethical challenges. *PLoS Medicine, 15*(11), e1002689. doi:10.1371/journal.pmed.1002689 PMID:30399149

Venugopalan, J., Tong, L., Hassanzadeh, H. R., & Wang, M. D. (2021). Multimodal deep learning models for early detection of Alzheimer's disease stage. *Scientific Reports*, *11*(1), 3254. doi:10.1038/s41598-020-74399-w PMID:33547343

Verma, A. K., Pal, S., & Kumar, S. (2020). Prediction of skin disease using ensemble data mining techniques and feature selection method—A comparative study. *Applied Biochemistry and Biotechnology*, *190*(2), 341–359. doi:10.1007/s12010-019-03093-z PMID:31350666

Vijayalakshmi, P., Shankar, R., Karthik, S., & Bhambri, P. (2021). Impact of Work from Home Policies on Workplace Productivity and Employee Sentiments during the Covid-19 Pandemic. [The Maharaja Sayajirao University of Baroda.]. *Journal of Maharaja Sayajirao University of Baroda*, *55*(01(VI)), 1314–1331.

Visa, S. (2011). *Confusion Matrix-based Feature Selection*. Conference: Proceedings of the 22nd Midwest Artificial Intelligence and Cognitive Science Conference 2011, Cincinnati, OH, USA.

Vishwakarma, L. P., Singh, R. K., Mishra, R., & Kumari, A. (2023). Application of artificial intelligence for resilient and sustainable healthcare system: Systematic literature review and future research directions. *International Journal of Production Research*, 1–23. doi:10.1080/00207543.2023.2188101

Vuyk, J., Engbers, F. H. M., Bum, A. G. L., Vletter, A. A., & Bovill, J. G. (1995). Performance of Computer-Controlled Infusion of Propofol: An Evaluation of Five Pharmacokinetic Parameter Sets. *Anesthesia and Analgesia*, *81*, 1275–1282. PMID:7486116

Wang, A., Chen, G., Shang, C., Zhang, M., & Liu, L. (2016). Human activity recognition in a smart home environment with stacked denoising autoencoders. In *International conference on web-age information management* (pp. 29-40). Springer. 10.1007/978-3-319-47121-1_3

Wang, F., Casalino, L. P., & Khullar, D. (2019, March 1). Deep Learning in Medicine-Promise, Progress, and Challenges. *JAMA Internal Medicine*, *179*(3), 293–294. doi:10.1001/jamainternmed.2018.7117 PMID:30556825

Wang, H., Li, Y., & Fan, C. (2022). Internet of Things-Enabled Healthcare Systems: A Comprehensive Review. *Journal of Medical Systems*, *40*(12), 286.

Wang, L. L., Ge, L. Z., Li, R. F., & Fang, Y. (2017). Three-stream CNNs for action recognition. *Pattern Recognition Letters*, *92*, 33–40. doi:10.1016/j.patrec.2017.04.004

Wang, L., von Laszewski, G., Younge, A., He, X., Kunze, M., Tao, J., & Fu, C. (2010). Cloud Computing: A Perspective Study. *New Generation Computing*, *28*(2), 137–146. doi:10.1007/s00354-008-0081-5

Wang, Y., & Zhang, L. J. (2023). *The Routledge Handbook of Materials Development for Language Teaching*.

Wang, Z., Chen, L., Wang, L., & Diao, G. (2020). Recognition of audio depression based on convolutional neural network and generative antagonism network model. *IEEE Access : Practical Innovations, Open Solutions*, *8*, 101181–101191. https://ieeexplore.ieee.org/abstract/document/9103527/. doi:10.1109/ACCESS.2020.2998532

Wardana, A. A., Rakhmatsyah, A., Minarno, A. E., & Anbiya, D. R. (2019). *Internet of things platform for manage multiple message queuing telemetry transport broker server. Kinetik: Game Technology*. Information System, Computer Network, Computing, Electronics, and Control.

Wayne, B. (2002). *Process Control: Modeling, Design, and Simulation*. Prentice Hall PTR.

Weiss, J. C., Page, D., Peissig, P. L., Natarajan, S., & McCarty, C. (2012). Statistical relational learning to predict primary myocardial infarction from electronic health records. *Proceedings of the Innovative Applications of Artificial Intelligence Conference*, *2012*(2), 2341–2347. doi:10.1609/aaai.v26i2.18981 PMID:25360347

Wei, Z., Na, M., & Huisheng, S. (2009). Feature extraction of X-ray fracture image and fracture classification. *Proc. Int. Conf. Artif. Intell. Comput. Intell.*, (pp. 408–412). IEEE. 10.1109/AICI.2009.40

WHO. (2010). *Medical devices: managing the Mismatch An outcome of the Priority Medical Devices project.* WHO.

WHO. (2023). *Depression.* World Health Organization (WHO). https://www.thelancet.com/journals/lancet/article/PIIS0140-6736(07)61415-9/fulltext?pubType=related

WHO. (n.d.). *Diabetes Fact Sheet.* WHO. https://www.who.int/en/news-room/fact-sheets/detail/diabetes

Withey, D. J., & Koles, Z. J. (2008). A review of medical image segmentation: method and available software. International Journal of Bioelectromagnetism, 10(3).

World Health Organization (WHO). (2021). *Human papillomavirus and cervical cancer.* WHO. https://www.who.int/news-room/fact-sheets/detail/human-papillomavirus-(hpv)-and-cervical-cancer

World Health Organization. (2022). *Consolidated guidelines on HIV, viral hepatitis and STI prevention, diagnosis, treatment and care for key populations.* World Health Organization.

World Health Organization. (2023). *2023 emerging technologies and scientific innovations: a global public health perspective.* WHO.

World Robotics. (2020). *Report* [DB/OL]. World Robotics. https://ifr.org/news/record-2.7-million-robots-work-infactories-around-the-globe

Wright, L. G., Onodera, T., Stein, M. M., Wang, T., Schachter, D. T., Hu, Z., & McMahon, P. L. (2022). Deep physical neural networks trained with backpropagation. *Nature, 601*(7894), 549–555. doi:10.1038/s41586-021-04223-6 PMID:35082422

Wsy, A., & Syh, B. (2006). A process-mining framework for the detection of healthcare fraud and abuse. *ExpSystAppl, 31*(1), 56–68.

Xie, J., & Coggeshall, S. (2010). Prediction of transfers to tertiary care and hospital mortality: A gradient boosting decision tree approach. *Statistical Analysis and Data Mining, 3*(4), 253–258. doi:10.1002/sam.10079

Xue, Q., Wang, X., Meehan, S., Kuang, J., Gao, J. A., & Chuah, M. C. (2018). Recurrent neural networks based obesity status prediction using activity data. In *2018 17th IEEE International Conference on Machine Learning and Applications (ICMLA)* (pp. 865-870). IEEE. 10.1109/ICMLA.2018.00139

Yamashita, R., Nishio, M., Do, R. K. G., & Togashi, K. (2018, August). Convolutional neural networks: An overview and application in radiology. *Insights Into Imaging, 9*(4), 611–629. doi:10.1007/s13244-018-0639-9 PMID:29934920

Yang, J., & Zhang, B. (2019). Artificial intelligence in intelligent tutoring robots: A systematic review and design guidelines. *Applied Sciences (Basel, Switzerland), 9*(10), 2078. doi:10.3390/app9102078

Yang, M., Kiang, M. Y., & Shao, C. (2023). A Predictive Analytics Approach to Forecasting Rare Disease Cases at Healthcare Centers. *Information Sciences, 381*, 145–163.

Yaqoob, I., Ahmed, E., & Hashem, I. A. (2022). Enabling Real-Time Decision-Making in Telemedicine Systems: A Comprehensive Review. *IEEE Access : Practical Innovations, Open Solutions, 8*, 55629–55644.

Yaxue, Q. (2020). Convolutional Neural Networks for Literature Retrieval. *2020 International Conference on Computer Vision, Image and Deep Learning (CVIDL)*, (pp. 393-397). IEEE. 10.1109/CVIDL51233.2020.00-64

Yu, Z., Scherer, S., Devault, D., Gratch, J., Stratou, G., Morency, L.-P., & Cassell, J. (2013). Multimodal prediction of psychologicaldisorders: Learning verbal and nonverbal commonalities in adjacency pairs. *Semdial 2013 DialDam: Proceedings of the 17thWorkshop on the Semantics and Pragmatics of Dialogue*. ACM.

Yu, J., Yi, Z., & Zhou, J. (2010, October). Continuous Attractors of Lotka–Volterra Recurrent Neural Networks With Infinite Neurons. *IEEE Transactions on Neural Networks*, *21*(10), 1690–1695. doi:10.1109/TNN.2010.2067224 PMID:20813637

Zanella, A., Mason, F., Pluchino, P., & Cisotto, G. (2020). *Internet of Things for Elderly and Fragile People*. arXiv:2006.05709v1

Zhang, F., Li, Z., Zhang, B., Du, H., Wang, B., & Zhang, X. (2019). Multi-modal deep learning model for auxiliary diagnosis of Alzheimer's disease. *Neurocomputing*, *361*, 185–195. doi:10.1016/j.neucom.2019.04.093

Zhang, R., & Cui, J. (2020). Application of Convolutional Neural Network in multi-channel Scenario D2D Communication Transmitting Power Control. *2020 International Conference on Computer Vision, Image and Deep Learning (CVIDL)*, (pp. 668-672). IEEE. 10.1109/CVIDL51233.2020.000-3

Zhang, X., Zhang, S., & Wang, C. (2022). The Internet of Things in Healthcare: A Comprehensive Survey. *Journal of Healthcare Informatics Research*, *3*(1), 1–17. PMID:35419512

Zhang, Y., Liao, W., & Li, Y. (2019). Wearable Healthcare: Architectural Design and Impacts on the Public and Private Healthcare Systems. *Journal of Ambient Intelligence and Humanized Computing*, *10*(12), 4867–4877.

Zhao, Z., Li, X., Luan, B., Jiang, W., Gao, W., & Neelakandan, S. (2023). Secure internet of things (IoT) using a novel brooks Iyengar quantum byzantine agreement-centered blockchain networking (BIQBA-BCN) model in smart healthcare. *Information Sciences*, *629*, 440–455. doi:10.1016/j.ins.2023.01.020

Zheng, S. (2021). Network Intrusion Detection Model Based on Convolutional Neural Network. *2021 IEEE 5th Advanced Information Technology, Electronic and Automation Control Conference (IAEAC)*, 634-637. 10.1109/IAEAC50856.2021.9390930

Zhong, R., Li, M., Chen, Q., Li, J., Li, G., & Lin, W. (2019). The P300 event-related potential component and cognitive impairment in epilepsy: A systematic review and meta-analysis. *Frontiers in Neurology*, *10*, 943. doi:10.3389/fneur.2019.00943 PMID:31543861

Zhou, Z., Shuai, Y. U., & Chen, X. (2019). Edge intelligence:a new nexus of edge computing and artificial intelligence. *Big Data Res*, *5*(2), 53–63.

Zulpe, N. S. (2012). Level set and Thresholding for Brain Tumor Segmentation. *International Journal of Computer and Electrical Engineering*, *4*(1).

Zvikhachevskaya, A., & Sharipov, A. (2020). IoT-Based Wearables for Healthcare: Current State and Prospects. *Journal of Physics: Conference Series*, *1155*, 012013.

About the Contributors

Alex Khang, is a Professor in Information Technology, D.Sc. D.Litt., AI and data scientist, Software industry expert, and the chief of technology officer (AI and Data Science Research Center) at the Global Research Institute of Technology and Engineering, North Carolina, United States. ORCID: 0000-0001-8379-4659. He has more than 28 years of teaching and research experience in information technology at the universities and institutes of information technology in Vietnam, India, and United States. He has published 74 documents indexed by Scopus, 52 authored books, 3 authored books (software development), and authored/co-authored 10 papers, 50 book chapters. He has published 15 edited books, and calling for book chapters for 16 edited books in the fields of AI ecosystem. He has over 30 years of working experience as a software product manager, data engineer, AI engineer, cloud computing architect, solution architect, software architect, database expert in the foreign corporations of Germany, Sweden, the United States, Singapore, and multinationals (former CEO, former CTO, former Engineering Director, Product Manager, Senior Software Production Consultant, Data Product Manager).

* * *

Mohammed H. AlAqad is an assistant professor in the fields of translation, interpretation, and linguistics. He holds a PhD and MA in linguistics and translation studies from the top university in Malaysia, University of Malaya. Presently, Dr. AlAqad serves as an assistant professor of translation, interpreting, and linguistics at Management and Science University in Malaysia. His areas of expertise encompass Translation, Interpreting, and Linguistics Studies, as well as Legal Practicing. Dr. AlAqad has made significant contributions to the field through the publication of numerous scholarly papers and book chapters. Moreover, he has been recognized as an esteemed speaker and presenter, having participated in over 40 international conferences across various locations such as Hong Kong, Belgium, Palestine, the UK, Malaysia, Singapore, and many others.

Harishchander Anandaram completed a PhD in Bioengineering, a M.Tech, and a B.Tech in Bioinformatics from the Sathyabama Institute of Science and Technology, Chennai, in 2020, 2011, and 2009. In his bachelor's and master's theses, he worked on analysing resistance to HIV protease inhibitors based on molecular mechanics and machine learning studies, a collaborative project with IIT Madras. In his PhD thesis, he worked on pharmacogenomics and miRNA-regulated networks in psoriasis, a collaborative project with Georgetown University, USA, JIPMER, India, CIBA, India, and ILS, India. His thesis illustrated a multi-disciplinary approach by combining computational biophysics and molecular biology with machine learning. While doing a PhD, he had the opportunity to collaborate with international researchers and have publications in reputed international journals in bioinformatics and systems biology. He has received the prestigious "Young Scientist Award" from "The Melinda Gates Foundation" for his research abstract on "The Implications of miRNA Dynamics in Infectious Diseases". To date, he has reviewed more than 200 manuscripts in systems biology. He is now using computer methods to guess new lead molecules and biomarkers that can be used to target the inflammatory pathways that are linked to autoimmune and infectious diseases.

Pankaj Bhambri is affiliated with the Department of Information Technology at Guru Nanak Dev Engineering College in Ludhiana. Additionally, he fulfills the role of the Institute's Coordinator for the Skill Enhancement Cell and acts as the Convener for his Departmental Board of Studies. He possesses nearly two decades of teaching experience. Dr. Bhambri acquired a Master of Technology degree in Computer Science and Engineering and a Bachelor of Engineering degree in Information Technology with Honours from I.K.G. Punjab Technical University in Jalandhar, India, and Dr. B.R. Ambedkar University in Agra, India, respectively. Dr. Bhambri obtained a Doctorate in Computer Science and Engineering from I.K.G. Punjab Technical University, located in Jalandhar, India. Over an extended period, he fulfilled many responsibilities including those of an Assistant Registrar (Academics), Member (Academic Council/ BoS/DAB/RAC), Hostel Warden, APIO, and NSS Coordinator within his institution. His research work has been published in esteemed worldwide and national journals, as well as conference proceedings. Dr. Bhambri has made significant contributions to the academic field through his role as both an editor and author of various textbooks. Additionally, he has demonstrated his innovative thinking by filing several patents. Dr. Bhambri has received numerous prestigious awards from esteemed organizations in recognition of his exceptional achievements in both social and academic/research domains. These accolades include the ISTE Best Teacher Award in 2022 and 2023, the I2OR National Award in 2020, the Green ThinkerZ Top 100 International Distinguished Educators award in 2020, the I2OR Outstanding Educator Award in 2019, the SAA Distinguished Alumni Award in 2012, the CIPS Rashtriya Rattan Award in 2008, the LCHC Best Teacher Award in 2007, and several other commendations from various government and non-profit entities. He has provided guidance and oversight for numerous research projects and dissertations at the undergraduate, postgraduate, and Ph.D. levels. He successfully organized a diverse range of educational programmes, securing financial backing from esteemed institutions such as the All India Council for Technical Education (AICTE), the Technical Education Quality Improvement Programme (TEQIP), among others. Dr. Bhambri's areas of interest encompass machine learning, bioinformatics, wireless sensor networks, and network security. Dr. Bhambri possesses a wide array of professional responsibilities, encompassing the duties of an educator, editor, author, reviewer, expert speaker, motivator, and technical committee member for esteemed national and worldwide organizations.

Ahona Ghosh is a B.Tech., M.Tech. in CSE and presently is an AICTE Doctoral Fellow in the Department of Computer Science and Engineering, Maulana Abul Kalam Azad University of Technology, West Bengal (In house). Before joining Ph.D., she was an Assistant Professor in the Department of Computational Science, Brainware University, Barasat, Kolkata. She has published more than 20 papers in International conferences, Peer reviewed international journals and book chapters with IEEE, Springer, Elsevier, IGI Global, CRC Press etc. Her research interests include Machine Learning and Internet of Things.

Namria Ishaaq, a dedicated B.Tech Computer Science undergraduate at Jamia Hamdard, New Delhi, India, is driven by a profound interest in the intersection of technology and the biomedical field. Focused on the healthcare sector, Namria is passionately immersed in the application of computer science principles to advanced medical solutions. Currently pursuing her degree, she is building a strong foundation in both computer science and biomedical sciences, preparing to contribute to transformative developments in healthcare technology. Actively engaged in collaborative projects and staying abreast of emerging technologies, Namria aspires to bridge the gap between computing and healthcare, aiming to make impactful contributions to the biomedical field. With a commitment to excellence and a vision for innovative solutions, Namria Ishaaq is poised to play a significant role in shaping the future of healthcare through technology.

Anam Reyaz is a final-year B.Tech CSE student at Jamia Hamdard. She has honed her computer science fundamentals with guidance from dedicated professors. With a passion for deep learning, she aspires to specialize in this dynamic field. Anam's academic journey reflects resilience and curiosity, marked by active participation in research projects and competitions. She envisions contributing to groundbreaking advancements, fostering collaborative learning, and staying abreast of industry trends. Poised to graduate, Anam Reyaz represents a promising force in computer science, driven by a commitment to innovation and a focus on deep learning.

Sriparna Saha received her M.E. and Ph.D. degrees from Electronics and Tele-Communication Engineering department of Jadavpur University, Kolkata, India. She is currently an Assistant Professor (Stage-II) in the Department of Computer Science and Engineering of Maulana Abul Kalam Azad University of Technology, West Bengal, India. Prior to that, she was associated as a faculty with Jadavpur University and two other institutions. She has more than 8 years of experience in teaching and research. Her research area includes artificial intelligence, image processing, machine learning and recently she is giving more focus on deep learning. She has over 70 publications in IEEE, Elsevier, Springer, etc. She is the author of a book on Gesture Recognition published by Studies in Computational Intelligence, Springer. She is also the reviewer for many international journals. Her major research proposal is accepted for Start Up Grant under UGC Basic Scientific Research Grant. Not only that, she also got University seed money for setting up her laboratory.

Muthmainnah Yakin, Ph.D., an accomplished Assistant Professor at Universitas Al Asyariah Mandar in West Sulawesi, Indonesia, stands as a distinguished academician with a diverse and impactful professional portfolio. Her multifaceted career spans roles such as Chairman of the Indonesian Language Department, Public Relations Officer, Director of Women's Centre Studies, Deputy Director of Quality Assurance Unit, and her current position as Deputy Director of the Language and Character Development Institute. In addition to her administrative roles, Muthmainnah is a prolific author, contributing to the scholarly landscape with 58 national and international books. Her publications, hosted by prestigious publishers such as Springer, Emerald, IGI Global, Wiley, Routledge, and Taylor and Francis, underscore her commitment to advancing knowledge in various domains. Her profile of authored books is accessible via the Science and Technology Index (SINTA) portal: . Muthmainnah's global influence extends beyond her academic achievements. As an international board member for several scientific innovation research groups and a member of the United Nations Volunteers roster, she actively contributes to international research collaborations and initiatives. Her exceptional contributions have earned her over

100 international awards, including recognitions as Outstanding Professor, Outstanding Leadership, Best International Influencer, Best Emerging Professor of the Year, and the International Award for Working Women and SDGs Warrior. Notably, she holds an honorary doctorate degree from Layahe University and has been honored with the Doctor of Excellence award from the Philippines. Muthmainnah's dedication to education is further evidenced by her membership in the United Nations Volunteers' roster and her advisory role in the Indonesian Education Share to Care Volunteers. Her research interests encompass a broad spectrum, including the development of literary works, instructional teaching materials, Assurance of Learning (Assure), Teaching English to Speakers of Other Languages (TESOL), ICT in education, digital education, and cybergogy. Muthmainnah's scholarly impact is quantified by her Sinta score of 2052, h-index of 18, and her role as an External Examiner for Ph.D. students at three A+ accredited campuses in India and Australia. Her commitment to international collaboration and teamwork positions her as an ideal candidate for various academic and leadership roles.

Index

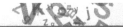
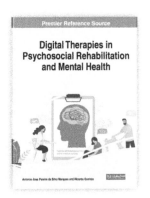
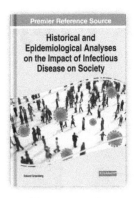
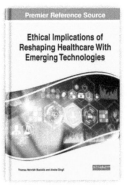
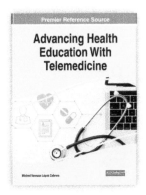
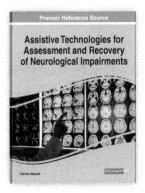
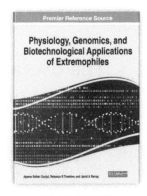
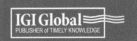

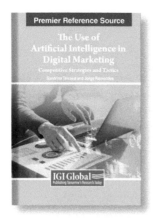
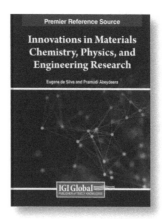
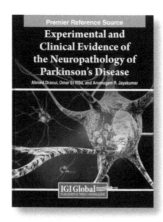
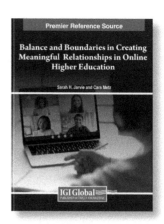

Submit an Open Access Book Proposal

Have Your Work Fully & Freely Available Worldwide After Publication

Seeking the Following Book Classification Types:

Authored & Edited Monographs • Casebooks • Encyclopedias • Handbooks of Research

Gold, Platinum, & Retrospective OA Opportunities to Choose From

Easily Track Your Work in Our Advanced Manuscript Submission System With **Rapid Turnaround Times**

Double-Blind Peer Review by Notable Editorial Boards (*Committee on Publication Ethics* (COPE) Certified

Publications Adhere to All **Current OA Mandates & Compliances**

Affordable APCs *(Often 50% Lower Than the Industry Average)* Including Robust Editorial Service Provisions

Direct Connections with **Prominent Research Funders** & OA Regulatory Groups

Institution Level OA Agreements Available (Recommend or Contact Your Librarian for Details)

Join a **Diverse Community of 150,000+ Researchers Worldwide** Publishing With IGI Global

Content Spread Widely to Leading Repositories (AGOSR, ResearchGate, CORE, & More)

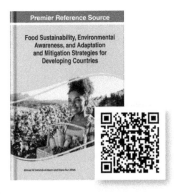

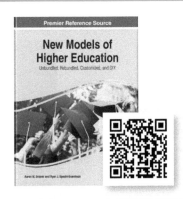

 DID YOU KNOW?

Retrospective Open Access Publishing

You Can Unlock Your Recently Published Work, Including Full Book & Individual Chapter Content to Enjoy All the Benefits of Open Access Publishing

Learn More

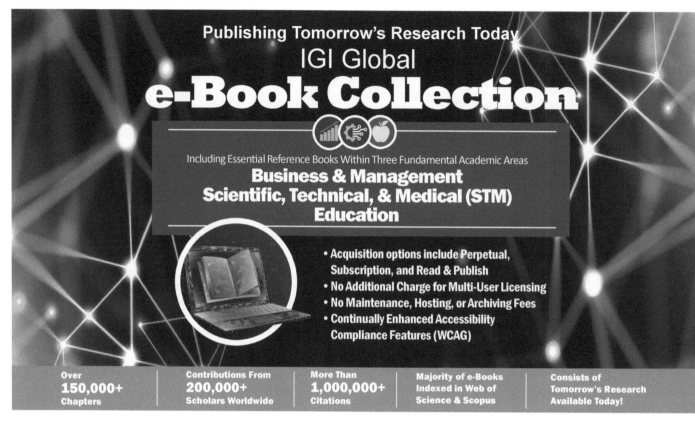
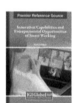
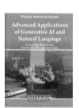
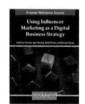
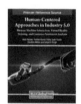
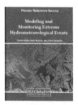
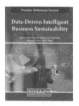
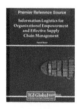
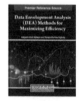

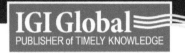

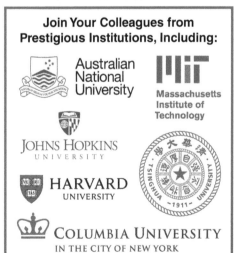

Individual Article & Chapter Downloads

US$ 37.50/each

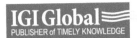
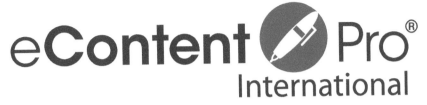

Milton Keynes UK
Ingram Content Group UK Ltd.
UKHW050820070324
438953UK00003B/26

9 798369 336793